made INCREDIBLY EASY!

Nutrition

Adapted for the UK by

Kathy Martyn, SRN, DIP.NS, BSc (Hons), BEd (Hons), MSc

Principal Lecturer
Brighton University

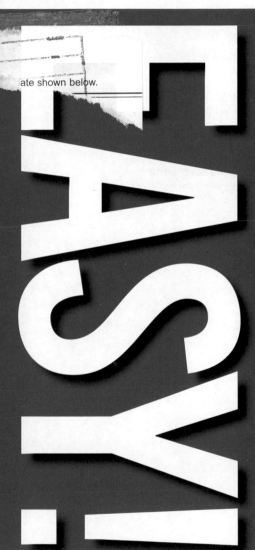

ate shown below.

First UK Edition

Lippincott Williams & Wilkins
a Wolters Kluwer business

Philadelphia · Baltimore · New York · London
Buenos Aires · Hong Kong · Sydney · Tokyo

Staff

Acquisitions Editor
Rachel Hendrick

Academic Marketing Executive
Alison Major

Production Editor
Kevin Johnson

Proofreader
Helena Engstrand

Illustrator
Bot Roda

Text and Cover Design
Designers Collective

Printed in the People's Republic of China.

Typeset by MPS Limited, a Macmillan Company

For information, write to Lippincott Williams & Wilkins, 250 Waterloo Road, London SE1 8RD

British Library Cataloging-in-Publication Data. A catalogue record for this book is available from the British Library

ISBN-13: 978-1-901831-17-7
ISBN-10: 1-901831-17-5

Contents

Appendices and index

Acknowledgements

Reviewers of the UK edition

Pat Berridge, MA (Ed), PG Dip Ed, BSc (Hons), RGN, RNT
Senior Lecturer, Deputy Programme Director (RTP)
Birmingham City University

Lynne Colagiovanni, RN, BSc
Consultant Nurse—Nutrition Support
Queen Elizabeth Hospital, Birmingham

Dr Stephanie A. Dillon, BSc, PhD
Lecturer in Nutrition,
Faculty of Science & Technology
University of Central Lancashire

Caroline Jane Dodd-Reynolds, BSc, MSc, PhD
Senior Lecturer and Programme Leader
BSc (Hons) Sport, Exercise and Nutrition
Department of Sport and Exercise Sciences,
Northumbria University

Tracey Lewarne, BSc, MPhil, R. Nutr.
Senior Lecturer in Nutrition
Department of Science,
Bath Spa University

Helen MCarthy, BSc (Hons), PhD, PgCHEP, RD
Lecturer (Dietetics), School of Biomedical Sciences
University of Ulster

Kate Pickering, RGN, Dip. N, BA Nursing
Lead nutrition Nurse Specialist
University Hospitals of Leicester

Andrew Scott, PhD, MSc, FHEA
Senior Lecturer,
Sport and Exercise Physiology
Department of Sport and Exercise Science,
University of Portsmouth

Trevor Simper, RPHNutr, MSc, PGCHE, BSc
Senior Lecturer, Food and Nutrition
Sheffield Hallam University

Collette Straughair, RN, Dip. NSc, RM, BSc Midwifery, MSc Practice, Education and Development
Senior Lecturer Pre-Registration Adult Nursing
School of Health, Community and Education
Studies, Northumbria University

Foreword

As you know, nutrition plays a major role in health promotion, disease prevention and treatment in a range of different settings including the NHS and private sector. To provide the best care and advice for people, you must have a sound knowledge of nutritional principles. You must also be able to apply that knowledge in your practice and care and impart that knowledge to both patients and individuals so that they can make healthier food choices for themselves. How do you do all of this? With the help of *Nutrition Made Incredibly Easy*, First UK edition—the resource that you need to take this challenging topic and make it more understandable, more practical, more digestible and more appetising! This book has been adapted from the original American text for the UK, drawing on the work of the Food Standards Agency, NICE and NHS guidelines.

Do you have complete confidence in the nutritional care you provide to your patients? If not, it's probably because the when taught in school seems very distant from practice and contained long words. Well, in this new edition of *Nutrition Made Incredibly Easy*, you won't find any drab drawings of chemical structures or drawn-out descriptions of complex gastrointestinal processes. You'll find only clear descriptions of nutrition-related topics, simply explained.

Nutrition is a complex subject. Understanding how to provide the best nutritional care requires you to learn many concepts. Because nutrients come from food, you need to learn what foods should be eaten, and how differing foods can make up a balanced diet and which portion sizes are appropriate. Your knowledge of anatomy and physiology is essential to helping you understand what happens to food in the digestive tract and how nutrients are absorbed and distributed throughout the body. You need to recall basic pathophysiology information to appreciate how diseases affect nutrition and how foods can be used in the treatment of various disorders. *Nutrition Made Incredibly Easy*, First UK edition, makes learning all of this information simple—and fun!

Offering comprehensive information on nutritional care throughout the lifespan, this one-of-a-kind reference is a fantastic tool for practitioners, students, faculty and anyone interested in diet and nutrition. The text is organised into three square servings. Part I, Introduction to nutrition, offers a concise yet hearty review of such topics as nutrition basics, digestion and absorption, and essential nutrients. Fully updated, this first edition includes the *dietary guidelines based on the Food Standards Agency's Eat Well, Be Well programme*, making links with its exciting online packages.

Part II brings the topic of nutrition a little closer to your practice. It thoroughly covers nutritional screening including identifying at-risk patients, taking a dietary history, evaluating weight and body size, and documenting nutritional screening findings. This section also has an entire chapter devoted to how nutritional considerations vary throughout the lifespan. In Part III, Clinical nutrition, you'll find coverage of not only common nutritional and GI disorders, such as obesity, anorexia, dysphagia, GORD and lactose intolerance, but also nutritional considerations for patients with cardiovascular, renal and neurologic disorders; diabetes; HIV disease and such special conditions as burns and trauma. In addition, you'll find the information on feeding patients that you'll need to use daily in your practice. Where applicable reference is made to referral to the registered dietitian for guidance and advice.

Sounds boring? Hardly! You'll find plenty of features in *Nutrition Made Incredibly Easy* that make the complex study of nutrition simple, interesting and fun. Characters that appear throughout the book reinforce important points and also spice up the text with a dash of humour. Objectives for each chapter help focus your study. In addition, special logos highlight important points and bolster learning throughout the book:

Lifespan lunchbox points out important age-related nutritional considerations.

Menu maven offers sample menus for special diets.

NutriTips gives pointers on nutritional care—many of which you can share with your patients.

Bridging the gap alerts you to practices and preferences of various cultures and ethnic groups that may affect your nutritional care.

Memory jogger provides mnemonics and other ways to help you understand and remember difficult concepts.

To people involved in education about health care or health promotion and who are interested in using a well-organised reference to help their students grasp important nutrition concepts and to students who are looking for nutrition to be boiled down to the basics, I would highly recommend *Nutrition Made Incredibly Easy*, First UK edition. What might have been intimidating has been dissected, simplified, streamlined and illustrated for easy application to daily practice. With the broad understanding of nutrition gained from this book, you'll be ready to make a valuable contribution to the nutritional health and well-being of the people you are involved with. Bon appétit!

Kathy Martyn, SRN, Dip. NS,
BSc (Hons), BEd (Hons), MSc
Principal Lecturer,
Brighton University

Contributors and consultants to the US edition

Liz Applegate, PhD, FACSM
Senior Lecturer, Nutrition Department
University of California, Davis

Jennifer Bueche, PhD, CDN, RD
Assistant Professor, Department of
Human Ecology
SUNY College at Oneonta, New York

Nancy Collins, PhD, LD/N, RD
Consultant Dietitian
Weston, Florida

Peggi Guenter, RN, PhD, CNSN
Managing Editor for Special Projects
American Society for Parenteral and
Enteral Nutrition
Silver Spring, Maryland

Alison H. Harmon, PhD, RD
Assistant Professor
Montana State University
Department of Health & Human
Development
Bozeman, Montana

Cristen L. Harris, MS, LD/N, RD
Nutrition Consultant
Ft. Lauderdale, Florida

Susan Luck, RN, BSN, MA, CCN, HNC
Clinical Nutritionist
Special Immunology Services
Mercy Hospital
Miami, Florida

Kathleen D. Meyer, LD, RD
Assistant Manager, Dietary
Fairfield Medical Center
Lancaster, Ohio

Sherry A. Parmenter, LD, RD
Clinical Dietitian
Fairfield Medical Center
Lancaster, Ohio

**Alison J. Rigby, MPH, MS, PhD,
CNSD, RD**
Stanford University School of Medicine
Pediatric Endocrinology and Diabetes
Stanford, California

Martine Scannavino, MS, LDN, RD
Assistant Professor
Associate Director—Allen Center for
Nutrition
Cedar Crest College
Allentown, Pennsylvania

Susan S. Swadener, PhD, RD
Dietetic Internship Director & Lecturer
California Polytechnic State University
San Luis Obispo, California

Kate Willcutts, MS, CNSD, RD
Assistant Nutrition Support Manager
University of Virginia Hospital
Instructor
School of Nursing
Charlottesville, Virginia

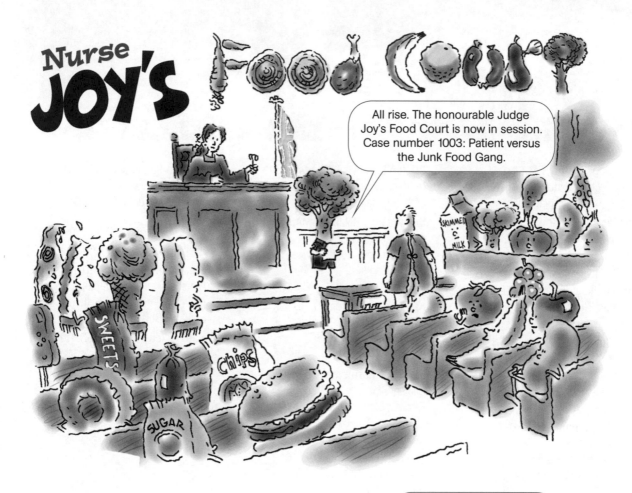

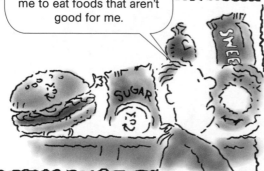

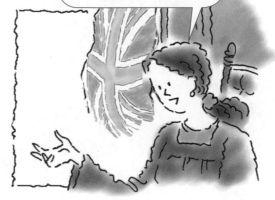

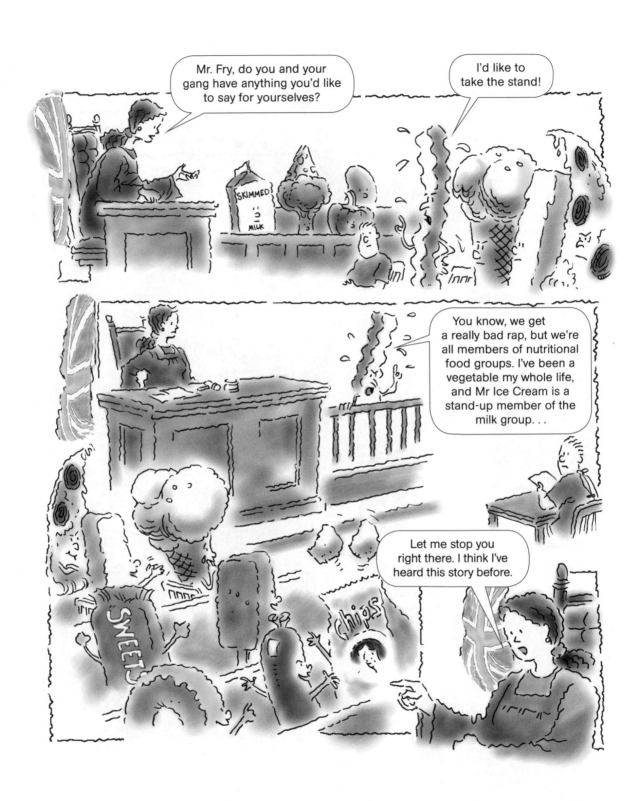

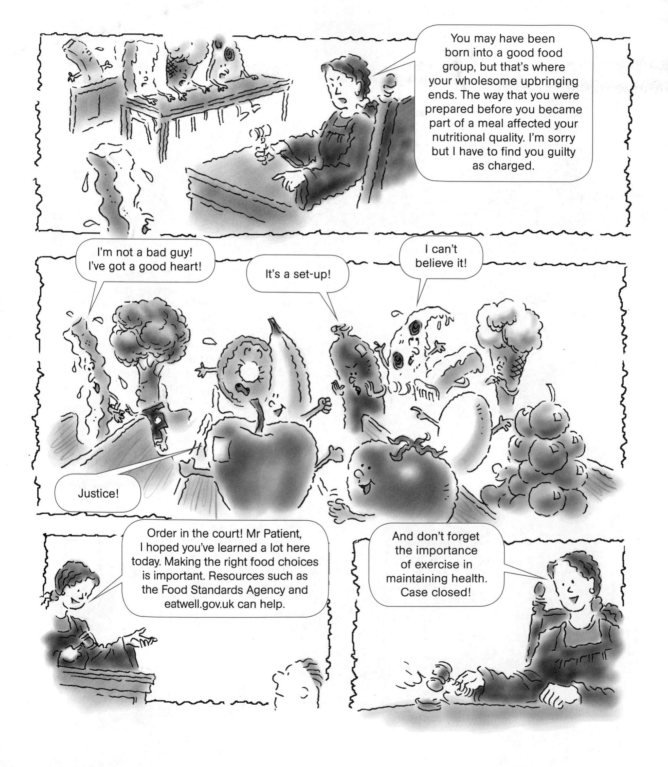

Part I

Introduction to nutrition

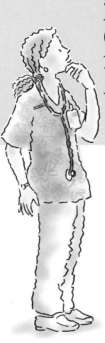

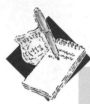

Just the facts

This chapter presents fundamental information about the key elements of nutrition. In this chapter, you'll learn:

♦ the role nutrients play in health promotion

♦ three levels of disease prevention

♦ the way to differentiate between good nutrition and poor nutrition

♦ techniques for ensuring that your patient eats a balanced diet

♦ the current nutrient standards for health promotion.

A look at nutrition

Nutrition refers to the processes by which a living organism ingests, digests, absorbs, transports, uses and excretes nutrients (food and other nourishing material). Nutrition as a clinical area is primarily concerned with the properties of food that build sound bodies and promote health.

More than just a pretty process

Because good nutrition is essential to good health and disease prevention, any person involved in health care needs a thorough knowledge of nutrition and the body's nutritional requirements throughout the life span. What's more, the study of nutrition must focus on health promotion.

Nutrients

For nutrition to be adequate, a person must receive certain *essential nutrients*—carbohydrates, fats, proteins, vitamins, minerals and water. These nutrients must be present for proper

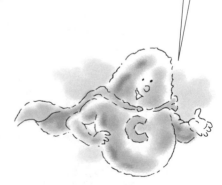

Each of us nutrients has his or her own special power, but we all work together to keep the body functioning.

growth and functioning; however, the body can't produce them on its own in adequate quantities, so they must be obtained through food. In addition, the digestive system must function properly to make use of these nutrients.

Each nutrient has a number of specific metabolic functions, but no nutrient works alone. Close metabolic relationships exist among all of the basic nutrients as well as with their metabolic products.

The non-essentials

A non-essential nutrient is one that isn't needed in the diet because it's manufactured by the body.

The nutrient breakdown dance

Nutrients can be used by the body for its immediate needs, or they can be stored for later use. The body breaks down food into simpler compounds for absorption in the stomach and intestines in two ways:
- mechanical breakdown, which begins in the GI tract with chewing
- chemical breakdown, which starts with salivary enzymes in the mouth and continues with acid and enzyme action through the rest of the GI tract.

The role of a lifeline

Nutrients play a vital role in maintaining health and wellness. They have several important functions:
- providing energy, which can be used for vital activities or stored in the body
- building and maintaining body tissue
- controlling metabolic processes, such as growth, cell activity, enzyme production and temperature regulation.

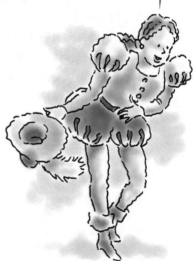

All the body's a stage...and all the nutrients play their roles, including providing energy, building tissue and controlling metabolism.

Metabolism

Regulated mostly by hormones, metabolism is a combination of several processes by which energy is extracted from certain nutrients (carbohydrates, proteins and fats) and then used by the body. Vitamins and minerals don't directly provide us with energy, but they are an important part of the metabolic process.

Metabolism can be broken down into two parts:
- *Catabolism* is the breakdown of complex substances into simpler ones, resulting in the release of energy. This process provides the energy necessary for tissue growth, maintenance and repair.
- *Anabolism* is the synthesis of simple substances into more complex substances.

Energy

Energy, in the form of adenosine triphosphate, is produced as a by-product of carbohydrate, fat and protein metabolism. The amount of energy in food products is measured in kilocalories, which is commonly referred to as *calories*.

Through the processes of digestion and absorption, energy is released from food into the body. Small amounts of energy are stored within cells for immediate use. Larger amounts of energy are stored in glycogen and fat tissue to fuel long-duration activities. (For more information, see Chapter 2.)

Balancing act

In a healthy adult, the rate of anabolism equals the rate of catabolism, and energy balance is obtained. In other words, energy balance occurs when the caloric intake from food equals the number of calories expended. These calories may be used for voluntary activities (such as physical activity) or involuntary activities (such as basal metabolism—the amount of energy used when the body is at rest).

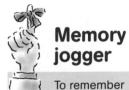

Memory jogger

To remember the difference between catabolism and anabolism, think **cat**abolism and **add** anabolism. Catabolism cuts, or breaks down, substances in the body, whereas anabolism adds, or synthesizes, new substances.

Nutrition and health promotion

Many people may consider themselves healthy because they don't feel sick. However, you must be concerned about a more holistic meaning of the term *health*—one that incorporates aspects of the person's internal and external environments—in order to best care for your patients.

For you, health promotion must consider all of a patient's needs, including physical, emotional, mental and social needs. Only when these needs are met can it be said that a person is healthy, or well. Furthermore, wellness implies a state of balance between a person's activities and goals. Maintaining this balance allows the person to maintain his or her vitality and ability to function productively in society.

A nutritional diet provides the basis for health promotion and disease prevention, making it an important part of caring for any patient.

Approaches to health promotion

There are two main approaches to health promotion:
• The *traditional approach* is reactive; it focuses on treating symptoms after they present.
• The *preventive approach* involves identifying and eliminating risk factors to stop health problems from developing.

The current public health movement in UK is grounded in the preventive approach, with individuals educating themselves about maintaining health and preventing illness and disease.

20/10 vision

The UK national health goals, which were published in the Department of Health, *White Paper (Choosing Health)*, published in November 2004, build on Our Healthier Nation and set out the key principles of supporting the public to make healthier and more informed choices in regards to their health. In February 2010 three independent reports have been published (DH 2010) which also reflect the preventive wellness philosophy. Prominent themes in the latest reports include:

- the role of the individual and the state in making healthier choices
- choosing a healthy diet
- maintaining weight control
- monitoring for and reducing high risk factors for disease.
- increasing activity levels.

Health promotion and disease prevention

Promoting health, establishing wellness and preventing disease is a three-part process. (See *Three parts to prevention*.)

Nutrition and a balanced diet

You're part of a health care team that's responsible for making sure the individual maintains optimal nutritional health, even though he or she may be battling illness or recovering from surgery. It's also your job to stress to the individual the importance of good nutrition in maintaining health and recovering from illness, so that he or she can continue sound nutritional practices when he or she is no longer under your care.

Nutritional status

You must use your knowledge of nutrition to promote health through education and counselling of sick and healthy people. This includes encouraging individuals to consume appropriate types and amounts of food. It also means considering poor food habits as a contributing factor in a patient with chronic illness. Therefore, assessing nutritional status and identifying nutritional needs to meet the requirements of a balanced diet are primary activities in planning patient care. (See *Religious practices and dietary restrictions*, page 8.)

Assessing nutritional status

A patient's nutritional status can influence the body's response to illness and treatment. Regardless of your patient's overall condition, an evaluation of his or her nutritional health is an essential part of your assessment. Assessment of the patient's nutritional status includes determining nutritional risk factors as well as individual needs.

How many ways can I serve it up? A nutritious diet provides the basis for health promotion and disease prevention.

Three parts to prevention

Health promotion and disease prevention efforts can be categorised into three groups.

 Primary prevention

Examples of primary prevention measures, which focus on health promotion, include:

- conducting classes that explore food and diet to promote healthy eating patterns
- modifying menus in restaurants and offering low-fat alternatives
- offering fresh fruit and vegetables in workplace cafeterias.

 Secondary prevention

Secondary prevention, which focuses on risk reduction, may include such measures as:

- screening for potential diseases (hypercholesterolemia, osteoporosis)
- nutritional counselling for people at risk for cardiovascular diseases and diabetes
- immunisations.

 Tertiary prevention

Examples of tertiary prevention measures, which focus on disease treatment and rehabilitation, include:

- physical rehabilitation for the stroke patient
- cardiac rehabilitation for the cardiac patient
- diabetes education classes for the patient with newly diagnosed type 1 or type 2 diabetes.

Memory jogger

To remember the three parts to prevention, think **PST:**

Primary = Health **P**romotion

Secondary = **S**creening

Tertiary = **T**reatment.

Balance is best! An assorted diet that provides all of the essential nutrients is a main ingredient of good nutrition.

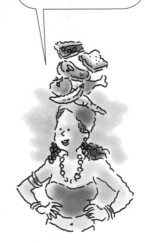

Good nutrition

Good nutrition, or optimal nutrition, is essential in promoting health, preventing illness, and restoring health after an injury or illness. To achieve optimal nutrition, a person must eat a varied diet containing carbohydrates, proteins, fats, vitamins, minerals, water and fibre in sufficient amounts. An excess of certain nutrients such as carbohydrates and fats can be detrimental to a person's health; however, it is important that the intake of essential nutrients is greater than the minimum requirements to provide stores for later use and to allow for variations in health.

Poor nutrition

Poor nutrition, or malnutrition, is a state of inadequate or excess nutritional intake. It's most common in people in lower socio-economic groups and those with greater nutritional need such as chronic illness, pregnant women, children and infants. It also occurs in hospitals and long-term care settings, because the patients in these situations have illnesses that place added stress on their bodies, raising nutritional requirements.

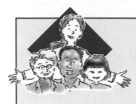

Bridging the gap

Religious practices and dietary restrictions

Religious beliefs can greatly impact dietary practices and, therefore, dietary nursing considerations. For example:

- Orthodox Jews who follow Kosher laws don't consume milk and other dairy products with meat or poultry.
- Many Seventh-Day Adventists are lacto-ovo vegetarians. Among those who do eat meat, pork is avoided.
- Hindus and Buddhists may also avoid consuming meat.

Don't underestimate undernutrition

Undernutrition occurs when a patient consumes fewer daily nutrients than his or her body requires, resulting in a nutritional deficit. Typically, undernourished patients are at greater risk for physical illnesses. They may also suffer from limitations in cognitive and physical status.

Undernutrition can result from:
- inability to metabolise nutrients
- inability to obtain the appropriate nutrients from food
- accelerated excretion of nutrients from the body
- illness or disease that increases the body's need for nutrients.

Don't overdo it

In contrast, overnutrition occurs when a patient consumes an excessive amount of nutrients. For example, overnutrition may occur in patients who overeat and in those who self-prescribe mega doses of vitamins and mineral supplements. These practices can result in damage to body tissue or obesity.

Nutrient standards

To maintain healthy populations, most developed countries have established nutrition standards for major nutrients. These standards serve as guidelines for nutrient intake based on the nutritional needs of most healthy population groups.

UK standards

The UK nutrient standards, called Recommended Intakes of Nutrients for the United Kingdom, were first published in 1969 as a guide for planning and acquiring food supplies and promoting good nutrition. To keep up with increasing scientific information and social concerns about nutrition and health, these standards have been revised and expanded.

> Most people need to step up their exercise. UK dietary guidelines include recommending 30 minutes of moderate physical activity almost every day for adults.

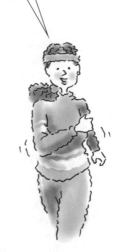

> ### Dietary Reference Values
>
> Dietary Reference Values (DRVs) comprise a set of three nutrient-based reference values being developed by the Panel on Dietary Reference Values of the Committee on Medical Aspects of Food Policy. A fourth value—Safe Intake—is set for those nutrients which are known to have important functions in humans, but where there is insufficient reliable evidence on human requirements. They include updated values for Estimated Average Requirement (EAR), Lower Reference Nutrient Intake (LRNI) and Reference Nutrient Intake (RNI).
>
> #### Estimated Average Requirement
>
> The EAR of a nutrient is the average daily dietary intake needed to meet the requirements of half of all healthy people in a given life stage or gender group. Determination of this value isn't based solely on preventing nutritional deficiencies but also includes concepts related to risk reduction and bioavailability of a given nutrient.
>
> #### Lower Reference Nutrient Intake
>
> The LRNI represents the lowest intakes which will meet the needs of some individuals within the group. Intakes below this level are almost certainly inadequate for most individuals.
>
> #### Reference Nutrient Intake
>
> The RNI will meet 97.5% of the populations needs. Intakes above this amount will almost be adequate for the majority of people in the UK.

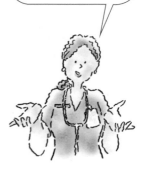

RNI...LRNI... No wonder I have a craving for alphabet soup!

Dietary Reference Values (DRVs) are the most recent version of the UK nutrient standards. Because DRVs consider an individual's sex and age group and aren't limited to preventing deficiency diseases, these standards are more comprehensive than the previous Recommended Daily Amounts (RDA's), in measuring a patient's nutritional status and long-term health. (See *Dietary Reference Values.*)

Other standards

The published standards of other countries, such as Canada and United States, are similar to British standards. In impoverished countries, where quality of food and nutrition are lacking, standards are set by the Food and Agriculture Organization and the World Health Organization. No matter who sets the standards, the goal is the same: to promote good health and prevent disease through sound nutrition.

Dietary guidelines

Dietary guidelines have been developed by governmental agencies, nutritionists and special groups to provide recommendations that promote healthy eating habits. The UK dietary guidelines recommend that people age 2 and older eat a healthy assortment of foods from the basic food groups. They also emphasise the importance of:

- choosing foods that are low in added sugars and saturated and trans fats
- eating reasonable portions.

When advising on diet, the guidelines also emphasise the importance of exercise and include getting at least 30 minutes of moderate physical activity on most days for adults (the guidelines for children recommend at least 60 minutes of physical activity on most days of the week).

Dietary guidelines for UK

The Department of Health and the Health Education Authority first released their Dietary Guidelines and Healthy Eating in 1991 to enable an individual to prepare a well-balanced diet through variety, balance and moderation of choices. These guidelines have been updated and modified to form the Eatwell Plate through the *Food Standards Agency* (*FSA*) and is linked to online advice and information. (See *Anatomy of the eatwell plate*.)

Anatomy of the eatwell plate—a guide to healthier eating

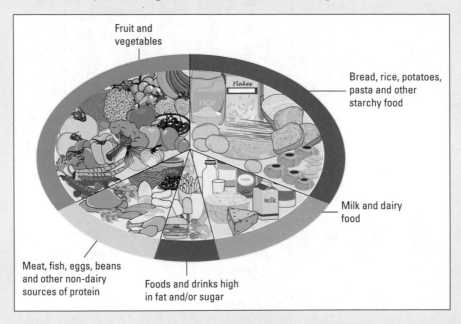

The *FSA* eatwell plate is designed to be simple and has been developed to remind consumers to make healthy food choices. The plate forms part of an integrated approach to healthy eating which includes physical activity and includes the eight steps to a healthier diet available online http://www.eatwell.gov.uk/healthydiet/eighttipssection/8tips/

Step 1. Base your meals on starchy foods

Starchy foods such as bread, cereals, rice, pasta and potatoes are a really important part of a healthy diet. Try to choose wholegrain varieties of starchy foods whenever you can.

Anatomy of the eatwell plate—a guide to healthier eating (continued)

Some people think starchy foods are fattening, but gram for gram they contain less than half the calories of fat.

You just need to watch the fats you add when cooking and serving these foods, because this is what increases the calorie content.

Wholegrain foods contain more fibre and other nutrients than white or refined starchy foods.

We also digest wholegrain foods more slowly so they can help make us feel full for longer.

Wholegrain foods include:

- wholemeal and wholegrain bread, pitta and chapatti
- wholewheat pasta and brown rice
- wholegrain breakfast cereals.

Step 2. Eat lots of fruit and veg

Most people know we should be eating more fruit and veg. But most of us still aren't eating enough.

Step 3. Eat more fish

Most of us should be eating more fish—including a portion of oily fish each week. It's an excellent source of protein and contains many vitamins and minerals.

Aim for at least two portions of fish a week, including a portion of oily fish. You can choose from fresh, frozen or canned—but remember that canned and smoked fish can be high in salt.

Step 4. Cut down on saturated fat and sugar

Fats

To stay healthy we need some fat in our diets. What is important is the kind of fat we are eating. There are two main types of fat:

- saturated fat—having too much can increase the amount of cholesterol in the blood, which increases the chance of developing heart disease
- unsaturated fat—having unsaturated fat instead of saturated fat lowers blood cholesterol

Try to cut down on food that is high in saturated fat and have foods that are rich in unsaturated fat instead, such as vegetable oils (including sunflower, rapeseed and olive oil), oily fish, avocados, nuts and seeds.

Sugar

Most people in the UK are eating too much sugar. We should all be trying to eat fewer foods containing added sugar, such as sweets, cakes and biscuits, and drinking fewer sugary soft and fizzy drinks.

Having sugary foods and drinks too often can cause tooth decay, especially if you have them between meals. Many foods that contain added sugar can also be high in calories so cutting down could help you control your weight.

Step 5. Try to eat less salt—no more than 6 g a day

Lots of people think they don't eat much salt, especially if they don't add it to their food. But don't be so sure!

Every day in the UK, 85% men and 69% women eat too much salt. Adults—and children over 11—should have no more than 6g salt a day. Younger children should have even less.

(continued)

Anatomy of the eatwell plate—a guide to healthier eating (continued)

Three-quarters (75%) of the salt we eat is already in the food we buy, such as breakfast cereals, soups, sauces and ready meals. So you could easily be eating too much salt without realizing it.

Eating too much salt can raise your blood pressure. And people with high blood pressure are three times more likely to develop heart disease or have a stroke than people with normal blood pressure.

Step 6. Get active and try to be a healthy weight

It's not a good idea to be either underweight or overweight. Being overweight can lead to health conditions such as heart disease, high blood pressure or diabetes. Being underweight could also affect your health.

Physical activity is a good way of using up extra calories, and helps control our weight. But this doesn't mean you need to join a gym.

Just try to get active every day and build up the amount you do. For example you could try to fit in as much walking as you can into your daily routine. Try to walk at a good pace.

Whenever we eat more than our body needs, we put on weight. This is because we store any energy we don't use up—usually as fat. Even small amounts of extra energy each day can lead to weight gain.

But crash diets aren't good for your health and they don't work in the longer term. The way to reach a healthy weight—and stay there—is to change your lifestyle gradually. Aim to lose about 0.5 to 1 kg (about 1 to 2 lbs) a week, until you reach a healthy weight for your height.

Step 7. Drink plenty of water

We should be drinking about 6 to 8 glasses (1.2 L) of water, or other fluids, every day to stop us getting dehydrated.

When the weather is warm or when we get active, our bodies need more than this. But avoid drinking soft and fizzy drinks that are high in added sugar.

Alcohol

There is nothing wrong with the occasional drink. But drinking too much can cause problems. Alcohol is also high in calories, so cutting down could help you control your weight.

Women can drink up to 2 to 3 units of alcohol a day and men up to 3 to 4 units a day, without significant risk to their health.

A unit is half a pint of standard strength (3% to 5% alcohol by volume (ABV)) beer, lager or cider, or a pub measure of spirit. A glass of wine is about 2 units and alcopops are about 1.5 units.

For good health, it's a good idea to spread your drinking throughout the week and avoid binge drinking. Drinking heavily over a long period of time can damage the liver.

Step 8. Don't skip breakfast

Breakfast can help give us the energy we need to face the day, as well as some of the vitamins and minerals we need for good health.

Some people skip breakfast because they think it will help them lose weight. But missing meals doesn't help us lose weight and it isn't good for us, because we can miss out on essential nutrients.

There is some evidence to suggest that eating breakfast can actually help people control their weight.

What's new?

The plate uses wedges of different widths and colours to represent the recommended amount of food a healthy adult person should choose from a food group.

Another new feature of eatwell is that it is supported by online information. The new online information also makes recommendations based on health needs for specific populations, such as children and adolescents, women of childbearing age, pregnant and breast-feeding women, older adults, people with hypertension, and overweight children and adults.

The rainbow of colours in the new eatwell plate represents one basic rule: make sure that your patient's plate has a lot of colour on it.

Food group recommendations

Each wedge on the eatwell plate represents one of the five food groups: starchy foods such as bread, rice, potatoes and pasta, fruits and vegetables, milk and dairy foods, meat and meat alternatives, foods and drinks high in fat or sugar. The wedges are wider at the top, indicating that not all food groups are of equal nutritional value. The following guidelines can help guide your patient to eat healthy.

Starchy foods group

Foods in the starch group are sources of complex carbohydrates, vitamins, minerals and fibre. To help your patient make healthy food choices from this food group, suggest that they follow these recommendations:

- Starchy foods should make up about a third of the food we eat. They are a good source of energy and the main source of a range of nutrients in our diet. As well as starch, these foods contain fibre, calcium, iron and B vitamins.

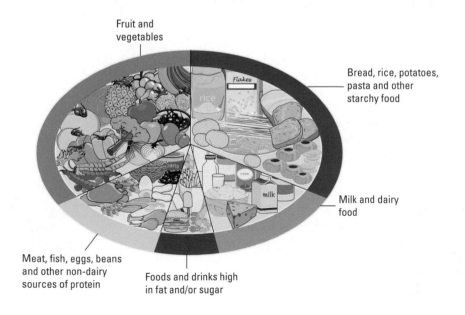

Fruit and vegetables

Bread, rice, potatoes, pasta and other starchy food

Milk and dairy food

Meat, fish, eggs, beans and other non-dairy sources of protein

Foods and drinks high in fat and/or sugar

- Select several servings of food made from whole grains to add fibre.
- Avoid baked grain products that are high in fat and sugar, such as cakes and biscuits.

Fruit and vegetable group

The fruit and vegetable group provides sources of many vitamin and minerals such as vitamin A, vitamin C and potassium. It is also a good source of fibre. The foods in this group are naturally low in fat and sodium. To help your patient make the right choices from the fruit and vegetable group, recommend that they follow these recommendations:

- Try to eat at least five portions of a variety of fruit and vegetables every day. It might be easier than you think.

They could try adding up their portions during the day.

For example you could suggest that they have:

- a glass of juice and a sliced banana with their cereal at breakfast
- a side salad at lunch
- a pear or apple instead of a pudding
- sliced carrots or cucumber as an afternoon snack
- a portion of peas or other vegetables with their evening meal.

They can choose from fresh, frozen, tinned, dried or juiced, but remember potatoes count as a starchy food, not as portions of fruit and vegetables.

Meat and meat alternatives group

Foods in the meat and meat alternatives group provide protein, vitamins and minerals. To help your patient make healthy food choices from this group, suggest that he or she follow these recommendations:

- Consume low-fat or lean meats and poultry.
- Eat meats that are boiled, steamed or grilled.
- Vary selections among fish, beans, peas, nuts and seeds.
- Trim away visible fat.

Milk and dairy foods group

Foods in the milk group provide protein, vitamins and minerals. To help your patient make healthy choices from this group, suggest that he or she follow these recommendations:

- Choose reduced-fat hard cheeses, which usually contain between 10 and 16 g fat per 100 g. A few cheeses are even lower in fat (3 g fat per 100 g or less), including reduced-fat cottage cheese and Quark.
- Pick low-fat or fat-free milk, yogurt and other milk products.
- Choose other calcium sources, such as fortified foods, if the patient doesn't or can't have milk.

Foods and drinks high in fat or sugar group

Try to eat these sorts of foods less often or in small amounts:

- meat pies, sausages and meat with visible white fat
- full fat cheese
- butter and lard
- pastry

Be sure to tell your patient to choose low-fat or fat-free milk and milk products.

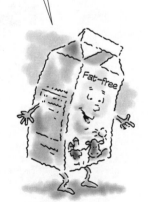

- readymade meals such as pizza or pies
- cakes and biscuits
- cream, soured cream and crème fraîche
- coconut oil, coconut cream or palm oil.

For a healthy choice, use just a small amount of vegetable oil or a reduced-fat spread instead of butter, lard or ghee. And when you are having meat, try to choose lean cuts and cut off any visible fat. Use only one half of the fat suggested when baking cakes or using cake mixes.

Vegetarian diets

For various reasons, including religious, environmental, ethical and health reasons, people may choose to follow vegetarian diets. Typically, vegetarian diets are lower in saturated fat and cholesterol and higher in fibre, carbohydrates, magnesium, boron, folate, antioxidants, carotenoids and phytochemicals. Vegetarians having a balanced diet have a lower risk of obesity, cancer, heart disease, hypertension, dementia, type 2 diabetes mellitus and, possibly, kidney disease, gallstones and diverticular disease. On the other hand, vegetarians are at risk for protein, iron and vitamin B_{12} deficiencies. If they avoid dairy products, they are also at risk for calcium and vitamin D deficiencies.

The three basic types of vegetarian diets vary according to the needs or beliefs of the person following the diet:

- Lacto-ovo vegetarians include dairy products and eggs in their diet.
- Lacto-vegetarians include only dairy products as an animal food source in their diet.
- Vegans include no animal food sources in their diet. For patients on such a diet, the use of soybeans and its by-products, along with plant foods, can help provide a balanced diet.

Well-planned vegetarian diets can be nutritionally balanced diets for any patient, including a pregnant or nursing woman. (See *Tips for the vegetarian* and *Nutrient concerns for vegetarians*, page 16.)

NutriTips

Tips for the vegetarian

If your patient is a vegetarian, suggest these tips to help ensure that he or she is meeting his or her daily protein requirements:

- Eat a variety of foods from all food groups, being sure to include all nutrients.
- Consume adequate calories for your lifestyle to prevent your body from using amino acids for fuel.
- Use low-fat or non-fat products and moderately consume nuts and seeds to maintain a low-fat diet.
- Select whole grains whenever possible to increase fibre and iron content.
- Include a vitamin C source at every meal to aid iron absorption.
- If a strict vegan your patient may need additional vitamin B_{12} (for strict vegans).

Nutrient concerns for vegetarians

It's important to emphasise to vegetarians that they include all nutrients in their diet. Here are some nutrients that are commonly lacking in vegetarian diets that are not well balanced, as well as suggestions for incorporating them into the diet.

Calcium

In a balanced diet calcium intake is comparable to or higher than that of the non-vegetarian diet. Found in dairy products and dark leafy vegetables, calcium can also be obtained by consuming calcium-fortified products, such as orange juice, or calcium supplements.

Iron

Iron can be incorporated into the diet through the consumption of fortified breads or grains, legumes and soy products.

Iron deficiency anaemia isn't prevalent in the vegan population. This may be because vegans consume large amounts of vitamin C, which enhances iron absorption.

Linolenic acid

Linolenic acid is a dietary fatty acid that aids tissue strength, muscle tone, blood clotting, cholesterol metabolism and heart function. Usually obtained in fish or eggs, linolenic acid can also be obtained in walnuts, flaxseeds and soybean and canola oils.

Vitamin B_{12}

Vitamin B_{12} occurs naturally only in animal products. In the UK it is commonly added to fortified breakfast cereals or it may be taken as a supplement.

Vitamin D

Vitamin D intake is typically low in the vegan diet because of the lack of milk and milk products; vitamin D can't be obtained in adequate quantities in plants alone. Milk is the largest source of vitamin D because it is fortified with the vitamin.

Vitamin D can also be found in fortified soy milk and ready-to-eat cereal. In healthy people most vitamin D can be obtained by spending about 10 minutes in the sun each day.

Zinc

Vegetarians typically eat fewer foods that contain zinc. Despite this, most maintain adequate levels in the body because there are some plant sources of zinc. The zinc found in plants isn't as easily absorbed as zinc from animal sources. Zinc can also be found in whole grains, soy products, nuts and seeds.

To help a vegetarian patient meet all the nutrition recommendations of the *Food Standards Agency*, offer the following suggestions:

- Eat a variety of foods to meet caloric needs.
- Plan meals around sources of protein that are low in fat. This includes beans, lentils and rice. Avoid using cheeses that are high in fat to replace meat.
- If they are not consuming cow's milk, suggest they increase calcium intake by using calcium-fortified, soy-based beverages, which are typically low in fat and cholesterol.
- Prepare food dishes that are usually made with meat or poultry, such as lasagne or pizza, as vegetarian dishes. This increases the number of servings of vegetables while reducing saturated fat and cholesterol.
- Consider vegetarian products that look, and often taste, like meat dishes, such as soy-based sausages and 'veggie burgers'. These vegetable products are usually low in saturated fat and cholesterol free.

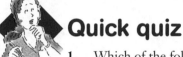

Quick quiz

1. Which of the following activities would be considered a secondary prevention measure?
- A. Promotion of health behaviours
- B. Implementation of screenings for disease
- C. Conduction of classes for patients with diabetes
- D. Rehabilitation of a stroke patient

Answer: B. Secondary prevention focuses on risk reduction, which may include screening for disease.

2. Through metabolism, energy is extracted from which nutrients?
- A. Carbohydrates, proteins and fats
- B. Carbohydrates, fats and sodium
- C. Fats, adenosine triphosphate and minerals
- D. Vitamins, minerals and electrolytes

Answer: A. Energy is produced through the metabolism of carbohydrates, proteins and fats.

3. Essential nutrients are supplied to the body by:
- A. Vitamin or mineral supplements.
- B. Certain food combinations
- C. Body functions
- D. Food in many different combinations

Answer: D. Essential nutrients are supplied by the many combinations of food consumed.

4. Which of the following populations is most at risk for poor nutrition?
- A. Young adults
- B. Adult men
- C. Adult women
- D. Elderly people

Answer: D. Elderly people are a high-risk population for poor nutrition due to the ageing process.

> If you thought this chapter was tasty, wait 'til you feast on Chapter 2!

Scoring

⭐⭐⭐ If you answered all four questions correctly, treat yourself to a fresh salad or a juicy apple! You've earned a tasty reward for knowing the basics of nutrition so well.

⭐⭐ If you answered three questions correctly, good for you! You have a well-balanced knowledge of nutrient essentials.

⭐ If you answered fewer than three questions correctly, don't give up! There's still plenty of time to climb the food guide pyramid and energise your nutrient know-how.

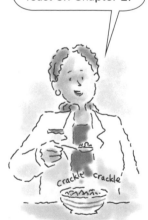

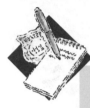

2 Digestion and absorption

Just the facts

The processes of digestion and absorption are fundamental to nutrition. In this chapter, you'll learn:

♦ the purpose of digestion and absorption

♦ structures of the GI tract wall, digestive organs and accessory organs as well as their functions in digestion and absorption

♦ the mechanical and chemical processes of digestion.

Chew on this fact: digestion, absorption and excretion of waste products are the GI tract's major functions.

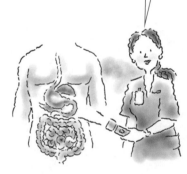

A look at digestion and absorption

The basic purpose of digestion and absorption is to deliver essential nutrients to the cells in order to sustain life. To break food down into these essential nutrients, the body sends it through various mechanical and chemical processes in the gastrointestinal (GI) tract, or *alimentary canal*. Successful digestion and absorption depend on the coordinated function of the GI tract wall's muscles and nerves, the GI tract organs and the accessory organs of digestion. (See *Structures of the GI system*.)

GI tract wall structures

The wall of the GI tract consists of four major layers:

 visceral peritoneum

 tunica muscularis

 submucosa

 mucosa.

Structures of the GI system

The GI system includes the alimentary canal (pharynx, oesophagus, stomach and small and large intestines) and the accessory organs (liver, biliary duct system and pancreas).

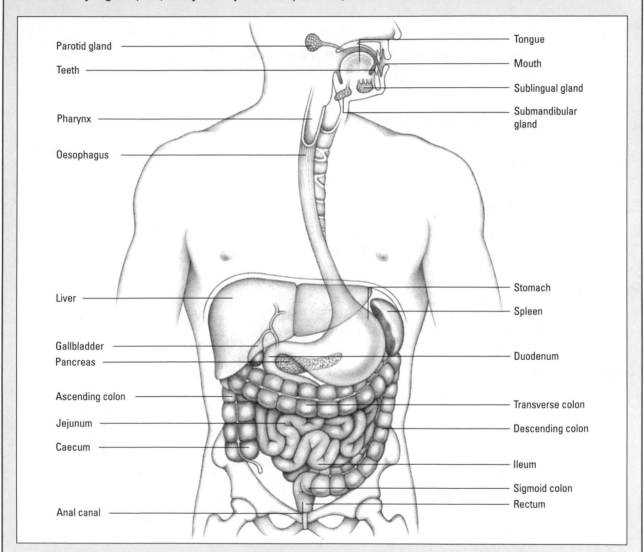

Parotid gland

Teeth

Pharynx

Oesophagus

Liver

Gallbladder

Pancreas

Ascending colon

Jejunum

Caecum

Anal canal

Tongue

Mouth

Sublingual gland

Submandibular gland

Stomach

Spleen

Duodenum

Transverse colon

Descending colon

Ileum

Sigmoid colon

Rectum

Visceral peritoneum

The *visceral peritoneum* is the GI tract's outer covering. It covers most of the abdominal organs and lies next to an identical layer, the *parietal peritoneum*, which lines the abdominal cavity.

To serve and protect

The main job of this outer layer of the GI tract wall is to protect the blood vessels, nerves and lymphatics. It also attaches the jejunum, ileum and transverse colon to the posterior abdominal wall to prevent twisting.

Many names, one layer

The visceral peritoneum has many names. In the oesophagus and rectum, it's called the *tunica adventitia*. Elsewhere in the GI tract, it's called the *tunica serosa*.

Tunica muscularis

The *tunica muscularis*, which lies within the visceral peritoneum, is a layer composed of skeletal muscle in the mouth, pharynx and upper oesophagus.

Elsewhere in the tract …

The tunica muscularis is made up of longitudinal and circular smooth-muscle fibres. At points along the tract, circular fibres thicken to form sphincters.

Pucker pouches

In the large intestine, these fibres gather into three narrow bands (*taeniae coli*) down the middle of the colon and pucker the intestine into characteristic pouches (*haustra*).

Nerve network

Between the two muscle layers lies a nerve network—the *myenteric plexus*, also known as *Auerbach's plexus*. The stomach wall contains a third muscle layer made up of oblique fibres.

Submucosa

The *submucosa*, also called the *tunica submucosa*, lies under the tunica muscularis. It's composed of loose connective tissue, blood and lymphatic vessels, and another nerve network called the *submucosal plexus*, or *Meissner's plexus*.

Mucosa

The *mucosa*, the innermost layer of the GI tract wall, is also called the *tunica mucosa*. This layer consists of epithelial and surface cells and loose connective tissue. Villi from surface cells secrete gastric and protective juices and absorb nutrients.

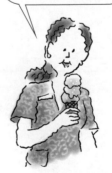

Past the lips, past the gums… look out mucosa, here it comes!

GI tract wall functions

The nerves and muscles of the GI tract wall work jointly to ensure that food moves spontaneously through the digestive system (motility). GI tract functions include innervation and secretion.

GI tract innervation

Distension of the submucosal plexus in the submucosa or myenteric plexus in the tunica muscularis stimulates transmission of nerve signals to the smooth muscle, which initiates contraction and relaxation of these muscles, or *peristalsis*. During peristalsis, longitudinal fibres of the tunica muscularis shorten the lumen length and circular fibres reduce the lumen diameter.

GI tract secretion

Five major substances secreted by the GI tract contribute to the chemical process of digestion:

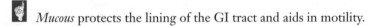 *Mucous* protects the lining of the GI tract and aids in motility.

Enzymes are proteins that break down nutrients.

Acid and various buffer ions contribute to the level of alkalinity or acidity (pH) needed to activate digestive enzymes.

Electrolytes and water carry nutrients through the GI tract and aid in the absorption process.

Bile emulsifies fat to promote intestinal absorption of fatty acids, cholesterol and other lipids.

How digestion and absorption work

The organs of the GI tract play a major role in mechanical and chemical digestion and absorption of food and fluid. (See *Functions of the digestive system organs*, page 22.) Aided by the GI tract wall and accessory organs, the organs of the GI tract process nutrients in three phases of digestion:

 cephalic

 gastric

 intestinal.

Functions of the digestive system organs

This chart lists the digestive system organs and their primary functions.

Organ	Function
Mouth	• Breaks down food into smaller particles • Releases saliva to promote chewing and swallowing • Secretes amylase (ptyalin) to begin breaking down starch
Oesophagus	• Propels food downwards into the stomach
Stomach	• Acts as a food reservoir • Mixes food with gastric secretions (hydrochloric acid, pepsin, mucous, intrinsic factor) • Begins protein digestion • Absorbs water, alcohol and some drugs
Liver	• Produces bile • Metabolises carbohydrate, protein and fat • Stores nutrients • Detoxifies drugs and waste products
Gall bladder	• Concentrates and stores bile • Releases bile into the duodenum
Pancreas	• Produces and secretes insulin and glucagon • Produces and secretes digestive enzymes: proteases, lipase and amylase
Small intestine	• Secretes hormones to stimulate the secretion of pancreatic juices, bile and intestinal enzymes • Secretes digestive enzymes: peptidases and disaccharidases • Absorbs iron, magnesium and calcium (duodenum) • Absorbs water-soluble vitamins and simple sugars (jejunum) • Absorbs amino acids, peptides, fat-soluble vitamins, fats, cholesterol, bile salts and vitamin B_{12} (ileum)
Large intestine	• Absorbs water, sodium, potassium and vitamin K formed by colonic bacteria • Eliminates solid waste

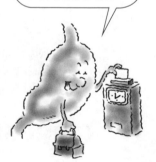

I'd better punch in! All of us GI organs have a lot of work to do.

Cephalic phase

The cephalic phase of digestion uses the GI tract organs of the mouth, pharynx and oesophagus to begin the mechanical processes of digestion. It begins as soon as you see, smell or begin to think about food. Mechanical chewing breaks down food into smaller particles, which increases the surface area on which digestive enzymes can work.

Mouth

Digestion begins in the mouth (also called the *buccal cavity* or *oral cavity*). Ducts connect the mouth with the three major pairs of salivary glands:
- parotid
- submandibular
- sublingual.

These glands secrete the enzyme *ptyalin* (a salivary amylase) to moisten food during chewing (mastication) and begin breaking down starch into maltose. (See *Causes of dry mouth in older adults*.)

Pharynx

The *pharynx* is a cavity extending from the base of the skull to the oesophagus. It aids swallowing by grasping food and propelling it towards the oesophagus.

Oesophagus

A muscular tube, the *oesophagus* extends from the pharynx through the mediastinum to the stomach.

Down the hatch

When a person swallows, the cricopharyngeal sphincter in the upper oesophagus relaxes, allowing food to enter the oesophagus. In the oesophagus, the glossopharyngeal nerve activates peristalsis, which moves the food bolus down towards the stomach.

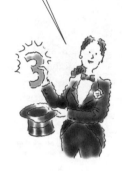

And the magic number is…3. The three major pairs of salivary glands are the parotids, submandibulars and sublinguals.

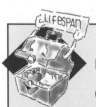

Lifespan lunchbox

Causes of dry mouth in older adults

As people age, salivation decreases, leading to dry mouth and a reduced sense of taste. Certain drugs, such as anticholinergics, antihistamines, tricyclic antidepressants, phenothiazines, clonidine and opioid analgesics, can also decrease salivation. Be sure to take a medication history for older adults. Other causes of dry mouth in older adults include facial nerve paralysis, salivary duct obstruction, Sjögren's syndrome and radiation of the mouth or face.

One slippery bolus

As food passes through the oesophagus, glands in the oesophageal mucosal layer secrete mucous, which lubricates the bolus and protects the mucosal membrane from damage caused by poorly chewed foods.

Stomach express

Because food is in the mouth only for a short time, digestion of starch is limited. The salivary amylase that's swallowed continues to work for another 15 to 30 minutes in the stomach before it's inactivated by gastric acids. By the time the food bolus is travelling towards the stomach, the stomach has begun secreting digestive juices (hydrochloric acid [HCl] and pepsin).

Gastric phase

When food enters the stomach, the gastric phase of digestion begins.

Stomach

Chemical digestion, which occurs as food mixes with digestive enzymes, begins in the stomach. The stomach acts, in part, as a temporary storage area for food and has four main regions:

 cardia

 fundus

 body

 antrum.

Cardia
The *cardia* lies near the junction of the stomach and oesophagus. Relaxation of the cardiac sphincter in this region allows food to pass from the oesophagus to the stomach.

Fundus
The *fundus* is an enlarged portion above and to the left of the oesophageal opening into the stomach. Continued peristaltic activity in this region propels the intact food bolus towards the stomach body.

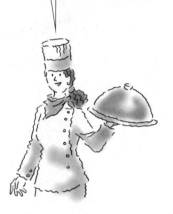

Digestive juices are secreted in response to stimuli aroused by smelling, tasting, chewing or thinking about food.

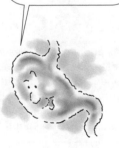

I can't help it. Just thinking about food makes me gush!

Body

The *body* is the middle portion of the stomach. In this region, distension of the stomach wall due to the food bolus stimulates secretion of gastrin.

Gassing up with gastrin

Gastrin, in turn, stimulates the stomach's motor functions and release of digestive secretions by the gastric glands. Highly acidic (pH of 0.9 to 1.5), these secretions consist mainly of HCl, intrinsic factor (which helps the body absorb vitamin B_{12}) and proteolytic enzymes (which help the body use proteins). (See *GI system changes in older adults* and *Sites and mechanisms of gastric secretion*, page 26.)

HCl helps absorb calcium and iron and activates gastric enzymes that kill most foodborne bacteria. HCl is also needed to convert the enzyme pepsinogen into pepsin.

Enzyme with pep

Pepsin, a major protein-splitting enzyme, activates the secretion of the gastric mucous that protects the gastric lining. The mucous also helps move the food bolus along the path to the small intestine.

Not much at all but alcohol

Normally, except for alcohol, little food absorption occurs in the stomach. Peristaltic contractions in the stomach body churn the food into tiny particles and mix it with gastric juices, forming *chyme*.

Antrum

The *antrum* is the lower portion of the stomach, lying near the junction of the stomach and duodenum. Stronger peristaltic waves move the chyme from the stomach body into the antrum. Here, it backs up against the pyloric sphincter before being released into the small intestine and triggering the intestinal phase of digestion. (See *Stomach emptying*, page 27.)

Intestinal phase

The majority of absorption occurs during the intestinal phase of digestion, which involves the small and large intestines.

Small intestine

The longest organ of the GI tract, the *small intestine* is a tube measuring about 20 in. (6 m) long. It performs most of the work of digestion and absorption. (See *Digestion and absorption in the small intestine*, page 27.)

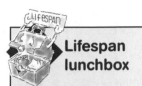

Lifespan lunchbox

GI system changes in older adults

Age-related changes in the GI system can lead to conditions that impact nutrition. Reduced gastric acid secretion in older adults can result in pernicious anaemia, iron deficiency anaemia and reduced calcium absorption. Reduced production of bile acid, enlargement of the common bile duct and increased output of cholecystokinin can lead to biliary stasis, cholelithiasis and reduced appetite. Reduced synthesis of intrinsic factor will also inhibit vitamin B_{12} absorption.

Sites and mechanisms of gastric secretion

Between the lower oesophageal sphincter (LES), or cardiac sphincter, and the pyloric sphincter lie the fundus, body, antrum and pylorus of the stomach. These areas have a rich variety of mucosal cells that help the stomach carry out its tasks.

Glands and gastric secretions

Cardiac, pyloric and gastric glands secrete 2 to 3 L of gastric juice daily through the stomach's gastric pits.

- Both the cardiac gland (near the LES) and the pyloric gland (near the pylorus) secrete thin mucous.
- The gastric gland (in body and fundus) secretes hydrochloric acid (HCl), pepsinogen, intrinsic factor and mucous.

Protection from self-digestion

Specialised cells line the gastric glands, gastric pits and surface epithelium. Mucous cells in the necks of the gastric glands produce thin mucous. Mucous cells in the surface epithelium produce an alkaline mucous. Both substances lubricate food and protect the stomach from self-digestion by corrosive enzymes.

Other secretions

Argentaffin cells produce gastrin, which stimulates gastric secretion and motility. Chief cells produce pepsinogen, which breaks down proteins into polypeptides.

Large parietal cells scattered throughout the fundus secrete HCl and intrinsic factor. HCl degrades pepsinogen, maintains an acid environment and inhibits excess bacteria growth. Intrinsic factor promotes vitamin B_{12} absorption in the small intestine.

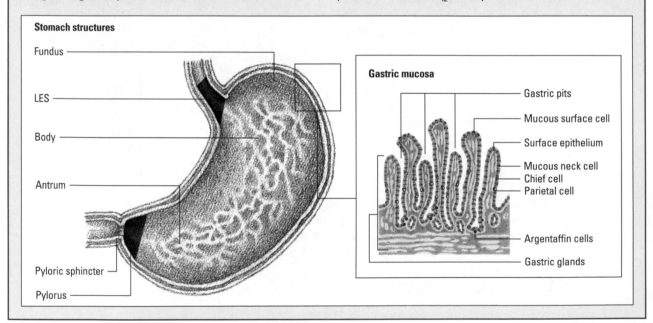

Stomach structures

- Fundus
- LES
- Body
- Antrum
- Pyloric sphincter
- Pylorus

Gastric mucosa

- Gastric pits
- Mucous surface cell
- Surface epithelium
- Mucous neck cell
- Chief cell
- Parietal cell
- Argentaffin cells
- Gastric glands

The small intestine has three major divisions:
- The *duodenum* is the first part of the small intestine and is about 25 cm long.
- The *jejunum*, the middle portion, is about 2.5 m long.
- The *ileum* is the last portion and is between 2 and 4 m long.

Stomach emptying

The rate of stomach emptying depends on several factors, including gastrin release, neural signals generated when the stomach wall distends and the *enterogastric reflex*.

Enterogastric reflex

The enterogastric reflex is a response in which the duodenum releases secretin and gastric-inhibiting peptide, and the jejunum secretes cholecystokinin. Both reactions decrease gastric motility.

Break it down, please

In the small intestine, intestinal wall contractions and digestive enzymes break down carbohydrates, proteins and fats so the intestinal mucosa can facilitate absorption of these nutrients into the bloodstream (along with water and electrolytes). These nutrients are then available for use by the body.

Digestion and absorption in the small intestine

The small intestine performs most of the work of digestion and absorption. Here's a summary of the small intestine's major tasks.

Mechanical digestion

- Small muscles mix chyme.
- Peristaltic motions propel the food mass over the length of the intestine.
- Surface villi mix chyme at the intestinal wall, enhancing absorption.
- Long muscle moves the food mass in a circular motion, providing new surface sites for absorption.
- Segmentation rings from circular muscle mix the food into soft masses and then mix it with secretions.

Chemical digestion

- Lipase breaks fats into fatty acids and glycerides.
- Amylase converts starch to the disaccharides maltose and sucrose.
- Enterokinase activates trypsinogens, which become trypsin.
- Trypsin and chymotrypsin split protein molecules into small peptides and then into individual amino acids.
- Disaccharidases convert their respective disaccharides to monosaccharides.
- Bile from the liver helps to digest and absorb fat.
- Carbohydrate foods are changed into simple sugars.
- Fats are changed into fatty acids and glycerides.
- Proteins are changed into amino acids.
- Vitamins and minerals are also released.

Absorption

- Microvilli, villi and mucous absorb essential nutrients.
- Absorption is controlled by diffusion—passive for the small materials and carrier assisted for larger items.
- Digestive contents are mostly water soluble and can be absorbed directly into the circulation.
- Fatty contents aren't water soluble; they must pass through the villi, then into the lymph system and finally into the bloodstream.

The great intestinal wall

The intestinal wall has structural features that significantly increase its absorptive surface area. These features include:

- *plicae circulares*—circular folds of the intestinal mucosa, or mucous membrane lining
- *villi*—fingerlike projections on the mucosa
- *microvilli*—tiny cytoplasmic projections on the surface of epithelial cells.

Secretion police

The small intestine also releases hormones that help control the secretion of bile, pancreatic juice and intestinal juice.

Large intestine

The main tasks of the large intestine are absorption of body water and elimination of digestive waste. In addition, the large intestine harbours the bacteria *Escherichia coli*, *Enterobacter aerogenes*, *Clostridium perfringens* and *Lactobacillus bifidus*. All of these bacteria help synthesize vitamin K and break down cellulose into usable carbohydrates. Bacterial action also produces *flatus*, which helps propel stool towards the rectum.

Protection from bacterial action

The mucosa of the large intestine also produces *alkaline secretions* from tubular glands composed of goblet cells. This alkaline mucous lubricates the intestinal walls as food pushes through, protecting the mucosa from acidic bacterial action.

The *large intestine* extends from the ileocaecal valve (the valve between the ileum of the small intestine and the first segment of the large intestine) to the anus. The large intestine has five segments:

 caecum

 ascending colon

 transverse colon

 descending and sigmoid colons

rectum and anus.

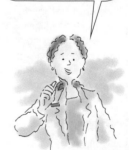

There's nothing small about the job of the small intestine. It does most of the digesting and absorbing!

Caecum

The *caecum*, a saclike structure, makes up the first few inches of the large intestine. The caecum is connected to the ileum of the small intestine by the ileocaecal pouch.

Ascending colon

The *ascending colon* rises on the right posterior abdominal wall, and then turns under the liver at the hepatic flexure. By the time chyme passes through the ileocaecal valve and enters the ascending colon of the large intestine, it has been reduced to mostly indigestible substances.

Transverse colon

The *transverse colon* is located above the small intestine, passing horizontally across the abdomen and below the liver, stomach and spleen. It proceeds to turn downwards at the left colic flexure. Through blood and lymph vessels, the large intestine absorbs all but about 100 ml of water from the chyme by the time it leaves the transverse colon. It also absorbs large amounts of sodium and chloride at this point.

Got to have your fibre

Because dietary fibre isn't digested, it travels through the large intestine unabsorbed and contributes to the formation of faeces. It also helps to keep the colon healthy by supporting a healthy population of bacteria.

Descending and sigmoid colons

The *descending colon* starts near the spleen and extends down the left side of the abdomen into the pelvic cavity. The *sigmoid colon* descends through the pelvic cavity, where it becomes the rectum. The descending and sigmoid colons are responsible for evacuation. Contents move slowly along the tract, enabling water and electrolytes to be absorbed.

Rectum

The rectum, the last few inches of the large intestine, terminates at the anus.

Mass movement

In the lower colon, long and relatively sluggish contractions cause propulsive waves, or *mass movements*. Normally occurring several times per day, these movements propel intestinal contents into the rectum and produce the urge to defecate.

Accessory organs of digestion and absorption

Accessory organs of the digestive system—the liver, biliary duct system and pancreas—contribute hormones, enzymes and bile vital to digestion and absorption.

Liver

The body's largest gland, the highly vascular liver, is enclosed in a fibrous capsule in the right upper quadrant of the abdomen.

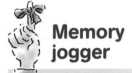

Memory jogger

To remember the five segments of the large intestine, think **C**ookies **A**lways **Tra**vel **D**own **R**ight:

Caecum

Ascending colon

Transverse colon

Descending and sigmoid colons

Rectum and anus.

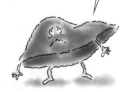

Accessory? But I'm the largest gland in the body!

The *lesser omentum*, a fold of peritoneum, covers most of the liver and anchors it to the lesser curvature of the stomach. The *hepatic artery* and *hepatic portal vein* as well as the common bile duct and hepatic veins pass through the lesser omentum.

Functioning features

The liver's functional unit, the *lobule*, consists of a plate of hepatic cells, or *hepatocytes*, that encircle a central vein and radiate outwards. Separating the hepatocyte plates from each other are *sinusoids*, the liver's capillary system. Reticuloendothelial macrophages (Kupffer cells) lining the sinusoids remove bacteria and toxins that have entered the blood through the intestinal capillaries.

Go with the blood flow

The sinusoids carry oxygenated blood from the hepatic artery and nutrient-rich blood from the portal vein. Deoxygenated blood leaves through the central vein and flows through hepatic veins to the inferior vena cava.

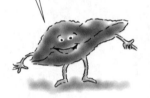

My role in carbohydrate metabolism is very important. I also detoxify plasma.

All that and a bag of chips

The liver performs many important functions in the processes of digestion and absorption. The liver:
- aids in carbohydrate metabolism
- detoxifies various endogenous and exogenous toxins, such as drugs and alcohol
- synthesizes plasma proteins, non-essential amino acids and vitamin A
- stores essential nutrients, such as vitamins K, D, and B_{12} and iron
- removes ammonia from body fluids, converting it to urea for excretion in urine
- converts glucose to glycogen and stores it as fuel for the muscles
- produces and secretes bile to aid in digestion
- stores fats and converts the excess sugars to fats to store in other parts of the body
- removes naturally occurring ammonia from body fluids, converting it to urea for excretion in the urine.

Biliary duct system

The biliary duct system consists of a network of ducts and includes the gall bladder.

Ducts

Think of ducts as a subway system transporting bile through the GI tract. *Bile* is a greenish liquid composed of water, cholesterol, bile salts and phospholipids. From the liver, bile travels via the common bile duct to the small intestine, entering through the duodenum.

When bile salts are missing

When bile salts are absent from the intestinal tract, lipids are excreted and fat-soluble vitamins are absorbed poorly.

Report on bile production

The liver recycles about 80% of bile salts into bile, combining them with bile pigments (biliverdin and bilirubin, the breakdown products of red blood cells) and cholesterol. The liver secretes this alkaline bile continuously. Bile production may increase from stimulation of the vagus nerve, release of the hormone secretin, increased blood flow in the liver and the presence of fat in the intestine. (See *GI hormones: Production and function*.)

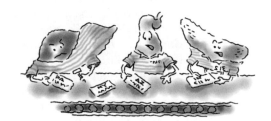

They got us on charges of accessories to digestion. Who says chyme doesn't pay?

Gall bladder

The *gall bladder* is a pear-shaped organ joined to the ventral surface of the liver by the cystic duct. The gall bladder:
- stores and concentrates bile produced by the liver
- releases bile into the common bile duct for delivery to the duodenum in response to the contraction and relaxation of the sphincter of Oddi.

The secretion of the hormone cholecystokinin causes the gall bladder to contract. This allows the release of bile into the common bile duct for delivery to the duodenum.

GI hormones: Production and function

When stimulated, GI structures secrete four hormones. Each hormone plays a different part in digestion.

Hormone and production site	Stimulating factor or agent	Function
Gastrin Produced in pyloric antrum and duodenal mucosa	• Pyloric antrum distension • Vagal stimulation • Protein digestion products • Alcohol	• Stimulates gastric secretion and motility
Gastric inhibitory peptides Produced in duodenal and jejunal mucosa	• Gastric acid • Fats • Fat digestion products	• Inhibits gastric secretion and motility
Secretin Produced in duodenal and jejunal mucosa	• Gastric acid • Fat digestion products • Protein digestion products	• Stimulates secretion of bile and alkaline pancreatic fluid
Cholecystokinin Produced in duodenal and jejunal mucosa	• Fat digestion products • Protein digestion products	• Stimulates gall bladder contraction and secretion of enzyme-rich pancreatic fluid

Pancreas

The *pancreas* is a somewhat flat organ that lies behind the stomach. Its head and neck extend into the curve of the duodenum and its tail lies against the spleen. The pancreas performs both exocrine and endocrine functions.

Exocrine function

The pancreas's exocrine function involves scattered cells that secrete more than 1,000 ml of digestive enzymes every day. Lobules and lobes of the clusters (*acini*) of enzyme-producing cells release their secretions into ducts that merge into the pancreatic duct. The pancreatic duct runs the length of the pancreas and joins the bile duct from the gall bladder before entering the duodenum. The vagus nerve stimulates the production and release of secretin and cholecystokinin, which are the two hormones responsible for regulating the rate and amount of pancreatic secretions.

Endocrine function

The endocrine function of the pancreas involves the islets of Langerhans. Two types of cells formulate the islets of Langerhans, alpha and beta cells.

The ABCs of alpha and beta cells

Over 1 million of these alpha and beta cells are in the islets. Alpha cells secrete *glucagon*, a hormone that stimulates glycogenolysis in the liver; beta cells secrete *insulin* to promote carbohydrate metabolism. Both hormones flow directly into the blood. Their release is stimulated by blood glucose levels.

Pancreatic duct

Running the length of the pancreas, the *pancreatic duct* joins the bile duct from the gall bladder before entering the duodenum. Vagal stimulation and release of the hormones secretin and cholecystokinin control the rate and amount of pancreatic secretion.

Memory jogger

To remember the difference between exocrine and endocrine, just remember that **exo**crine refers to **ex**ternal, so **endo**crine refers to **in**ternal.

Quick quiz

1. Which of the following functions is characteristic of the stomach?
   A. Breaks down carbohydrates for absorption
   B. Mixes food with gastric secretions
   C. Completes food digestion
   D. Helps synthesize vitamin K

   Answer: B. The stomach mixes food with gastric secretions to aid digestion.

2. Which of the following GI hormone stimulates gastric secretion and motility?
   A. Gastrin
   B. Gastric inhibitory peptides

    C. Secretin
    D. Pepsinogen

Answer: A. Gastrin is produced in the pyloric antrum and duodenal end mucosa and stimulates gastric secretion and motility.

3.   In which of the following phases of digestion does the stomach secrete the digestive juices hydrochloric acid and pepsin?
    A. Cephalic
    B. Gastric
    C. Intestinal
    D. Mastication

Answer: A. By the time the food is travelling towards the stomach, the cephalic phase—during which the stomach secretes digestive juices—has begun.

Scoring

☆☆☆   If you answered all three questions correctly, bravo! You've passed through the GI system and absorbed this material with the greatest of ease.

☆☆   If you answered two questions correctly, super! You've chewed the fat of this system, and it's time to move on.

☆   If you answered fewer than two questions correctly, keep at it! Take a few more minutes to digest this material.

3 Carbohydrate

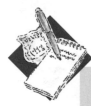

Just the facts

This chapter reviews carbohydrate, one of the essential nutrients that must be consumed in the diet. In this chapter, you'll learn:

♦ classification of carbohydrates

♦ carbohydrate functions

♦ the ways in which carbohydrates are digested, absorbed and metabolised

♦ food sources of carbohydrates.

A look at carbohydrates

Carbohydrates are organic compounds of carbon, hydrogen and oxygen that are stored in muscles and in the liver and can be converted quickly when the body needs energy. Carbohydrates are made through photosynthesis—the process by which the sun's energy allows chlorophyll-containing plants to take in carbon dioxide through their roots and release oxygen into the air. Carbon and water that remain in the plant form carbohydrates.

> Carbohydrates are organic compounds that can be quickly converted to energy.

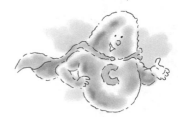

Classification of carbohydrates

Carbohydrates are classified according to the number of sugar units, or *saccharides,* that make up their structure:

• Simple carbohydrates are sugars with a simple structure of one (*monosaccharides*) or two (*disaccharides*) sugar units.

• Complex carbohydrates, or starches, consist of many sugar units (*polysaccharides*).

Singled out

Monosaccharides, also known as *simple sugars*, are carbohydrates that can be absorbed through the small intestine into the blood, where they then travel to the liver. Monosaccharides aren't broken down in the digestive process.

Examples of monosaccharides include:
- glucose (dextrose), which comes from the digestion of starch and circulates in the blood; it's the primary fuel for cells
- fructose (fruit sugar), which is found in fruits and in honey and is the sweetest of the sugars
- galactose, which comes from the digestion of lactose.

Two sweet

Disaccharides consist of two monosaccharides (one of which is glucose) minus a water molecule. These simple carbohydrates must first be digested into their component monosaccharides before being absorbed.

Important disaccharides include:
- sucrose, a common table sugar that occurs naturally in minimal amounts in some fruits and vegetables
- lactose, a non sweet sugar found in milk that aids calcium absorption and helps manufacture bacteria that are necessary for vitamin K production in the intestines
- maltose, a sugar found in germinating grains that's also a by-product of stomach digestion.

Poly want a cracker?

Polysaccharides, or complex carbohydrates, consist of larger, more complex molecules of carbohydrates that contain many sugar units. Polysaccharides are ingested and broken down into simple sugars so that they can later be used as fuel.

Examples of polysaccharides include:
- starch, which is found primarily in plant foods and is most abundant in grains, legumes and starchy vegetables (such as potatoes)
- glycogen, which is formed within the body's tissues as a store of carbohydrate energy and is then converted as needed to glucose for metabolism and energy balance

Non–starch polysaccharides (NSPs)

These are commonly referred to as *fibre or roughage*, which is found in fruits, vegetables, legumes and grains (it can't be digested and, therefore, is vital to good dietary health). Insoluble NSPs include cellulose, the outer part of grain such as bran, and are important for defecation. Soluble NSPs include gum from fruits and vegetables and are important for the health of the colon. (See *Poor oral health effects in older adults*.)

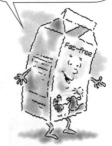

The lactose found in milk aids calcium absorption and vitamin K production.

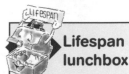

Lifespan lunchbox

Poor oral health effects in older adults

Older adults with dental problems or ill-fitting dentures might have trouble chewing fruits, vegetables and wholegrains, and their diet may be imbalanced as a result. Older adults who avoid these foods are at increased risk for nutritional deficiencies. Poor oral health may result in ineffective chewing, increasing the risk of gum disease. A lack of NSPs in the diet can increase the risk of constipation.

Functions of carbohydrates

The metabolic processes of anabolism and catabolism keep the body's carbohydrate supply in constant flux, ensuring that adequate supplies are available for both energy needs and the production of other necessary compounds.

Other functions of carbohydrates include:
- conserving protein during energy production
- helping to burn fats more efficiently and completely
- providing a quick source of energy (glucose)
- aiding in the normal functioning of the intestines (fibre)
- providing laxative action and aiding in the absorption of calcium (lactose).

Although the body can make glucose from amino acids and glycerol, carbohydrates serve as the body's primary energy source. The Dietary Reference Value is based on the role of carbohydrates as a primary energy source for the brain. The percentage of carbohydrates for energy nutrients is based on the role of carbohydrates as a source of calories to maintain body weight and to reduce the risk of chronic disease. The intake of carbohydrates should be no more than 50% of total calories.

Function 1: Energy

The primary function of carbohydrates is to meet the body's specific needs for energy. Each gram of carbohydrate yields 4 kilocalories (kcal) of energy. Because glucose burns more efficiently and completely than protein or fat and because the end products are easily eliminated, it's the body's primary fuel source. Within cells, glucose molecules are partially broken down to produce energy in the form of adenosine triphosphate (ATP). To function properly, the body must have a continuous supply of glucose available to all cells. (See *Tracking the glucose pathway*.)

Brains constantly crave carbs

Carbohydrates are also the primary source of energy for the central nervous system, especially the brain. Because the brain can't store carbohydrates, it must have an uninterrupted source of carbohydrates to function properly.

Preventing the misappropriation of protein

Adequate carbohydrate intake is also essential to preserve protein function. To meet the high energy demands of the body, dietary protein is converted to glucose when the supply of carbohydrates is inadequate. Protein used for energy is then unavailable for other protein functions, such as replenishing

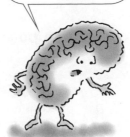

If you want me to function properly, keep the carbs coming!

Tracking the glucose pathway

All ingested carbohydrates, except NSPs, are converted to glucose, the body's main energy source. Glucose catabolism generates energy in three phases: glycolysis, the Krebs cycle and the electron-transport chain. The flow chart shown here summarises the first two phases.

Glycolysis

Glycolysis, the first phase, breaks apart one molecule of glucose to form pyruvate, which yields energy in the form of adenosine triphosphate (ATP) and acetyl coenzyme A (acetyl CoA).

Krebs cycle

The second phase, the Krebs cycle, continues carbohydrate metabolism. Fragments of acetyl CoA join to oxaloacetic acid to form citric acid. The CoA molecule breaks off from the acetyl group and may form more acetyl CoA molecules. Citric acid is first converted into intermediate compounds, and then back into oxaloacetic acid. The Krebs cycle also liberates carbon dioxide (CO_2).

Electron-transport chain

In the third phase of glucose catabolism, molecules on the inner mitochondrial membrane attract electrons from hydrogen atoms and carry them through oxidation–reduction reactions in the mitochondria. The hydrogen ions produced in the Krebs cycle then combine with oxygen (O_2) to form water (H_2O).

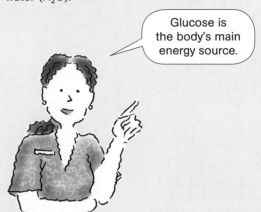

Glucose is the body's main energy source.

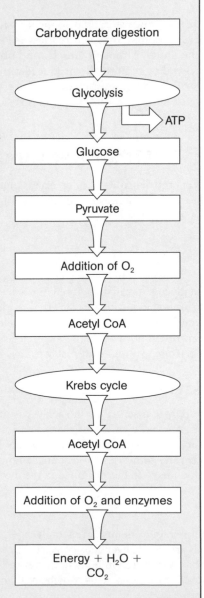

Carbohydrate digestion

Glycolysis

→ ATP

Glucose

Pyruvate

Addition of O_2

Acetyl CoA

Krebs cycle

Acetyl CoA

Addition of O_2 and enzymes

Energy + H_2O + CO_2

enzymes, hormones and blood cells. When the supply is extremely low, the body begins to break down its own protein tissue. This results in the production of energy as well as a reduction in energy needs. Adequate carbohydrate intake is especially important when the body's protein needs are high, such as in trauma and sepsis, for wound healing, in acute illness and during pregnancy and breast-feeding.

Fat's not good

The body also breaks down stored fat to meet its fuel needs when carbohydrate levels are low. When stored fats are used for energy ketones accumulate in the blood. Although muscles and other body tissues can use ketones for energy, they're normally produced only in small quantities. Rising ketone levels lead to ketosis, which may result in fatigue, nausea and lack of appetite. If the condition becomes severe, coma and death may result.

Function 2: Other compounds

After the body's energy demands are met, excess glucose can be converted to glycogen, used to produce non-essential amino acids and other compounds, or converted to fat and stored.

Conversion version

Liver and muscle cells pick up unused glucose molecules and join them together to form glycogen, which is stored in the liver and in muscles. Liver glycogen stores can quickly be converted to glucose in times of need. Between meals, glycogen breaks down and releases glucose into the bloodstream to maintain normal blood glucose levels and provide fuel for tissues. Muscle glycogen stores are available for use only by the muscles.

Essentials of non-essentials

If an adequate supply of essential amino acids is available, the body can use them and glucose to make non-essential amino acids. Non-essential amino acids are necessary for protein synthesis and metabolism (tissue and cellular). Because the body can synthesise non-essential amino acids with the use of nitrogen, they don't have to be consumed in the diet.

Fat figures

When body energy requirements are met, glycogen reserves are full and body compounds are made, liver cells convert the remaining glucose into triglycerides, which are stored in body fat. Liver cells do so by combining acetate molecules to form fatty acids, which are then combined with glycerol to make triglycerides.

How the body handles carbohydrates

Carbohydrates move through the body via the processes of digestion, absorption and metabolism.

Digestion

Monosaccharides are the only carbohydrates that the body can absorb intact. All other forms of digestible carbohydrates must be broken down into monosaccharides before they can be absorbed:
• Disaccharides must be split, in one step, into their two component sugar molecules for digestion.
• Starches require a step-by-step breakdown of complex sugar molecules into simple ones for digestion.

Too much to swallow?

Carbohydrate digestion begins in the mouth, where food is chewed and broken down into smaller particles, before entering the stomach. The food mass, now known as *chyme*, is moved by peristalsis to the small intestines, where most carbohydrate digestion occurs. In the small intestine, pancreatic amylase breaks down complex carbohydrates into disaccharides. Disaccharide enzymes (maltase, isomaltase, sucrase and lactase) finish digestion by splitting maltose, isomaltose, sucrose and lactose into monosaccharides, which are the only form of carbohydrates the body can absorb. (See *Carbohydrate digestion*, page 40.) Some people do not secrete the enzyme lactase and are unable to digest lactose, they are lactose intolerant (See *Lactose intolerance link to race*, page 40)

Fibre foibles

The GI tract lacks the enzymes to digest fibre; however, fibre is important because it can speed up the digestive process. Insoluble fibre isn't soluble and can't be dissolved in water; soluble fibre dissolves or forms a gel in water. Soluble fibres delay gastric emptying. Most fibres are fermented by bacteria in the

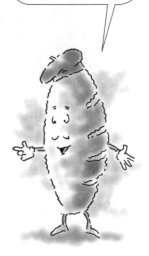

Zut alors! In order for the starches found in me to be absorbed, they must first be broken down into simple sugars.

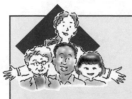

Bridging the gap

Lactose intolerance link to race

The highest rates tend to be found in South America, Africa and Asia, with approximately 50% of the population affected and almost 100% in some Asian countries. When caring for patients from these ethnic groups, ask about a family history of lactose intolerance and question them about its signs and symptoms.

Carbohydrate digestion

This chart explains how carbohydrates are digested in the body.

Organ	Action
Mouth	• Chewing action breaks down food into smaller particles. The salivary enzyme amylase acts on starch to break it down first into dextrin and then into maltose.
Stomach	• Peristalsis mixes food particles with gastric secretions.
Small intestine	• The pancreatic enzyme amylase continues the breakdown of starch to maltose. • The intestinal enzyme sucrase acts on sucrose to produce fructose. • The intestinal enzyme lactase acts on lactose to produce galactose. • The intestinal enzyme maltase acts on maltose to produce glucose. • The intestinal enzyme isomaltase acts on maltose and isomaltose to produce glucose.

large intestine to form gas, water, short-chain fatty acids and other compounds. Short-chain fatty acids are an energy source for the mucosal lining of the colon.

Absorption

The monosaccharides glucose, fructose and galactose are absorbed through the intestinal mucosa and travel to the liver through the portal vein. Small amounts of starch and fibre that haven't been fully digested are excreted in faeces. Soluble fibre slows the absorption of glucose, delaying the rise in serum glucose that occurs after eating.

Metabolism

In the liver, fructose and galactose are converted to glucose. The liver then releases glucose into the bloodstream, where its level is maintained by the actions of hormones. A rise in serum blood glucose stimulates insulin, which moves glucose out of the bloodstream and into the cells.

Levelling off

Eventually, the body uses up the energy from the most recent meal and blood glucose levels start to fall. Even a slight drop in glucose stimulates the pancreas to release glucagon, which causes the liver to release glucose from its supply of glycogen. The result is that blood glucose levels again rise to normal.

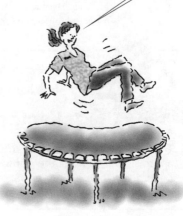

What goes up must come down. Insulin and glucagon regulate rising and falling glucose levels.

Sources of carbohydrates

Carbohydrates are found in all of the food groups. The amounts and types of carbohydrates vary considerably between food groups and among selections within each group.

> The best place to find me is in breads, cereals, rice and pasta.

Starch group

This group includes potatoes and grains including bread, cereal, rice and pasta. They provide complex carbohydrates and some protein; some grain selections also contain fat. Fibre content is low in refined products, moderate in wholegrains and highest in bran products. At least half of the recommended servings of grains should be wholegrains. Starch-containing foods represent the foundation of a healthy diet.

For many selections in this group, one serving provides approximately 15 g of carbohydrates. A serving is equal to:
• one slice of bread
• 50 g uncooked pasta or rice
• 50 g uncooked cereal.

Fruit and vegetable group

Most of the carbohydrates in the vegetable group are found in starchy vegetables, such as peas, corn and legumes.

The useable carbohydrates found in fruit are mostly sugar, fructose (a disaccharide). Dried fruits have a higher sugar content than fresh fruits because the removal of water increases the sugar concentration. In addition, eating whole fruits rather than drinking fruit juice increases fibre intake and moderates fructose intake.

> There's at least one of us in every group. Most of the carbs in the vegetable group are found in starchy vegetables such as potatoes.

Milk group

The milk, yogurt and cheese (or dairy) group contains the sugar lactose. Dairy products such as chocolate milk, strawberry yogurt and ice cream are flavoured or have added sugar, which increases the amount of carbohydrates per serving. Hard cheese, however, is a selection from the dairy group that's low in lactose and, therefore, low in carbohydrates.

Meat and beans group

The foods in the meat and beans group are mostly protein. However, dried beans, which are a plant source of protein, are also high in carbohydrates, such as starch and fibre. In addition, the majority of the calories in nuts come from fats, but most varieties of nuts have some carbohydrates.

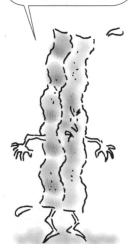

Legumes belong to both the vegetable and the meat and bean group because they contain protein and are high in fibre.

Carbohydrates in health promotion

Carbohydrates should provide up to 50% of the total calories in a person's diet, with the majority coming from complex carbohydrates (starches). Foods with added sugar, such as soft drinks, sweets, biscuits, fruit drinks and fruit juices, should be limited. The carbohydrates on your plate should make up about one-third of the food you eat.

Balancing act

Each type of carbohydrate has its own benefits to a person's health. The key to a healthy diet is balance, consuming selections from each food group in moderation. Eating enough carbohydrate is necessary to prevent the physical symptoms of ketosis and muscle wasting.

Fibre

Fibre, which has numerous health benefits, is an NSP that may be soluble or insoluble:
• Soluble fibre dissolves in water and forms a gel. It's primarily found in fruits, vegetables, oats, barley and legumes and the grain psyllium. Soluble fibre binds bile acids so they can't be reabsorbed in the colon, which aids in their excretion. This reduces serum cholesterol, a risk factor for cardiovascular disease. Soluble fibre also helps regulate blood glucose concentration by slowing glucose absorption in the small intestine.
• Insoluble fibre doesn't dissolve in water. It is found primarily in the bran layers of cereal grains and in certain vegetables (such as cabbage and brussel sprouts). Insoluble fibre increases faecal bulk and decreases free radicals in the GI tract.
    Eating five portions of fruits and vegetables each day will help you to have enough fibre in your diet. A portion of fruit or vegetables is 80 g or approximately what you can hold in one hand. (See *Tips for increasing fibre intake* and *Constipation in older adults*.)

Fantastic fibre facts

Because humans lack the enzymes necessary to digest fibre, it can't be broken down by the body for fuel. However, this inability to be digested gives fibre unique benefits, including:
• preventing or relieving constipation (insoluble)
• protecting against colon and rectal cancer (insoluble)
• preventing diverticulitis (insoluble)

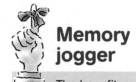

Memory jogger

The benefits of fibre are easy to 'C'. It prevents:

Constipation

Cancer

Colonic diverticulitis.

It also **C**auses a feeling of fullness and reduces **C**holesterol.

Up to 50% of a healthy person's total caloric intake should come from carbohydrates.

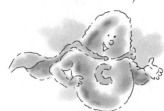

NutriTips

Tips for increasing fibre intake

Here are some easy ways to increase your daily fibre intake:

- Choose whole fruits or vegetables over fruit juice.
- Eat a variety of fruits and vegetables daily—the more colours, the better.
- Eat foods with wholegrains instead of refined grains, such as wholemeal breads, brown rice and wholemeal pasta.
- Read the fibre content on cereal boxes and choose one that has at least 5 g of fibre per serving.
- Eat foods that include beans, such as chilli and minestrone soup.

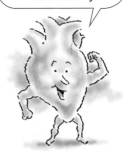

Increasing fibre intake helps to reduce cholesterol levels and keeps a heart healthy!

- reducing serum cholesterol (soluble)
- aiding weight management by causing a feeling of fullness, which leads to reduced intake (insoluble)
- decreasing blood glucose (soluble).

Sugar

Sugar is commonly used in drinks, such as tea, coffee and fruit squashes, and sweet foods. Limiting sugar intake is advised as part of a healthier diet. People with diabetes mellitus, obesity or cardiovascular disease may need to limit their intakes as it can provide extra calories without beneficial nutrients. Excess sugar intake is associated with an increased risk of dental caries, which may be a predictor of heart disease.

How much is enough?

Added sugars provide minimal or no essential nutrients. They include the sugars and syrup added to foods and beverages that are not naturally occurring. (See *Recognizing added sugars*, page 44.) Encourage people to select foods without added sugars to meet their nutritional needs while reducing the amount of calories. Reducing intakes of alcohol can also help to reduce calorie intakes.

The Food Standards Agency recommends that we should all be eating less sugary, refined foods such as sweets, cakes and fizzy drinks.

Here are some tips you can give people to help decrease their daily sugar intake:

- Have fewer sugary drinks and snacks.
- Instead of sugary fizzy drinks and juice drinks, go for water or unsweetened fruit juice (remember to dilute these for children). If you like fizzy drinks, then try diluting fruit juice with sparkling water.

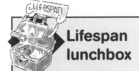

Lifespan lunchbox

Constipation in older adults

Constipation is a concern in as much as 20% of adults over the age of 65. Encourage older adults to eat foods high in dietary fibre, such as fresh fruits and vegetables, breakfast cereals such as bran flakes and other wholegrain products. Recommend that they drink plenty of fluids each day unless contraindicated by a medical condition. Also be sure to emphasise the importance of regular exercise.

- Instead of cakes or biscuits, try having a scone or some malt loaf with low-fat spread.
- If you take sugar in hot drinks, or add sugar to your breakfast cereal, gradually reduce the amount until you can cut it out altogether.
- Rather than spreading jam, marmalade, syrup, treacle or honey on your toast, try a low-fat spread, sliced banana or low-fat cream cheese instead.
- Check food labels to help you pick the foods with less added sugar or go for the low-sugar version.
- Try halving the sugar you use in your recipes. It works for most things except jam, meringues and ice cream.
- Choose tins of fruit in juice rather than syrup.
- Choose wholegrain breakfast cereals rather than those coated with sugar or honey.

Sugar substitutes

Sugar alcohols, such as sorbitol, mannitol and hydrogenated starch hydrolyses, are low-calorie alternatives to sugar. Non-nutritive sweeteners, such as saccharin, aspartame and sucralose, have virtually no calories and are much sweeter than sugar, requiring smaller amounts for flavour. However, people with phenylketonuria should avoid all foods containing aspartame because they can't metabolise the phenylalanine it contains, which increases the risk of toxic blood levels. People should limit their intakes of artificially sweetened foods as they can have a laxative effect.

Recognising added sugars

Help your patient avoid added sugars in foods by teaching him or her to look for 'hidden' sources of sugar on food labels. Examples include:

- corn sweetener
- corn syrup (especially high in fructose often used to sweeten processed foods)
- dextrose
- fructose
- fruit juice concentrates
- glucose
- honey
- lactose
- maltose
- malt syrup
- molasses
- sucrose
- sugar (brown, invert, raw)
- syrup

Although I may go by a pseudonym to disguise my identity on food labels, sugar is still sugar.

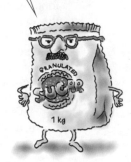

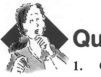

Quick quiz

1. Carbohydrates are composed of all of the following elements except:
   A. Carbon
   B. Hydrogen
   C. Nitrogen
   D. Oxygen

Answer: C. Carbohydrates are organic compounds that are composed of carbon, hydrogen and oxygen.

2. Which substance is a type of carbohydrate?
   A. Monosaccharide
   B. Amino acid
   C. Lipid
   D. Albumin

Answer: A. Monosaccharides, or simple sugars, are carbohydrates that aren't broken down in the digestive process.

3. Which hormone regulates the blood glucose level?
   A. Insulin
   B. Cortisol
   C. Adrenalin
   D. Thyroxine

Answer: A. Insulin is the only hormone that significantly reduces blood glucose by aiding glucose entry into the cells, stimulating glycogenesis and promoting glucose catabolism.

4. Carbohydrates are found in which of the following food groups?
   A. Vegetable
   B. Milk
   C. Starch
   D. All of the above

Answer: D. Carbohydrates can be found in all food groups.

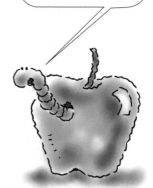

Don't try to worm your way out of reading the next chapter. It's packed with protein power!

Scoring

★★★ If you answered all four questions correctly, excellent! It looks like you've been carb-loading the right information.

★★ If you answered three questions correctly, you're getting the essentials! Move on to the next chapter.

★ If you answered fewer than three questions correctly, don't worry! Your body is just craving more carbohydrates. Go back and review the chapter.

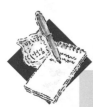

(4) Protein

Just the facts

This chapter explains the importance of the essential nutrient protein to the body. In this chapter, you'll learn:

♦ the classification of protein

♦ protein functions

♦ the ways in which proteins are digested, absorbed and metabolised

♦ food sources of protein.

A look at proteins

Proteins, which are components of every living cell, are large, complex molecules composed of individual building blocks known as *amino acids*. Like carbohydrates, amino acids are organic compounds made from carbon, hydrogen and oxygen atoms. Unique to amino acids is their nitrogen component, which distinguishes them from other energy nutrients. Proteins come in various sizes and shapes and are composed of different amino acids joined in various proportions and sequences. The shape of a protein molecule determines how it functions.

Protein is required for normal growth and development and provides some of our energy each day. It's broken down by the body in greater amounts as a source of energy when the supply of carbohydrates and fats is inadequate. Protein is found in muscle, bone, blood, skin, cartilage and lymph.

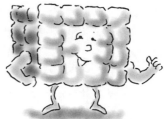

Protein is the body's backup generator. I'm used for energy after carbs and fats.

Amino acids

All amino acids have a carbon atom core with four bonding sites: one site holds a hydrogen atom, one an amino group (NH_2) and one an acid group (COOH). Attached to the fourth bonding site is a side group (R group), which contains the atoms that give each amino acid its distinct identity.

Essential and non-essential amino acids

Amino acids are the structural units of proteins. There are more than 20 amino acids that make up the human body. Here is a list of the common 21 amino acids required by the body. They're divided into two classes: essential (can't be synthesised and must be obtained from the diet) and non-essential (can be synthesised and therefore don't need to be obtained from the diet).

Essential	Non-essential
• Histidine	• Alanine
• Isoleucine	• Asparagine
• Leucine	• Aspartic acid
• Lysine	• Cystine
• Methionine	• Glutamic acid
• Phenylalanine	• Glutamine
• Threonine	• Glycine
• Tryptophan	• Hydroxylysine
• Valine	• Hydroxyproline
	• Proline
	• Serine
	• Tyrosine

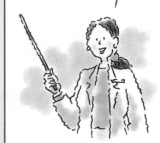

There are 21 common amino acids: 9 essential and 12 non-essential.

Reviewing the essentials

There are 21 common amino acids. Nine of them are classified as essential amino acids because they can't be made by the body and therefore must be consumed through food. The remaining 12 are non-essential amino acids because they can be synthesised in the liver if nitrogen and other precursors are available. (See *Essential and non-essential amino acids*.)

Classification of food protein

Food proteins are classified as complete or incomplete. This classification depends on their amino acid compositions.

Complete proteins

Complete proteins are foods that contain all of the essential amino acids in the correct proportions. They must contain enough of each amino acid to meet the body's needs. Meat, milk, cheese and eggs are considered complete proteins. Soy is the only plant source that's considered a complete protein.

Incomplete proteins

If a food source is deficient or has limited amounts of one or more essential amino acids, it's considered an incomplete protein. With the exception of soybeans, all plant proteins are incomplete.

The buddy system

It's possible to combine two different incomplete proteins to make a complete protein. In other words, one source may be lacking a particular amino acid; if that amino acid is found in another source, together they can create a complete protein. Examples of foods that contain complementary proteins include:

- breakfast cereal and milk
- beans on toast
- pea soup with toast
- ham sandwich
- cheese on toast
- vegetable quiche.

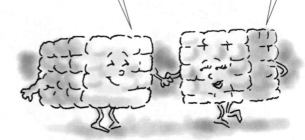

Two incomplete proteins that can be combined to obtain sufficient quantities and proportions of all essential amino acids are called complementary proteins.

That's what friends are for!

Functions of protein

Protein performs many functions in the body:
- The primary function of protein is the growth, repair and maintenance of body structures and tissue. The body's cells are always making proteins to replace those that are broken down from normal wear.
- Proteins are involved in the manufacture of hormones, such as insulin and adrenalin (epinephrine).
- Proteins may act as enzymes that help bring about certain chemical reactions, such as digestion or protein synthesis.
- Plasma proteins (such as albumin) aid in maintaining fluid and electrolyte balance by attracting water and causing changes in osmotic pressure.
- Amino acids contain an acid and a base; therefore, they can neutralise excesses of either acids or bases in the body, thereby maintaining a normal pH.
- Proteins help transport other substances through blood. For example haemoglobin transports oxygen and lipoproteins transport lipids.

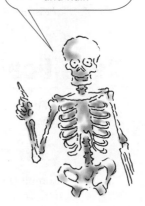

A continuous supply of protein maintains body structures, such as bones, muscles, tendons, skin and hair.

• Proteins function within the immune system by helping to create lymphocytes and antibodies that protect the body from infection and disease.
• Protein is a component of numerous body compounds, including thrombin, which helps blood to clot.
• Proteins can be used as a source of energy (providing 4 kcal/g) when intake of carbohydrates and fats is inadequate.

How the body handles protein

Protein moves through the body via the processes of digestion, absorption and metabolism.

Digestion

The digestion of protein begins in the stomach, where hydrochloric acid (HCl) works on protein to make it more susceptible to the action of enzymes. HCl converts pepsinogen to the enzyme pepsin. Pepsin begins to break down proteins into smaller polypeptides and some amino acids.

The bulk of protein digestion takes place in the small intestines with the help of enzymes secreted by the pancreas. These pancreatic enzymes (trypsin, chymotrypsin and carboxypeptidase) are responsible for breaking down proteins into simpler substances (tripeptides, dipeptides and amino acids). Enzymes located on the surface of the intestinal wall (amino peptidase and dipeptidase) complete the digestive process. (See *Protein digestion*.)

Memory jogger

To remember the enzymes active in protein digestion, think **T**eeth **C**an't **C**ut it **A**fter **D**inner:

Trypsin

Chymotrypsin

Carboxypeptidase

Aminopeptidase

Dipeptidase.

Protein digestion

Active enzymes in the stomach and intestine break protein down into various substances, as shown below.

Organ	Active enzymes	Digestive action
Stomach	Pepsin	• Breaks down protein into polypeptides
Intestine	Trypsin–pancreatic enzyme	• Breaks down protein and polypeptides into tripeptides and dipeptides
	Chymotrypsin–pancreatic enzyme	• Breaks down protein and polypeptides into tripeptides and dipeptides
	Carboxypeptidase	• Breaks down polypeptides into simpler peptides and amino acids
	Aminopeptidase	• Breaks down polypeptides into peptides, dipeptides and amino acids
	Dipeptidase	• Breaks down dipeptides into amino acids

Absorption

Amino acid absorption takes place in the mucosa of the small intestines through active transport, with the aid of vitamin B_6. Intestinal cells release amino acids into the bloodstream for transport to the liver through the portal vein.

Metabolism

Protein metabolism is a constant two-part process. Proteins are broken down by the body into amino acids through the process of catabolism and then resynthesised into tissues as needed through anabolism. This continuous conversion is needed to maintain overall protein balance within the body.

Leave it to liver

The liver serves many important functions related to protein metabolism:
• It uses the amino acids that it needs and releases those that aren't needed elsewhere.
• It retains amino acids to make liver cells, non-essential amino acids and plasma proteins, such as heparin, prothrombin and albumin.
• It regulates the release of amino acids into the bloodstream and removes excess amino acids from the circulation.
• It regulates energy metabolism by removing nitrogen from amino acids so that they can be burned for energy and by converting amino acids into glucose or fat, as necessary.

> I regulate the release of amino acids in the bloodstream and remove excess amino acids from the circulation.

Waiting pool

Unlike excess glucose and fat, the body can't store excess protein for later use. However, a limited supply of free amino acids exists within cells in a metabolic pool that accepts and donates amino acids as needed. This metabolic pool is constantly changing in response to the ongoing build-up and breakdown of body proteins and the influx of amino acids from food.

Neutral nitrogen balance is best

When the amount of protein made is equal to the amount used, as in healthy adults, the body has a neutral nitrogen balance. If protein synthesis exceeds protein breakdown, such as during growth, pregnancy or recovery from injury, a positive nitrogen balance exists. A negative nitrogen balance exists when protein breakdown exceeds protein synthesis, such as during starvation or acute illness.

Protein turnovers

The body's supply of amino acids comes from food (exogenous) and its own protein tissue (endogenous). Amino acids released from protein breakdown may be recycled to build new proteins or burned for energy. This continuous process of protein synthesis and breakdown is called *protein turnover*.

The rate of turnover varies throughout the body. For example turnover in the GI system (pancreas, liver and stomach) is rapid, and turnover in muscles is slower.

Sources of protein

Proteins can be found in both plant and animal sources. In each food group, the protein quantity and quality vary among the items, with the meat and meat alternative group (chicken, dry beans, steak and peanut butter) and milk and dairy product group (cottage cheese, yogurt and hard cheese) having the greatest amounts of protein. The starch group (potatoes, rice, pasta and wholegrain bread) and fruit and vegetable group (dark green and deep yellow vegetables) contain lesser amounts of protein. Fruits contain minimal amounts of protein.

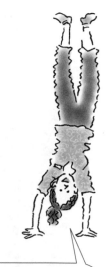

Protein synthesis and breakdown happens continuously in a process called protein turnover.

Proteins in health promotion

The Dietary Reference Value (DRV) of protein in a healthy diet is 0.8 g/kg of recommended body weight per day, or approximately 10% of total recommended daily calories. This protein allowance is based on the minimum requirements needed to maintain nitrogen balance and the mixed quality of proteins typically consumed. The recommended protein allowance per kilogram of body weight is higher for children (from infancy to adolescence) and for pregnant and breast-feeding women.

Other factors also determine how much protein the body needs. Emotional or physical stress, infection and high environmental temperatures increase protein needs. Protein requirements also increase during times when the body must heal itself, such as after surgery, trauma or burn injuries.

Building up the body

Protein needs are also higher for people with large muscle mass because muscle tissue is metabolically active and requires protein to maintain itself. Many bodybuilders believe that consuming large amounts of protein will help increase their muscle strength and size. Some even utilise protein supplements. It's important to remind your patient that muscles are built and maintained through a combination of caloric intake and strength

Supplement setbacks

Single amino acid supplements can offer more of one amino acid than another. When this occurs, it may have adverse effects on the body. For example an excess of the amino acid tryptophan, which promotes sleep, has been linked to cases of permanent brain damage and even death.

If your patient is a bodybuilder, advise him not to use supplements to build and maintain muscle mass; instead, suggest that he:

consume tuna, eggs and milk as protein sources rather than protein powders and liquids to provide an adequate supply of protein in the diet

drink adequate fluids because exercise increases the body's fluid requirements

eat a variety of foods from all food groups

consume calories appropriate for his lifestyle, which may mean larger or more frequent meals.

Building muscle requires adequate amounts of carbohydrates and proteins.

training. (See *Supplement setbacks*.) A bodybuilder should consume 60% to 65% of his total calories as carbohydrates and should consume adequate amounts of protein, 1 to 1.5 g of protein per kilogram of body weight.

Hi-pro, hi-pro...

Despite the importance of protein in forming muscle, protein intake shouldn't exceed twice the DRV, or 1.6 g/kg of body weight for adults. High protein intake:
• increases the excretion of calcium, which may increase the risk of osteoporosis
• increases excretion of nitrogen by the kidneys, which may play a role in the loss of renal function
• increases the risk of atherosclerosis and colon and prostate cancers.

Vegetarian variations

For most people in the UK, protein intake isn't a concern because the amounts of proteins and calories consumed are more than adequate. Most vegetarian diets also meet or surpass the DRV for protein; however, these diets contain less protein than nonvegetarian diets. To obtain adequate daily protein intake, a vegan should consume adequate amounts of the essential amino acids from plants. Soy protein, which is found in such foods as tempeh (fermented soybeans), tofu (soybean curd), textured soy products (soy flour altered to look like minced beef on rehydration) and meat analogues (soy sausages), is a meat alternative that's also a good source of protein.

Although most vegetarian diets aren't lacking in protein, some don't meet the minimum requirements for other important nutrients. For example calcium, iron, linolenic acid, vitamins B_{12} and D and zinc are important nutrients that can't be obtained in adequate quantities from plants and, therefore, are commonly lacking in vegetarian diets.

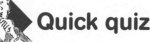

Quick quiz

1. Two incomplete proteins that combine to make a complete protein are known as:
   A. Combination proteins
   B. Complementary proteins
   C. Common proteins
   D. Core proteins

Answer: B. When two incomplete proteins combine to make a complete protein, they're known as complementary proteins. Examples include peanut butter sandwiches and beans on toast.

2. Essential amino acids are:
   A. The structural units of proteins that must be obtained from the diet
   B. The structural units of proteins that don't need to be obtained from the diet
   C. Organic compounds that don't dissolve in water but do dissolve in alcohol and other organic compounds
   D. Inorganic compounds

Answer: A. Essential amino acids are protein units that can't be synthesised in the body and therefore must be obtained from the diet.

3. The primary function of protein in the body is:
   A. Maintenance of fluid and electrolyte balance
   B. Transportation of lipids
   C. Growth, repair and maintenance of body structures and tissue
   D. Maintenance of normal pH

Answer: C. The primary function of protein is growth, repair and maintenance of body structures and tissues.

4. Which of the following hormones is protein responsible for manufacturing?
   A. Insulin
   B. Thyroxine
   C. Oxytocin
   D. Oestrogen

Answer: A. Protein is responsible for the manufacture of insulin for the body.

5. Which of the following amino acids is considered an essential amino acid?
  A. Cystine
  B. Glutamine
  C. Tyrosine
  D. Lysine

Answer: D. Lysine is an essential amino acid that can't be synthesised by the body and, therefore, must be obtained in the diet.

Scoring

☆☆☆ If you answered all five questions correctly, you're a protein pro! Don't be shy about moving on to the chapter about fat.

☆☆ If you answered four questions correctly, you don't have to worry about your protein intake. You've thoroughly digested the information in this chapter.

☆ If you answered fewer than four questions correctly, don't be discouraged. Go take a dip in your metabolic pool and then come back and review the chapter.

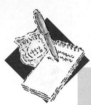

5 Fat

Just the facts

This chapter presents information about dietary fat. In this chapter, you'll learn:

♦ the classification of fat

♦ fat functions

♦ the ways in which fats are digested, absorbed and metabolised

♦ food sources of fat.

A look at fat

Fats (lipids) are organic compounds that dissolve in alcohol and other organic solvents but not in water. Fats are composed of the elements carbon, hydrogen and oxygen. Although these are the same elements that make up carbohydrates, the proportions of oxygen to carbon and hydrogen are lower in fats. Because fats have less oxygen, they provide more than double the amount of calories than provided by the same amount of carbohydrates. The body gets many fats from consumed food, but it also manufactures some fats.

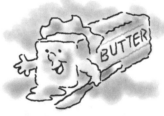

Fats are like supersized carbs—they're double the calorie count.

Classification of fat

There are three main types of fats: tricylglycerols, phospholipids and sterols.

Tricylglycerols

Tricylglycerols account for approximately 95% of the fat in foods and are the major storage form of fat in the body. The basic structural unit of tricylglycerols is one molecule of glycerol joined to three fatty acid chains.

The chain gang

A fatty acid is composed of a chain of carbon atoms with hydrogen and a few oxygen atoms attached. The fatty acid chains joined to the glycerol molecule vary in length and composition. The different taste, smell and physical appearance of each fat result from the variety of fatty acids and their physical arrangements in the fat molecule. The length of the chain, which can be between 2 and 24 carbon atoms long, determines how the body transports and absorbs the fat. Short-chain fatty acids have 2 to 4 carbon atoms, medium-chain fatty acids contain 6 to 12 carbon atoms and long-chain fatty acids include more than 12 carbon atoms. Long-chain fatty acids are found in most food fats.

Saturation explanation

Saturation of fatty acids depends on how many hydrogen atoms bond to the four potential bonding sites of each carbon atom. If two sites have a hydrogen atom bond, it's *saturated*. Because all of the carbon atoms are bonded to as many hydrogen atoms as they can hold, no double bonds between carbon atoms exist.

Saturated fats are found in meat, poultry, full-fat dairy products and tropical oils, such as palm and coconut oils. Most saturated fats:
- originate from animal sources
- remain solid at room temperature
- have high melting points
- are less likely to become rancid.

Unsaturation explanation

An *unsaturated* fatty acid isn't completely filled with all the hydrogen atoms it can hold. This results in the formation of double bonds between carbon atoms.

In general, unsaturated fats:
- originate from plant fat and oils
- are soft or liquid at room temperature
- have lower melting points than saturated fats
- can become rancid when exposed to extended periods of light and oxygen.

There are two types of unsaturated fatty acids: monounsaturated fatty acids (MUFA) and polyunsaturated fatty acids (PUFA). MUFA are found mostly in vegetable oils, such as olive, canola and peanut oils. PUFA are found in nuts and vegetable oils, such as sunflower, safflower and soybean oils, and in fatty fish. (See *Comparing saturated and unsaturated fats*.)

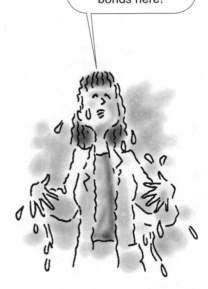

I'm saturated! I guess that means all of my carbon atoms are bonded to hydrogen atoms. No double carbon bonds here!

Comparing saturated and unsaturated fats

The saturation of fatty acids depends on how many hydrogen atoms bond to the four potential bonding sites of each carbon atom and the number of resulting double carbon bonds.

Saturated

A saturated fatty acid has no carbon–carbon double bonds.

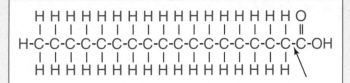

Unsaturated

A monounsaturated fatty acid has only one double carbon bond.

A polyunsaturated fatty acid has more than one double carbon bond.

Trans fats

In a process called *hydrogenation*, manufacturers add hydrogen to polyunsaturated oils to make them solid at room temperature. The hydrogenation process improves the shelf life of foods, making them less likely to become rancid. Oils that are lightly hydrogenated remain liquids but are more stable than polyunsaturated fats because they don't have as many double carbon bonds. Partially hydrogenated oils, however, are solid at room temperature.

Factory fat

Trans fat is produced by the hydrogenation process and is found in vegetable fat, certain margarines, crackers, biscuits, snack foods and other foods made with hydrogenated oils. Small amounts of trans fat occur naturally, mostly in dairy products but also in some meats and other animal foods.

Phospholipids

Phospholipids are a group of compound fats that are similar to tricylglycerols. They contain a glycerol molecule but only two fatty acid chains. Instead of the third fatty acid, phospholipids have a phosphate group and another nitrogen-containing compound. Phospholipids occur naturally in almost all foods.

Sterols

Sterols are complex molecules in which carbon atoms form four cyclic structures attached to various side chains. Sterols don't contain glycerol or fatty acid molecules. Cholesterol is one example of a sterol.

Cholesterol

Cholesterol, the most common sterol, is a fatlike substance that's manufactured daily by the body. The liver produces cholesterol and filters out excess cholesterol to eliminate it from the body. Cholesterol also is a component of the foods that we eat. It occurs naturally in all animal foods.

Cholesterol has several important functions:
- It's a vital component of bile salts that help in fat digestion.
- It's an essential part of all cell membranes. It's also found in brain and nerve tissue and in the blood.
- It's necessary for the production of several hormones, including cortisone, adrenaline, oestrogen and testosterone.

Functions of fat

Most people are all too aware that fats contribute flavour, satiety and palatability to food in the diet. They also supply texture to food, intensify its flavour and enhance its odour. Different fats have specific functions in the body. For example phospholipids work as emulsifiers to keep fats suspended in the blood and in body fluids. They also serve as an integral part of cell membranes and help to transport nutrients, metabolites and fat-soluble substances across cell membranes.

Fats perform six general functions in the body:
- providing energy for the body
- facilitating absorption of fat-soluble vitamins
- supplying essential fatty acids

- supporting and protecting internal organs
- aiding in temperature regulation
- lubricating body tissue.

Fat as fuel

Fat is a concentrated form of energy that provides 9 kcal/g—double the amount of calories of either a carbohydrate or a protein. Yet fat isn't the body's preferred fuel source because it's more difficult to metabolise. Stored fat in adipose cells represents the body's largest and most efficient energy reserve. Adipose cells have a virtually limitless capacity to store fat.

Taking in your vitamins

Dietary fat facilitates the absorption of fat-soluble vitamins—A, D, E and K.

Suppliers of essential fatty acids

Dietary fat supplies the essential fatty acids: linoleic acid and alpha-linolenic acid. These are considered essential fatty acids because the body can't manufacture them. Essential fatty acids are important for maintaining healthy skin, promoting normal growth in children and maintaining healthy immune function. They may also play a role in the prevention of age-related chronic diseases, such as heart disease and Alzheimer's disease.

People padding

Fatty tissue cushions and protects vital organs by providing a supportive fat pad that absorbs mechanical shocks. Examples of organs supported by fat are the eyes and kidneys.

Body insulation

Fat layers insulate the skin, helping to protect the body from excessive heat or cold. A sheath of fatty tissue surrounding nerve fibres provides insulation to help transmit nerve impulses.

Pretty slick

Fats also lubricate the body tissue. The human body manufactures oil in structures called *sebaceous glands*. Secretions from sebaceous glands lubricate the skin to slow the loss of body water to the outside environment.

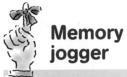

Memory jogger

To remember the fat-soluble vitamins **(A, D, E and K)**, think:

All

Dieters

Enjoy

Kale.

It may not be true, but it will help you remember!

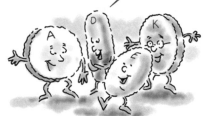

Dietary fat helps us become absorbed.

How the body handles fat

Fat moves through the body via the processes of digestion, absorption and metabolism. To be transported throughout the body, most fats must combine with plasma proteins to form lipoproteins.

Digestion

A minimal amount of fat digestion occurs in the mouth and stomach. General muscle action mixes the fat with the stomach contents. As fat enters the duodenum, it stimulates the release of the hormone cholecystokinin, which stimulates the gall bladder to release bile. Bile is an emulsifier that breaks fat into small particles and reduces the surface tension so that enzymes can penetrate the fat and work more effectively.

The pancreas provides a punch

Most fat digestion occurs in the small intestine. Pancreatic lipase, a powerful fat enzyme, breaks off one fatty acid at a time from the tricylglycerol molecule until only two free fatty acids and a monoglyceride are left. Each step of this process requires more energy. The end products of digestion are mostly monoglycerides with free fatty acids and some glycerol, which are absorbed into the intestinal cells. Small amounts of fat escape digestion and are excreted in the faeces.

The digestion of phospholipids is similar; however, the end products are two free fatty acids and a phosphorous fragment. Cholesterol isn't digestible; rather, it's absorbed unaltered.

Absorption

In the duodenum and jejunum, 95% of consumed fat is absorbed. Small fat particles are absorbed directly through the mucosal cells into the capillaries leading to the portal vein and liver.

Back to the beginning

Larger fat particles (monoglycerides and long-chain fatty acids) are dissolved into a compound called *micelles*, which are created from the bile salts that encircle the fat particles to aid their diffusion into the intestinal cells. After delivering the fat to the intestinal cells, the released bile salts are reabsorbed in the terminal ileum, travel back to the liver and are then recycled. Once inside the intestinal cells, monoglycerides and long-chain fatty acids combine to form tricylglycerols. These tricylglycerols, along with phospholipids and cholesterol, become encased in proteins to form chylomicrons (a class of lipoproteins). Chylomicrons transport absorbed fats from the intestinal cells through the lymph system and eventually into the bloodstream for distribution throughout the body.

Metabolism

In the bloodstream, tricylglycerols in the chylomicrons are broken down into glycerol and fatty acids by lipoprotein lipase, a fat-digesting enzyme located on the surface of adipose cells and other body cells. These fatty acids and glycerol enter cells, where they can be broken down for energy or rebuilt into tricylglycerols for storage. Fat metabolism is regulated by the hormones adrenocorticotropin, epinephrine (adrenalin), glucagon, glucocorticoids and thyroxin, which also promote fat mobilisation (catabolism). Insulin, another hormone, stimulates fat synthesis (anabolism).

Until required for use as energy fuel, lipids are stored in adipose tissue within cells. When needed for energy, each fat molecule is hydrolysed to glycerol and three molecules of fatty acids. Glycerol can be converted to pyruvic acid and then to acetyl coenzyme A (CoA), which enters the Krebs cycle.

Ketone body formation

The liver normally forms ketone bodies from acetyl CoA fragments, derived largely from fatty acid catabolism. Acetyl CoA molecules yield three types of ketone bodies:

acetoacetic acid—results from the combination of two acetyl CoA molecules and subsequent release of CoA from these molecules

beta-hydroxybutyric acid—forms when hydrogen is added to the oxygen atom in the acetoacetic acid molecule; *beta* indicates the location of the carbon atom containing the hydroxyl (OH) group

acetone—forms when the carboxyl (COOH) group of acetoacetic acid releases carbon dioxide; muscle tissue, brain tissue and other tissues oxidise these ketone bodies for energy.

More than enough

Under certain conditions, the body produces more ketone bodies than it can oxidise for energy. Such conditions include fasting, starvation and uncontrolled diabetes (in which the body can't break down glucose). The body must then use fat instead of glucose as its primary energy source.

Ketone cops

Use of fat instead of glucose for energy leads to an excess of ketone bodies. This condition disturbs normal acid–base balance and homeostatic mechanisms, leading to ketosis.

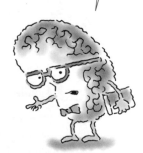

Along with other tissues, I oxidise ketone bodies for energy.

Lipid formation from proteins and carbohydrates

Excess amino acids can be converted to fat through keto acid–acetyl CoA conversion. Glucose may be converted to pyruvic acid and then to acetyl CoA, which is converted into fatty acids and then fat (in much the same way that amino acids are converted into fat).

Lipid carriers

Lipoproteins are a group of compounds made by the body that transport lipids through the bloodstream to various parts of the body. All lipoproteins contain both lipids and protein but in different ratios. Cholesterol is carried by the lipoproteins, and lipoproteins are often referred to as lipoprotein cholesterol. As the protein concentration increases, the density of the lipoprotein increases. There are four types of lipoproteins:

 very low density lipoproteins (VLDL cholesterol)

low-density lipoproteins (LDL cholesterol)

high-density lipoproteins (HDL cholesterol)

chylomicrons.

Each type of lipoprotein has a different function. (See *Types of lipoproteins*.)

Sources of fat

The type and amount of fat in each food group vary. Some fat is visible, such as butter and the fat surrounding a piece of steak. However, most fat is invisible, such as the fat in milk, cheese and nuts, and the fat that's intertwined in the steak. Animal sources account for approximately 57% of total fat intake; plant sources account for the rest.

The top five sources of saturated fat in the diet of an adult living in the UK are:

 beef

butter or margarine

salad dressings, including mayonnaise

cheese

 milk.

Major sources of trans fat in the diet include crisps, shop-bought cakes and other commercially fried foods. Other sources of trans fat include biscuits, crackers and other baked goods.

> Most of the fat we consume is invisible. Too bad it shows up later!

Types of lipoproteins

The various types of lipoproteins are detailed here.

Very low density lipoproteins (VLDLs)

VLDLs are produced and secreted by the liver cells. They contain 50% tricylglycerols, some cholesterol, phospholipids and protein. They transport the lipids made in the liver to body tissues. They also lose tricylglycerols to body cells and gain cholesterol from other body tissues. When present in large concentration, VLDLs may increase the risk of atherosclerosis.

Low-density lipoproteins (LDLs)

LDLs are the major carriers of cholesterol in the blood. They contain 50% cholesterol, lesser amounts of protein and phospholipids and a small amount of tricylglycerols. LDLs are responsible for transporting cholesterol from the liver to the tissues. Commonly called 'bad' cholesterol, LDLs are the major contributor to atherosclerosis.

High-density lipoproteins (HDLs)

Referred to as 'good' cholesterol, HDLs are made by the liver and contain 50% protein, with lesser amounts of cholesterol, phospholipids and tricylglycerols. HDLs carry cholesterol from body tissues to the liver, where it's recycled or degraded. High HDL levels decrease the risk of atherosclerosis.

Chylomicrons

Chylomicrons are composed of tricylglycerols absorbed from food and contain little protein, phospholipids and cholesterol. They transport dietary fats from the intestine to the liver and other body cells. Chylomicrons are the least dense and the largest of the lipoproteins.

Starch group

Starch-containing foods such as grains naturally contain very little fat. However, prepared foods within this group, such as granola cereals, pancakes, doughnuts, cakes, pizza and pies, contain significant added fat. These foods may also be sources of trans fat. Most people in the UK do not eat large amounts of trans fat. In the UK we eat a lot more saturated fat (see *Reducing your intake of saturated fat*, page 64).

Vegetable and fruit groups

With the exception of avocado, coconut and olives, fruits don't contain appreciable amounts of fat. Unadulterated vegetables contain little or no fat. Vegetables that are fried, creamed, served with cheese or mixed with mayonnaise contain significantly more fat.

Milk group

Items within the milk group come in fat-free, reduced-fat and whole-fat varieties. To reduce your patient's risk of high fat intake among foods in this group, advise him or her to read labels and compare different varieties and brands.

Meat and beans group

The plant items in this group (beans) are cholesterol free and contain little or no saturated fat. In general, untrimmed meats are higher in fat than lean portions, and white meat (chicken) is lower in fat than dark meat (beef). Shellfish, such as crab, lobster and shrimp, are high in cholesterol but low in fat and saturated fat. (See *Don't eat too much fish*.)

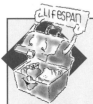

Lifespan lunchbox

Don't eat too much fish

Although most people should be eating more fish for their health, there are maximum levels recommended for oily fish and crab (and some types of white fish).

Oily fish can contain low levels of pollutants that can build up in the body. The pollutants found in oily fish include dioxins and PCBs (polychlorinated biphenyls). Dioxins and PCBs tend to be found in all foods containing fats. They have no immediate effect on health, but can be harmful because they build up in our bodies over time. Also, again for health reasons, adults should have no more than one portion of swordfish, shark or marlin a week. This is because these fish could contain high levels of mercury.

The recommended maximums for oily fish are lower for most girls and women because high levels of dioxins and PCBs in the diet could affect the development of a baby in the future.

If a woman changes her diet when she becomes pregnant, or when she starts trying for a baby, this won't change the levels of dioxins and PCBs that are already in her body. So it's a good idea to limit the amount of oily fish eaten from a young age.

Omega-3 fatty acids are good for a baby's development, so pregnant women shouldn't stop eating oily fish.

So remember, don't give up eating oily fish because the health benefits outweigh the risks as long as you don't eat more than the recommended maximums.

Adapted from FSA *Eat well be well*. Helping you to make healthier choices [Online]. http://www.eatwell.gov.uk/healthydiet/nutritionessentials/fishandshellfish/oilyfishshellfishandomega3/

Fat in health promotion

The National Service Frameworks (NSF), Diabetes UK and the British Heart Foundation all suggest that consumers choose diets low in fat, saturated fat, trans fat and cholesterol, and moderate in total fat.

The *Food Standards Agency (FSA)* also recommends a diet low in saturated fat, (See *Maximum daily amounts of saturated fat*, page 66.) trans fat and cholesterol, and moderate in total fat. However, this diet isn't recommended for everyone, particularly children and people who need to consume calorie-dense foods, such as elderly patients and those with chronic renal failure. (See *Fat intake for children*.)

Don't spend your fat allowance all in one place

For healthy adults, the *FSA* recommends that you choose lower-fat options, with most fat calories coming from polyunsaturated and monounsaturated fats. To help your patient meet this recommended guideline, make the following suggestions:
• Grill, bake, poach or steam food, rather than frying or roasting, so you don't need to add any extra fat.

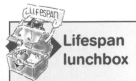

Lifespan lunchbox

Fat intake for children

The FSA recommends no restriction of fat or cholesterol for children aged 2 years and younger, when rapid growth and development require high energy levels. The majority of fats should come from polyunsaturated and monounsaturated fats. Children under the age of 2 should not be given skimmed or semi-skimmed milk as this reduces their intake of vitamin A.

As children begin to consume fewer calories from fat, they should replace these calories by eating more grain products, fruits, vegetables, low-fat milk products or other calcium-rich foods, beans, lean meat, poultry and fish or other protein-rich foods.

> ## Maximum daily amounts of saturated fats
>
> Most people in the UK eat too much saturated fat—about 20% more than the recommended maximum amount.
>
> The average man should have no more than 30 g saturated fat a day.
>
> The average woman should have no more than 20 g saturated fat a day.
>
> Children should have less saturated fat than adults. But remember that a low-fat diet isn't suitable for children under age 5.
>
> Adapted from FSA *Eat well be well*. Helping you to make healthier choices [Online]. http://www.eatwell.gov.uk/healthydiet/nutritionessentials/fishandshellfish/oilyfishshellfishandomega3/

- Trim visible fat and skin off meat before cooking.
- When you're shopping, compare the labels, so you can pick those with less fat and saturated fat.
- Choose lower-fat dairy products when you can.
- Put more vegetables or beans in casseroles, stews and curries, and a bit less meat—and skim the fat off the top before serving, if you can.
- Measure oil for cooking with tablespoons, rather than pouring it straight from a container—this will help you use less.
- If you do choose something high in fat to eat, pick something low in fat to go with it—for example you could swap deep-fried chips for a jacket potato.
- When you're making sandwiches, try leaving out the butter or spread— you might not need it if you're using a moist filling. When you do use spread, go for a reduced-fat variety and choose one that is soft straight from the fridge so it's easier to spread thinly.

Stress to your patient that a low-fat diet needs to be centred on the right types of fat. For example high levels of polyunsaturated fats have been shown to lower 'good' and 'bad' cholesterol levels. High levels of monounsaturated fats and low levels of saturated and trans fats in the diet may produce the right changes in HDL and LDL levels; however, if the diet is too high in fat, weight gain may result, increasing the risk of heart disease.

Read the writing

The FSA introduced food labelling laws in 1996 to require food to be marked or labelled with certain requirements such as:
- the name of the food
- a list of ingredients (including food allergens)
- the amount of an ingredient which is named or associated with the food
- an appropriate durability indication (e.g. 'best before' or 'use by')
- any special storage conditions or instructions for use
- the name and address of the manufacturer, packer or retailer
- the place of origin (where failure to do so might mislead).

(See *Understanding nutrition labelling*.)

Understanding nutrition labelling

The 1996 Food Labelling Regulations Act and its amendments provide the regulations for food labelling in the UK and are available on the Web from the Office of Public Sector Information (OPSI) site. The Food Standards Agency (FSA), formed in April 2000, is now responsible for proposing legislation on food labelling and for participating in negotiations at a European Community level.

The legal requirement is to specify quantities '**per 100 g**' (or 100 ml). The regulations also permit quantity per serving if the number of servings is specified. In this case, the serving is the whole pack of two sandwiches and data is given '**per pack**'.

In January 2007 the FSA recommended the use of its 'traffic lights' approach to simplify food labelling, agreeing the nutritional criteria for six out of seven food groups. This is a voluntary scheme and has not been adopted by all food manufacturers.

Food labelling is currently being reviewed by member states of the EU.

Nutrition		
Typical values	per pack	per 100g
Energy	1310kJ	736kJ
	312kcal	175kcal
Protein	16.6g	9.3g
Carbohydrate	32.6g	18.3g
of which sugars	4.1g	2.5g
Fat	12.8g	7.2g
of which saturates	3.0g	1.7g
Fibre	6.4g	3.6g
Sodium	0.72g	0.40g

per pack 312 calories
12.8g fat 1.8g salt

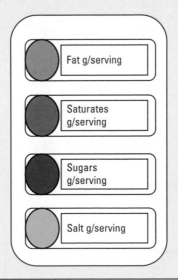

Fat g/serving

Saturates g/serving

Sugars g/serving

Salt g/serving

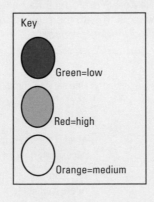

Key

Green=low

Red=high

Orange=medium

Check the label for saturated fat

Look out for the figure for 'saturates' or 'sat fat' on the label because this tells you how much saturated fat is in the food.

High is more than 5 g sat fat per 100 g.

Low is 1.5 g sat fat per 100 g.

If the amount of sat fat per 100 g is inbetween these figures, then that is a medium level. Some foods have 'traffic light' labels on the front of the pack. These show you if a food is high, medium or low in fat, sat fat, sugars and salt.

Red = high

Amber = medium

Green = low

Try to choose foods that are low in sat fat as often as you can, or go for medium. If foods are high in sat fat, try not to have them too often, or eat them in smaller amounts. (See *Tips for reducing dietary fat*.) When you're shopping, compare similar foods—there can be a big difference in how much sat fat they contain. And choose the option that is lower in sat fat. (See *Translating fat terminology*.)

> Not enough room to work? That's what fat can do to arteries— plaques of fat narrow artery lumens, reducing blood flow.

Translating fat terminology

In December 2006, a regulation on the use of nutrition and health claims for foods was adopted by the Council and Parliament of the EU. This regulation lays down harmonised rules for the use of health or nutritional claims (such as 'low fat', 'high fibre' and 'helps lower cholesterol') on foodstuffs based on nutrient profiles. Here's a guide you can give your patients to help them decipher terms used to describe the amount and type of fats listed in food products.

Terms	
Saturated fat free	One serving containing less than 0.5 g of fat, with the level of trans-fatty acids not exceeding 1% of total fat
Low fat	3 g or less of fat
Reduced or less saturated fat	At least 25% less fat than the reference food (but not necessarily 'low fat')
Light	One-third fewer calories or 50% less fat than the reference food
Low cholesterol	20 mg or less of cholesterol and 2 g or less of saturated fat
Reduced or less cholesterol	At least 25% less cholesterol than the reference food and less than 2 g of saturated fat

NutriTips

Tips to reduce dietary fat

Here are top 10 tips that can help your patient reduce the saturated fat in his or her diet:

Choose lower-fat dairy products. Try 1% skimmed milk and low-fat yoghurts. Look out for cheese that is lower in fat.

Grate cheese instead of slicing—this can help you eat less of it. And when you're shopping, compare the labels on different cheeses to see which contain less fat.

Eat chicken without the skin. And when you're cooking chicken, go easy with the creamy sauces—try a bit of lemon and some herbs instead.

Use leaner mince. Check the labels on minced beef and choose the option that is lower in fat. Or try using turkey mince, which is even leaner.

Trim the fat off meat. And try grilling meat instead of frying.

Compare labels and choose the option that is lower in saturated fat.

Eat less pastry. Pastry is high in saturated fat, so try not to have pies, pastries and sausage rolls too often. Also, go for pies with just a lid or a base.

When you're cooking, use unsaturated oils such as sunflower, olive and rapeseed, instead of butter, lard and ghee.

Eat healthier snacks when you're on the go. Many snacks can be high in saturated fat, so pick up an apple, some dried fruit or another healthy option. Check the label and choose food that is lower in saturates.

Eat more balanced meals. To get the balance right, eat lots of fruits and vegetables and plenty of bread, rice, potatoes, pasta and other starchy foods. These are low in saturated fat, so they help to make your meals healthier.

Calling in the swaps

Simply swapping one food for an healthier option can help patients to reduce their saturated fat intake.

Instead of	Try
Streaky bacon	Back bacon
Croissant with butter	Toasted bagel with low-fat soft cheese
Sausages	A lean cut of meat or chicken
Mashed potato with butter and whole milk	Mashed potato with lower-fat spread and skimmed milk
Cream	Reduced-fat Greek yoghurt
Creamy or cheese sauce	Tomato or vegetable sauce
Ice cream	Frozen yoghurt
Butter on bread	Low-fat spread on bread

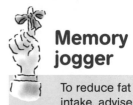

Memory jogger

To reduce fat intake, advise your patient not to fry foods. Instead, encourage him or her to remember the **BBG** of cooking:

Bake

Boil

Grill.

Disease prevention

More than any other nutrient, fat is identified as playing a leading role in several chronic diseases. Evidence is overwhelming that high-fat diets increase the risk of cardiovascular disease, obesity and certain cancers.

Cardiovascular disease

Coronary artery disease caused by atherosclerosis is the leading cause of death among people in the UK. In this condition, fatty fibrous plaques progressively narrow the coronary artery lumens, reducing the volume of blood that can flow through them. Plaque develops as a result of a complex series of events that seem to be initiated by increased amounts of LDLs. Eating a diet high in saturated fats, trans fats and cholesterol raises LDL level, increasing the risk of heart disease.

Obesity

Obesity—which is defined as a body mass index greater than 30—occurs from taking in more calories than the body requires. Fats contribute more calories to the diet than carbohydrates and proteins, which the body can burn more easily. Weight gain results when excess fats are stored.

Cancer

Although dietary fat hasn't been shown to cause cancer, it may help promote certain cancers. Cancer Research UK guidelines state that being obese and consuming a high-fat diet can increase the risk of colon, rectal, prostate and endometrial cancers.

Quick quiz

1. Fat is composed of all of the following elements except:
    A. Carbon
    B. Oxygen
    C. Hydrogen
    D. Potassium

Answer: D. Fats are organic compounds that are composed of carbon, hydrogen and oxygen.

2. An unsaturated fat is:
    A. A fatty acid that isn't completely filled with hydrogen atoms.
    B. A fatty acid that's completely filled with hydrogen atoms.
    C. A fatty acid that's highly concentrated and heavy.
    D. A fatty acid that originates from animals.

Answer: A. An unsaturated fatty acid isn't completely filled with hydrogen atoms and, therefore, is less concentrated and lighter.

3.   In which organ does the digestion of fats primarily occur?
    A.   Stomach
    B.   Large intestine
    C.   Liver
    D.   Small intestine

Answer: D. Fat digestion occurs in the small intestine, where the enzymatic processes occur.

4.   Which lipoprotein contributes to the development of atherosclerosis and is termed the 'bad' cholesterol?
    A.   LDL
    B.   HDL
    C.   VLDL
    D.   Chylomicrons

Answer: A. LDL levels contribute to atherosclerosis. They're the major source of cholesterol in the blood.

5.   When using the Nutrition Fact labels to make healthy food selections, choose foods with:
    A.   The lowest amount of saturated fat and trans fat
    B.   The highest percentage daily value of cholesterol
    C.   The lowest percentage daily value of trans fat
    D.   The highest amount of total fat

Answer: A. To select healthy foods, choose foods with the lowest amount of saturated fat and trans fat.

Scoring

☆☆☆   If you answered all five questions correctly, way to go! You're saturated with information on fats!

☆☆   If you answered four questions correctly, good job! Your mind bonded with the information on fats.

☆   If you answered fewer than four questions correctly, don't worry! You apparently didn't absorb fats well. That isn't always a bad thing, but you should probably look over the chapter again.

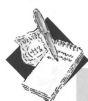

Just the facts

This chapter presents essential information about vitamins and minerals. In this chapter, you'll learn:

♦ the classification of vitamins and minerals

♦ the functions of vitamins and minerals

♦ the ways in which vitamins and minerals are digested, absorbed and metabolised

♦ food sources of vitamins and minerals.

A look at vitamins

Vitamins are organic compounds of carbon, hydrogen, oxygen and, occasionally, nitrogen or other elements that are needed in small quantities for normal metabolism, growth and development. Because they're needed only in small quantities, they're referred to as micronutrients. With few exceptions, the body can't produce vitamins, so they must be consumed in the diet.

Contrary to popular belief, vitamins don't directly provide energy to the body. As catalysts, they're part of the enzyme system that's required to release energy from protein, fat and carbohydrates. Vitamins are also needed to form red blood cells, hormones and genetic material and to maintain proper functioning of the nervous system. Many vitamins exist in more than one active form, and each of these forms has a different function in the body.

Classification of vitamins

Vitamins are classified as water-soluble or fat-soluble. (See *Guide to vitamins*.)

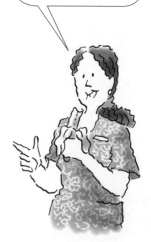

Eat up! Vitamins are essential in the diet because they can't be made by the body or are produced by the body in inadequate amounts.

Guide to vitamins

Good health requires intake of adequate amounts of vitamins to meet the body's metabolic needs. A vitamin excess or deficiency, although rare, can lead to various disorders. The chart below reviews major functions and food sources of vitamins.

Vitamins	Major functions	Food sources
Water-soluble vitamins		
Vitamin B_1 (thiamin)	Appetite stimulation, blood building, carbohydrate metabolism, circulation, digestion, growth, learning ability, muscle tone maintenance	Meat, fish, poultry, pork, molasses, brewer's yeast, brown rice, nuts, wheat germ, wholegrains and enriched grains
Vitamin B_2 (riboflavin)	Antibody and red blood cell (RBC) formation, energy metabolism, cell respiration, and epithelial, ocular and mucosal tissue maintenance	Meat, fish, poultry, milk, molasses, brewer's yeast, eggs, fruit, green leafy vegetables, nuts, whole grains
Vitamin B_3 (niacin)	Circulation, cholesterol-level reduction, growth, hydrochloric acid production, metabolism (carbohydrate, protein, fat), sex hormone production	Eggs, lean meat, milk products, offal, peanuts, poultry, seafood, whole grains
Vitamin B_6 (pyridoxine)	Antibody formation, digestion, deoxyribonucleic acid and ribonucleic acid synthesis, fat and protein utilisation, amino acid metabolism, haemoglobin production	Meat, poultry, bananas, molasses, brewer's yeast, desiccated liver, fish, green leafy vegetables, peanuts, raisins, walnuts, wheat germ, whole grains
Vitamin B_{12} (cobalamin)	Blood cell formation, cellular and nutrient metabolism, iron absorption, tissue growth, nerve cell maintenance	Beef, eggs, fish, milk products, offal, pork
Vitamin C (ascorbic acid)	Collagen production, digestion, fine bone and tooth formation, iodine conservation, healing, RBC formation, infection resistance	Fresh fruits and vegetables, especially citrus fruits and green leafy vegetables
Biotin	Cell growth, fatty acid production, metabolism, vitamin B utilisation, and skin, hair, nerve and bone marrow maintenance	Egg yolks, legumes, offal, whole grains, yeast, milk and seafood
Folate (folic acid)	Cell growth and reproduction, hydrochloric acid production, liver function, nucleic acid formation, protein metabolism and RBC formation	Citrus fruits, eggs, green leafy vegetables, milk products, offal, seafood, whole grains
Pantothenic acid	Antibody formation, cortisone production, growth stimulation, stress tolerance, vitamin utilisation, conversion of carbohydrates, fats and protein	Eggs, legumes, mushrooms, offal, salmon, wheat germ, wholegrains, fresh vegetables, yeast

(continued)

Guide to vitamins (continued)

Vitamins	Major functions	Food sources
Fat-soluble vitamins		
Vitamin A (retinol)	Body tissue repair and maintenance, infection resistance, bone growth, nervous system development, cell membrane metabolism and structure	Fish, green and yellow fruits and vegetables, milk products
Vitamin D (calciferol)	Calcium and phosphorus metabolism (bone formation), myocardial function, nervous system maintenance, normal blood clotting	Bone meal, egg yolks, offal, butter, cod liver oil, fatty fish
Vitamin E (tocopherol)	Ageing retardation, anticoagulation, diuresis, fertility, lung protection (antipollution), male potency, muscle and nerve cell membrane maintenance, myocardial perfusion, serum cholesterol reduction	Butter, dark-green vegetables, eggs, fruits, nuts, offal, vegetable oils, wheat germ
Vitamin K (menadione)	Liver synthesis of prothrombin and other blood-clotting factors	Green leafy vegetables, soybean oil, yogurt, liver, molasses

Daily duty

Water-soluble vitamins are absorbed into the bloodstream directly and move freely within cells. Because storage of these vitamins in the body is limited, they must be consumed daily in the diet. When excess amounts are consumed, they're excreted in urine.

Examples of water-soluble vitamins are:
- vitamin B_1 (thiamin)
- vitamin B_2 (riboflavin)
- vitamin B_3 (niacin)
- vitamin B_6 (pyridoxine)
- vitamin B_{12} (cobalamin)
- vitamin C (ascorbic acid)
- biotin
- folate (folic acid)
- vitamin B_5 (pantothenic acid).

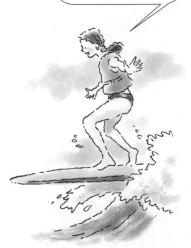

Zowee! Excess water-soluble vitamins are excreted in urine...

On layaway

Fat-soluble vitamins are absorbed with fat into the lymphatic system and the bloodstream. Once in the bloodstream, these vitamins need to attach to lipoproteins to be transported. Excess amounts of fat-soluble vitamins are stored in the liver and adipose tissue; therefore, these vitamins don't need to be consumed daily in the diet.

The fat-soluble vitamins are:
- vitamin A (retinol)
- vitamin D (calciferol)
- vitamin E (tocopherol)
- vitamin K (menadione).

Functions of vitamins

Vitamins have four main functions. They may work as:
- antioxidants
- coenzymes
- food additives
- pharmacologic agents.

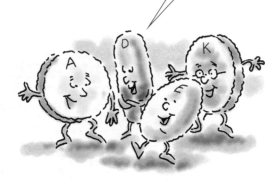

...while excess fat-soluble vitamins are stored in the liver and adipose tissue.

Fighting free radicals

Some vitamins function as antioxidants, which help protect the body from the instability of free radicals. Free radicals are unstable molecule fragments with one or more unpaired electrons that are produced in cells as they burn oxygen during metabolism. Other factors, such as ultraviolet radiation, smoking and air pollution, can also create free radicals in the body. Each of these free radicals attempts to become stable by gaining an electron. While doing so, they cause damage by oxidising body cells and deoxyribonucleic acid. These damaged cells are believed to contribute to ageing and such health problems as cancer and heart disease.

Antioxidants are substances that yield electrons to free radicals, helping to stabilise them and protect cells from damage. Vitamin C, vitamin E and beta-carotene (a precursor to vitamin A) are all important antioxidants. Because antioxidants complement each other and each antioxidant has a slightly different role, an excess or deficiency of one may impair the action of others.

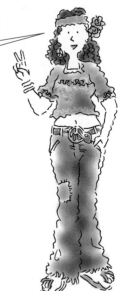

Radical, man! Some vitamins are antioxidants, which donate electrons to free radicals to stabilise them.

Catalysts for change

Enzymes are proteins that catalyse chemical reactions within the body without changing themselves in the process. Many enzymes aren't active without a coenzyme, an organic molecule that makes up the nonprotein portion of the enzyme. Vitamins work as coenzymes, facilitating many important chemical reactions throughout the body.

Food boosters

Vitamins are also used as additives in some foods to boost their nutritional content. Examples include vitamin-fortified breakfast cereals and juices. As additives, vitamins may also be used to preserve foods, such as fish, luncheon meats and oils.

Vitamins as therapy

Certain vitamins have been found to have pharmacologic uses. For example large doses of niacin have been used to help lower the levels of serum cholesterol, low-density lipoproteins and triglycerides in patients with elevated levels. In addition, retinoic acid, a form of vitamin A, has been used to treat acne vulgaris.

How the body handles vitamins

Vitamins move through the body via the processes of digestion, absorption and metabolism.

Digestion

Digestion of vitamins occurs mainly in the small intestine and requires the breakdown of food into its constituent parts. Contractions of the intestinal wall and the secretion of digestive enzymes break down food to facilitate absorption of nutrients through the intestinal wall.

Absorption

Absorption of vitamins is accomplished through active transport and diffusion across cell membranes. A number of vitamins require a specific carrier or transport system. For example vitamin B_{12} isn't absorbed in the absence of intrinsic factor, which is secreted by the parietal cells of the stomach.

Fat-soluble vitamins are absorbed in different portions of the small intestine. For example vitamin A is absorbed in the duodenal and upper jejunal areas of the small intestine. The process of their absorption is similar to that of fats and, like fats, these vitamins can be stored in the body. Consequently, excessive intake of fat-soluble vitamins can be fatal.

Water-soluble vitamins are generally absorbed throughout the GI tract. For example folic acid is absorbed in the ileum. Because excess amounts of water-soluble vitamins are typically excreted in urine, one of these vitamins is less likely to be toxic to the body.

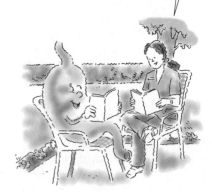

Don't you find the process of absorption so, well, absorbing?

Metabolism

All vitamins are metabolised independently of one another. The process differs for each vitamin.

Sources of vitamins

Vitamins can be found in all the major food groups:
• Bread, cereal, rice and pasta may be enriched with niacin, riboflavin and thiamin and fortified with folic acid. Wholegrain items also contain vitamin E.
• Fruits and fruit juices, particularly orange and grapefruit juices, are high in vitamin C and beta-carotene and are also significant sources of folate. Some juices are also fortified with calcium. Juices that contain 100% fruit juice are recommended.
• Vegetables are good sources of beta-carotene, vitamin C, folic acid and vitamin K. Because cooking and soaking can destroy vitamins, minimal preparation of vegetables is recommended.
• Milk, yogurt and cheese may contain riboflavin, some B vitamins and vitamins A and D.
• Meat contains niacin, riboflavin and vitamins B_6 and B_{12}; pork is also rich in thiamin. Dry beans contain folate, nuts and seeds supply vitamin E and eggs are good sources of vitamin A.
• Vegetable oils supply vitamin E. Margarine contains vitamins A, D and E. A basic principle of the *FSA Eat well be well* is that vitamins should come mainly from foods. (See *Nutritional needs of breast-feeding vegans*.)

Vitamins in health promotion

The recommended dietary intake necessary to meet the nutrient requirements of adults varies for each vitamin. (See *Vitamin requirements, deficiencies and toxicities*, page 78.)

Recently, an intensive consumer interest in vitamin therapy and supplementation has grown in conjunction with public interests in defying ageing and changing eating patterns.

Vitamin supplements

Vitamin supplements can prevent such deficiency diseases as scurvy and beriberi, which can occur when dietary intake is inadequate. Research is still needed, however, to determine if vitamin supplements can help prevent chronic disease.

Health and nutrition authorities agree that the best way to get nutrients is through food and not through supplements. Vitamin supplements are limited in what they offer and hardly compare with the array of vitamins, minerals and fibres found in foods. Vitamin supplements also lack the natural chemicals produced by plants needed to protect against bacteria, viruses and fungi.

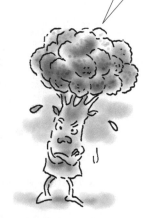

Boy, am I steamed! Overcooking us vegetables can cause our vitamins to vacate before we're even eaten.

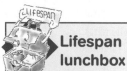

Lifespan lunchbox

Nutritional needs of breast-feeding vegans

Breast milk contains all the vitamins needed for an infant's growth and development. However, the milk of breast-feeding mothers who are vegans may be deficient in vitamin B_{12} and vitamin D. Breast-fed infants of these mothers may need vitamin B_{12} supplementation.

Vitamin requirements, deficiencies and toxicities

This table lists the daily requirements of common vitamins as well as the signs and symptoms of deficiency and toxicity for each.

Vitamins	Adult requirements	Signs and symptoms of deficiency	Signs and symptoms of toxicity
Water-soluble vitamins			
Vitamin B_1[†] (thiamin)	*Men:* 1.0 mg/day *Women:* 0.8 mg/day	Beriberi (fatigue, muscle weakness, confusion, oedema, enlarged heart, heart failure)	None
Vitamin B_2[†] (riboflavin)	*Men:* 1.3 mg/day *Women:* 1.1 mg/day	Ariboflavinosis (dermatitis, glossitis, photophobia)	None
Vitamin B_3 (niacin)[†]	*Men:* 17 mg/day *Women:* 13 mg/day	Pellagra (dermatitis, diarrhoea, dementia, death)	Flushing, gastric ulcers, low blood pressure, nausea, vomiting, diarrhoea, liver damage
(Vitamin B_5) Pantothenic acid*	3–7 mg/day	General failure of all body systems	None
Vitamin B_6 (pyridoxine)[†]	*Men:* 1.4 mg/day *Women:* 1.2 mg/day	Dermatitis, glossitis, seizures, anaemia	Depression, irritability, headaches, fatigue
Vitamin B_{12} (cobalamin)[†]	1.5 μg/day	Indigestion, diarrhoea or constipation, weight loss, macrocytic anaemia, fatigue, poor memory, irritability, paresthesia of the hands and feet	None
Vitamin C (ascorbic acid)[†]	*Men and women:* 40 mg/day	Scurvy (bleeding gums, delayed wound healing, haemorrhaging, softening of the bones, easy fractures)	Diarrhoea, nausea, headaches, fatigue, flushes, insomnia
Biotin*	10–20 μg	Anorexia, fatigue, depression, dry skin, heart abnormalities	None
Folate (folic acid)[†]	200 μg	Diarrhoea, macrocytic anaemia, confusion, depression, fatigue	Masks vitamin B_{12} deficiency
Fat-soluble vitamins			
Vitamin A (retinol)[†]	*Men:* 700 μg/day retinol equivalents *Women:* 600 μg/day retinol equivalents	Night blindness, bone growth cessation, dry skin, decreased saliva, diarrhoea	Headaches, vomiting, double vision, hair loss, liver damage
Vitamin D (calciferol)*	10 μg (>age 50)	Rickets (retarded bone growth, bone malformations, decreased serum calcium, abdominal protrusion), osteomalacia (softening of bones, decreased serum calcium, muscle twitching)	Kidney stones, kidney damage, muscle and bone weakness, excessive bleeding, headache, excessive thirst
Vitamin E (tocopherol)[†]	*Men:* above 4 mg/day *Women:* above 3 mg/day	Red blood cell haemolysis, oedema, skin lesions	None
Vitamin K (menadione)*	1 μg/kg/day	Haemorrhaging	None

*Safe intake   [†]Reference nutrient intake

Currently, there isn't a pill that can sufficiently substitute for a healthy diet, but while not recommended, taking a balanced multivitamin supplement that provides no more than 100% of the daily requirement for each vitamin should not cause harm. Some special populations and people whose food choices fall short of the ideal diet may benefit from taking a multivitamin. (See *Target populations for vitamin supplementation* and *Folic acid needs in women of childbearing age*.)

Target populations for vitamin supplementation

Even though vitamin supplements can't compete with the array of vitamins, minerals and fibres found in foods, special populations, such as those listed here, may benefit from vitamin supplements:

- Alcoholics—alcohol alters vitamin absorption, metabolism and excretion. Nutrients that may be affected include riboflavin, niacin, thiamin, folate and pantothenic acid.
- Elderly patients—vitamin requirements may be increased due to chronic disease, adverse effects of medication, illness, poor chewing and swallowing, physical limitations or a decreased sense of smell or taste. Absorption of vitamin B_{12} and synthesis of vitamin D decrease with ageing. Research has shown that a multivitamin and mineral supplement may improve immune function.
- Smokers—smokers require more vitamin C than non-smokers. If these patients consume an adequate amount of vitamin C in the diet, a supplement may not be needed.
- Dieters and particular eaters—if intake is less than 1,200 cal/day, it's difficult to obtain the necessary nutrients for a healthy diet. People who eliminate specific food groups from their diet, such as vegans and people with food intolerances or allergies, also may not obtain the needed nutrients.
- Pregnant and breast-feeding women and women of childbearing age—folate is vital to prevent neural tube defects. All childbearing women are encouraged to take synthetic folate through supplements or fortified foods.

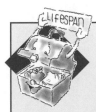

Lifespan lunchbox

Folic acid needs in women of childbearing age

Folate deficiency increases the risk of spina bifida and neural tube defects in unborn children. Therefore, women of childbearing age should consume 200 µg/day of synthetic folic acid from fortified foods and supplements, in addition to food forms of folate from a varied diet. Pregnant women should consume 400 µg/day of synthetic folic acid from fortified foods and supplements, in addition to food forms of folate from a varied diet. Rich sources of dietary folate include dark-green, leafy vegetables; dried peas; beans; citrus fruits; peanuts.

A look at minerals

Minerals are simple inorganic substances that are widely distributed in nature. They play a role in promoting growth and maintaining health. Minerals represent 4% of body weight and are found in all body fluids and tissues.

Classification of minerals

Minerals are classified as major minerals (macrominerals) or trace elements (microminerals). Major minerals are present in the body in amounts larger than 5 g (the equivalent of 1 tsp) and are needed in large quantities. Trace elements are present in the body in amounts less than 5 g and are needed only in small amounts.

Choose a major

There are seven major minerals:
- calcium
- chloride
- magnesium
- phosphorus
- potassium
- sodium
- sulphur.

Leaving a trace

Trace elements essential to health maintenance include chromium, cobalt, copper, fluoride, iodine, iron, manganese, molybdenum, selenium and zinc. (See *Guide to minerals*.)

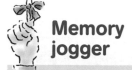

Memory jogger

To remember the seven major minerals, ask yourself, '**C**ould **C**ommon **M**inerals **P**ossibly **P**roduce **S**uch **S**afeguards?'

Calcium

Chloride

Magnesium

Potassium

Phosphorus

Sulphur

Sodium.

Functions of minerals

Minerals have many roles in the body, including:
- providing structure to body tissues
- regulating body processes.
  A disruption of the body's balance in any one mineral can be life threatening.

Structure

Minerals play a major role in several elements of body structure. For example calcium, phosphorus, magnesium and fluoride combine to give bones and teeth their hardness. Sulphur is a fundamental constituent of skin, hair and nails.

Guide to minerals

This chart reviews major functions and food sources of major and trace minerals.

Minerals	Major functions	Food sources
Major minerals		
Calcium	Blood clotting, bone and tooth formation, cardiac rhythm maintenance, cell membrane permeability, muscle growth and contraction, nerve impulse transmission	Bone meal, cheese, milk, molasses, yogurt, wholegrains, nuts, legumes, green leafy vegetables
Chloride	Fluid, electrolyte, acid–base and osmotic pressure balance	Fruits, vegetables, table salt
Magnesium	Acid–base balance, metabolism, protein synthesis, muscle relaxation, cellular respiration, nerve impulse transmission	Green leafy vegetables, nuts, seafood, cocoa, wholegrains
Phosphorus	Bone and tooth formation, cell growth and repair	Eggs, fish, grains, meats, poultry, yellow cheese, milk, milk products
Potassium	Muscle contraction, nerve impulse transmission, rapid growth, fluid distribution, osotic pressure balance, acid–base balance	Seafood, bananas, peaches, peanuts, raisins, oranges, tomatoes, peas, beans, green leafy vegetables, milk products
Sodium	Cellular fluid-level maintenance, muscle contraction, acid–base balance, cell permeability, muscle function, nerve impulse transmission	Seafood, cheese, milk, salt
Sulphur	Collagen synthesis, vitamin B formation, enzyme and energy metabolism, blood clotting	Milk, meats, legumes, eggs
Trace elements		
Chromium	Carbohydrate and protein metabolism, serum glucose level maintenance	Clams, meats, cheese, corn oil, whole grains
Cobalt	Vitamin B_{12} formation	Beef, eggs, fish, milk products, offal, pork
Copper	Bone formation, hair and skin colour, healing processes, haemoglobin and red blood cell formation, maintenance of nerve fibres, iron metabolism	Offal, raisins, seafood, nuts, molasses
Fluoride	Bone and tooth formation	Drinking water
Iodine	Energy production, metabolism, physical and mental development	Kelp, salt (iodised), seafood
Iron	Growth (in children), haemoglobin production, stress and disease resistance, cellular respiration, oxygen transport	Eggs, offal, poultry, wheat germ, liver, potatoes, enriched breads and cereals, green leafy vegetables

(continued)

Guide to minerals (continued)

Minerals	Major functions	Food sources
Trace elements (continued)		
Manganese	Enzyme activation, fat and carbohydrate metabolism, reproduction and growth, sex hormone production, vitamin B_1 metabolism, vitamin E utilisation	Bananas, egg yolks, green leafy vegetables, liver, soybeans, nuts, whole grains, coffee, tea
Molybdenum	Body metabolism	Wholegrains, legumes, offal
Selenium	Immune functions, mitochondrial adenosine triphosphate synthesis, cellular protection, fat metabolism	Seafood, meats, liver, kidneys
Zinc	Burn and wound healing, carbohydrate digestion, metabolism, prostate gland function, reproductive organ growth and development	Liver, mushrooms, seafood, soybeans, spinach, meat

Minerals are also components of vitamins, hormones and enzymes. Iodine, for example, becomes part of thyroid hormones.

Processes

Minerals also help to regulate various bodily processes. For example they help to maintain osmotic pressure in body compartments. Sodium, potassium and calcium have important functions in nerve cell transmission and muscle contraction. Sodium is also essential for maintaining fluid balance.

Potassium and phosphorus play a role in fluid and acid–base balance. Minerals also maintain normal haemoglobin levels, play a role in the function of the nervous system and are involved in hormone activity and skeletal development and maintenance.

> Ask the governator: minerals play an important role in muscle contraction.

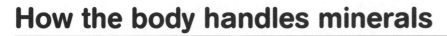

How the body handles minerals

Minerals move through the body via the processes of digestion, absorption and metabolism.

Digestion

Minerals must be digested in the GI tract by enzymes that split large units into smaller ones. The process, called *hydrolysis*, consists of a compound uniting with water and then splitting into simpler compounds. The smaller units are then absorbed from the small intestine and transported to the liver through the portal vein system.

Absorption

Minerals are absorbed in the small intestine. How much of a mineral is absorbed depends on three factors:

    tissue health—because tissue that's affected by disease has decreased absorptive capability

    food form—because minerals obtained from animal foods are more easily absorbed than those obtained from plant foods

    body requirements—because the body will absorb more of a mineral to compensate for a deficiency in that mineral.

    For some minerals, absorption isn't regulated, which can lead to problems. For example the body doesn't regulate sodium absorption, which can lead to sodium overload in patients who can't excrete the mineral properly.

Metabolism

Minerals are metabolised independently of one another. Metabolism occurs according to body need, and the process differs for each mineral. For example because calcium is absorbed according to body requirements and must be aided by vitamin D, calcium metabolism is hindered by excess fibre ingestion.

Sources of minerals

Minerals are obtained in a variety of ways. Most are found in unrefined or unprocessed foods. Trace minerals vary with the mineral content of the soil in which the food is grown. Processed foods are high in chloride and sodium. Drinking water contains different amounts of magnesium, calcium and other minerals. Sodium is added to soften the water, and fluoride can be an added or a natural component.

    Minerals are found in all the major food groups:
• Enriched and wholegrain breads and cereals provide magnesium, iron, chromium, and manganese. Bran contains potassium.
• Vegetables provide iron, potassium and magnesium. Green leafy vegetables provide calcium.
• Fruits aren't good sources of minerals, except for potassium, which is found in bananas and oranges.

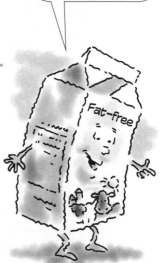

Got milk? Me and the guys in my gang are the richest sources of calcium you can find.

- Milk, yogurt and cheese may contain phosphorus and potassium. They're also the richest source of calcium.
- Animal proteins contain potassium, phosphorus, sulphur, zinc and iron. Dried peas and beans contain iron, potassium and calcium.
- Fats, oils and sugars contain almost no minerals.

Minerals in health promotion

The recommended dietary intake to meet the requirements of adults varies for each mineral. (See *Mineral requirements, deficiencies and toxicities*.)

Sodium is the mineral that causes the most health concerns. Most people in the UK consume more sodium than they need, which places them at risk for hypertension.

Mineral requirements, deficiencies and toxicities

This table lists the daily requirements of common minerals as well as the signs and symptoms of deficiency and toxicity for each.

Minerals	Adult requirements	Signs and symptoms of deficiency	Signs and symptoms of toxicity
Major minerals			
Calcium	700 mg/day	Arm and leg numbness, brittle fingernails, heart palpitations, insomnia, muscle cramps, osteoporosis	Renal calculi, impaired absorption of iron
Chloride	2.5 g	Disturbance in acid–base balance	None
Magnesium†	*Men:* 300 mg/day *Women:* 270 mg/day (ages 15–18) 270 mg/day (age >19)	Confusion, disorientation, nervousness, irritability, rapid pulse, tremors, muscle control loss, neuromuscular dysfunction	Cardiac rhythm disturbances, hypotension, respiratory failure
Phosphorus†	550 mg/day	Appetite loss, fatigue, irregular breathing, nervous disorders, muscle weakness	None
Potassium	3,500 mg/day	Muscle weakness; paralysis; anorexia; confusion; weak reflexes; slow, irregular heartbeat	Cardiac disturbances, paralysis
Sodium	1,600 mg/day	Appetite loss, intestinal gas, muscle atrophy, vomiting, weight loss	Oedema and elevated blood pressure
Sulphur	No recommended intake	None	None

*Adequate intake   †Reference nutrient intake

Mineral requirements, deficiencies and toxicities (continued)

Minerals	Adult requirements	Signs and symptoms of deficiency	Signs and symptoms of toxicity
Trace minerals			
Chromium*	>25 μg/day	Glucose intolerance (in diabetic patients)	None
Cobalt	Unknown	Indigestion, diarrhoea or constipation, weight loss, fatigue, poor memory	None
Copper†	1.2 mg/day	General weakness, impaired respiration, skin sores, bone disease	Vomiting, diarrhoea
Fluoride*	Infants only but adequate for adults 0.5 mg/kg/day	Dental caries	Mottling and pitting of permanent teeth, increased bone density and calcification
Iodine†	140 μg/day	Cold hands and feet, dry hair, irritability, nervousness, obesity, simple goitre	Enlarged thyroid gland
Iron†	*Men:* 8.7 mg/day *Women:* 14.8 mg/day (ages 19–50) 8.7 mg/day (age >50)	Brittle nails, constipation, respiratory problems, tongue soreness or inflammation, anaemia, pallor, weakness, cold sensitivity, fatigue	Abdominal cramps and pains, nausea, vomiting, haemosiderosis, haemochromatosis
Manganese*	>1.4 mg/day	Ataxia, dizziness, hearing disturbance or loss	Severe neuromuscular disturbances
Molybdenum*	50–400 μg/day	None	Headache, dizziness, heartburn, weakness, nausea, vomiting, diarrhoea
Selenium†	*Men:* 75 μg/day *Women:* 60 μg/day	None	Nausea, vomiting, abdominal pain, hair and nail changes, nerve damage, fatigue
Zinc†	*Men:* 9.5 mg/day *Women:* 7.0 mg/day	Delayed sexual maturity, fatigue, smell and taste loss, poor appetite, prolonged wound healing, slowed growth, skin disorders	Anaemia, impaired calcium absorption, fever, muscle pain, dizziness

*Adequate intake   †Reference nutrient intake

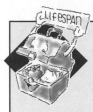

Lifespan lunchbox

Calcium consequence

Adequate calcium intake is important in all stages of life. During the first few decades of life, attaining maximum bone density is a safeguard against the inevitable net bone loss that occurs with ageing. After age 30, adequate calcium alone can't stop net bone loss, but it can slow the rate.

Calcium

Calcium is an important mineral throughout life. Adequate calcium intake may play a role in preventing hypertension and colon cancer and can slow the rate of bone loss. (See *Calcium consequence*.)

The latest recommendations for calcium intake are set at levels associated with maximum retention by the body. Many people in the UK have reduced vitamin D levels, which affects the absorption of calcium. They may take in enough to meet their requirement but fall short of the recommendation. Calcium supplements are appropriate for people who are deficient in vitamin D, or who can't or won't eat adequate calcium from foods alone.

People who take calcium supplements should:
• do so only in moderation (calcium is best absorbed when taken in amounts of 500 mg or less; if higher doses are needed, doses should be spread out throughout the day)
• know the kind of calcium they're taking and how it should be taken (calcium carbonate is best absorbed with food, and calcium citrate is best absorbed on an empty stomach)
• avoid taking it with iron (calcium can interfere with iron absorption)
• drink fluids (constipation is a common adverse effect of calcium supplements; drinking adequate amounts of fluids can reduce the risk)
• remember that supplements should add to what's already consumed (calcium supplements shouldn't be taken to replace dietary consumption of calcium).

Sodium

The *FSA* suggests limiting sodium intake by choosing and preparing foods with less salt. People in the UK are advised to limit their intake of salt to no more than 6 g/day. The Scientific Advisory Committee on Nutrition (2003) suggests that the average daily intake from food alone (not counting salt added at the table) is more than 9 g/day.

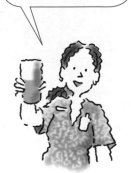

Drink up! Drinking adequate amounts of fluid can decrease the risk of constipation for patients taking calcium supplements.

High sodium intake is linked to high blood pressure, which can lead to stroke or heart attack. In order to help your patient limit his or her sodium intake, recommend the following actions:
• Reduce salt intake gradually in order to reduce the desire for salt.
• Read Food Facts labels to avoid or limit foods that contain too much sodium.
• Compare the labels of different brands of similar items to identify the product with the lowest salt content.
• Avoid processed foods.
• Be aware that high-sodium foods may not taste salty.
• Taste food before adding additional salt.
• Experiment with herbs, spices and vinegars as alternatives to salt.

Quick quiz

1. Which water-soluble vitamin requires intrinsic factor to be absorbed?
    A. Vitamin B_{12}
    B. Vitamin B_2
    C. Folate
    D. Biotin

Answer: A. Vitamin B_{12} requires the gastric protein intrinsic factor, the ingredient for absorption in the small intestine.

2. In which organ does the digestion of vitamins occur?
    A. Stomach
    B. Large intestine
    C. Small intestine
    D. Liver

Answer: C. Digestion of vitamins occurs in the small intestine.

3. The number of major minerals is:
    A. 4
    B. 6
    C. 7
    D. 10

Answer: C. There are seven major minerals: calcium, chloride, magnesium, phosphorus, potassium, sodium and sulphur.

4. Which mineral helps maintain osmotic balance?
    A. Phosphorus
    B. Thiamin
    C. Potassium
    D. Niacin

Answer: C. Potassium is the mineral that's needed to help regulate fluid distribution and osmotic pressure.

Scoring

☆☆☆   If you answered all four questions correctly, great job! You've certainly been fortified with all of your essential vitamins and minerals.

☆☆   If you answered three questions correctly, keep up the good work! It looks like traces of this chapter settled in your body.

☆   If you answered fewer than three questions correctly, don't worry! Maybe the information on water-soluble vitamins will make more sense after the next chapter—Fluids.

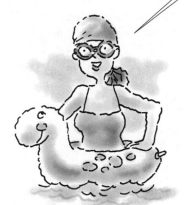

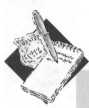

7 Fluids

Just the facts

This chapter presents the basics of fluids and fluid balance and explains their importance in body functioning. In this chapter, you'll learn:

♦ the importance of water in the body

♦ the way fluids move in the body

♦ factors that regulate fluid balance.

A look at fluids

A continual supply of water is one of our most basic nutritional needs. Without water, a person can survive no longer than a week. Ensuring balanced distribution of fluids to all body cells is an essential physiologic function.

A salute to solutes

Water makes up 50% to 80% of a person's total body weight. Body water contains solutes, or dissolved substances, that are necessary for physiologic functioning. Solutes include electrolytes, glucose, amino acids and other nutrients.

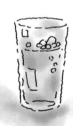

Fluid compartments

The body holds fluids in two basic areas, or compartments—inside the cells and outside the cells. Fluid inside cells is called *intracellular fluid* (ICF); fluid outside cells is called *extracellular fluid* (ECF). ICF and ECF are separated by capillary walls and cell membranes.

ECF consists of interstitial fluid, which surrounds the cells, and intravascular fluid or plasma (the liquid portion of blood). In an adult, interstitial fluid accounts for about 75% of ECF. Plasma accounts for the other 25%.

To maintain proper fluid balance, fluid distribution between ICF and ECF must stay relatively constant. In an adult, the total amount of ICF averages 40% of body weight, or about 28 L. The total amount of ECF averages 20% of body weight, or about 14 L.

Where's the water?

Skeletal muscle cells hold much of the body's water. Fat cells contain little water. That's why women, who normally have a higher ratio of fat to skeletal muscle than men, typically have lower relative water content. Likewise, an obese person may have a relative water content level as low as 45%. In an obese person, accumulated body fat increases weight without boosting the body's water content. Age also affects the proportion of water in the body. (See *Body water differences*.)

Functions of fluid

Fluid has many functions within the body. It:
- gives structure and shape to cells
- helps form the structure of large molecules, such as protein and glycogen
- serves as a lubricant (for example within the eyes and joints)
- helps regulate body temperature (for instance fluid absorbs the heat produced during a fever; blood then carries the excess heat to the skin, where it dissipates)
- acts as a solvent for minerals, vitamins, glucose, amino acids and other small molecules
- aids nutrient digestion and absorption
- transports nutrients to cells
- carries waste products away from cells through urine, faeces and expiration
- serves as a medium for all biochemical reactions in the body
- participates in chemical reactions, including the breakdown of proteins to amino acids and the synthesis of hormones and enzymes.

Water absorption and storage

A small amount of water can be absorbed into the bloodstream from the stomach. Over the course of 1 hour, roughly 1 L of water can be absorbed from the small intestine. Sodium and water are also absorbed from the large intestine, the colon. Water moves through the intestinal membrane by diffusion (a process we'll discuss later).

The body doesn't really store water. Instead, water moves continually from one compartment to another, and the body

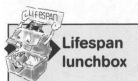

Lifespan lunchbox

Body water differences

Age affects the proportion of water in the body. Specifically, infants' bodies are 75% water, compared with 50% to 65% of adults' bodies. Preterm infants' bodies can be as much as 80% water by weight. Infants reach the adult proportion of water to weight between ages 9 and 12 months.

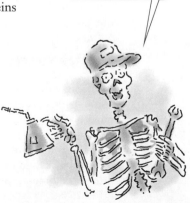

Keeping the joints lubricated is just one of the many functions fluid serves in the body.

often reuses it to perform different tasks. However, if a person's adaptive mechanisms are disrupted, water may be retained. Excessive fluid may accumulate between cells, causing a condition called *oedema*. This occurs in heart failure, hypothyroidism and certain kidney conditions. Water can also accumulate in cavities as in ascites commonly seen in the late stages of liver disease. Less commonly, the opposite occurs, with excessive fluid being dispersed throughout the body—a condition called *water intoxication*.

How fluids move in cells

Just as the heart beats constantly, fluids and solutes move constantly within the body. This movement allows the body to maintain homeostasis—the constant state of balance it seeks.

Solutes within the various compartments move through the membranes separating those compartments. The membranes are semipermeable, meaning they allow some solutes to pass through but not others. Solutes move through cell membranes by diffusion or active transport. Fluid moves by osmosis.

Diffusion

In diffusion, solutes move from an area of higher concentration to an area of lower concentration. Eventually, this movement results in equal distribution of solutes within the two areas. Diffusion is a form of passive transport. It requires no energy; it just happens. Like fish travelling downstream, the solutes simply go with the flow. (See *Diffusion: The power of passivity*.)

Active transport

In active transport, proteins within a semipermeable membrane move solutes from an area of lower concentration to an area of higher concentration. Think of active transport as swimming upstream. When a fish swims upstream, it has to expend energy. The energy a cell expends to move a solute against the concentration gradient comes from adenosine triphosphate (ATP), a substance stored in all cells. (See *Active transport: Swimming upstream*, page 92.)

Pump it up

Sodium and potassium move in and out of cells in a form of active transport fuelled by

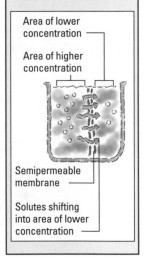

Diffusion: The power of passivity

In diffusion, solutes move from areas of higher concentration to areas of lower concentration until their concentration is equal in both areas.

Area of lower concentration

Area of higher concentration

Semipermeable membrane

Solutes shifting into area of lower concentration

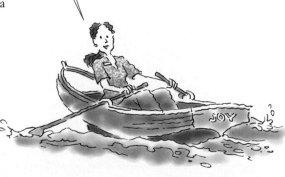

In active transport, solutes move from an area of lower concentration to an area of higher concentration.

ATP called the *sodium–potassium pump*. Keeping sodium out of cells and a balance between the sodium and potassium is important to keep cells, such as nerve cells, functioning. Other solutes that require active transport to cross cell membranes include calcium ions, hydrogen ions, amino acids and certain sugars.

Pin-up

An engulfing process called *pinocytosis* is a type of active transport used by larger particles, such as proteins and fats. In this process, tiny cavities called *vacuoles* take droplets of fluid containing dissolved substances into the cell. The engulfed fluid is then used in the cell. (See *Pinocytosis: When cells gulp up fluid*.)

Pinocytosis: When cells gulp up fluid

The illustrations below show the steps of pinocytosis, in which solutes encased in the microbody of a cell enter the cell's main body and are exposed to the cell enzymes for metabolism.

Large solutes attach to the cell body and membrane.

Solutes are engulfed by the cell become microbodies.

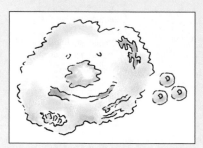

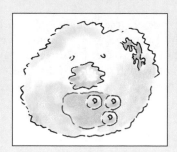

Microbodies are carried across the cell membrane and into the cell.

Once inside the cell, the microbodies open and solutes are metabolised by cells.

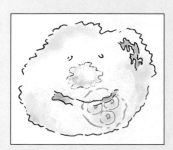

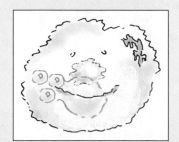

Active transport: Swimming upstream

During active transport, energy from a molecule called adenosine triphosphate (ATP) moves solutes from an area of lower concentration to an area of higher concentration.

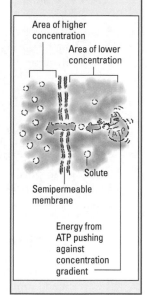

Area of higher concentration

Area of lower concentration

Solute

Semipermeable membrane

Energy from ATP pushing against concentration gradient

Understanding osmosis

In osmosis, fluid moves passively from areas with more fluid (and a lower solute concentration) to areas with less fluid (and a higher solute concentration). Remember that in osmosis, fluid moves, whereas in diffusion, solutes move.

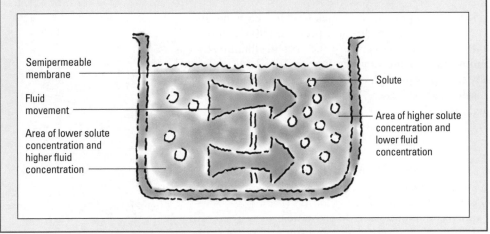

Semipermeable membrane

Fluid movement

Area of lower solute concentration and higher fluid concentration

Solute

Area of higher solute concentration and lower fluid concentration

Osmosis

Osmosis refers to passive movement of fluid across a membrane from an area of lower solute concentration and comparatively more fluid into an area of higher solute concentration and comparatively less fluid. Osmosis stops when enough fluid has moved through the membrane to equalise the solute concentration on both sides of the membrane. (See *Understanding osmosis*.)

How fluids move in the vascular system

In the vascular system, only capillaries have walls thin enough for solutes to pass through. Movement of fluids and solutes through capillary walls plays a key role in fluid balance.

May the force be with you

Fluid movement through capillaries—a process called *capillary filtration*—results from blood pushing against the capillary walls. That pressure, called *hydrostatic* (fluid-pushing) *pressure*, forces fluids and solutes through the capillary wall.

When hydrostatic pressure inside the capillary exceeds pressure in the surrounding interstitial space, fluids and solutes inside the capillary are forced out into the interstitial space. When pressure outside the capillary exceeds pressure within it, fluids and solutes move back into the capillary.

Fluid reabsorption

A process called *reabsorption* prevents too much fluid from leaving the capillaries—no matter how much hydrostatic pressure exists within them. When fluid filters through a capillary, the protein albumin remains behind in the diminishing volume of water. Because it's a large molecule, albumin normally can't pass through capillary membranes. As the albumin concentration inside a capillary rises, fluid starts to move back into the capillaries through osmosis.

H_2O attraction

Albumin acts as a water magnet. The osmotic, or pulling, force of albumin in the intravascular space is called *plasma colloid osmotic pressure*. In capillaries, this pressure averages about 25 mm Hg.

As long as capillary blood pressure (hydrostatic pressure) exceeds the plasma colloid osmotic pressure, water and solutes can leave the capillaries and enter the interstitial fluid. When capillary blood pressure falls below the plasma colloid osmotic pressure, water and diffusible solutes return to the capillaries.

Normally, blood pressure in a capillary exceeds plasma colloid osmotic pressure in the arteriole end and falls below it in the venule end. As a result, capillary filtration occurs along the first half of the vessel, and reabsorption, along the second half. As long as capillary blood pressure and plasma albumin levels remain normal, the amount of water that moves into the vessel equals the amount that moves out. When albumin levels in the blood are low, the patient develops oedema.

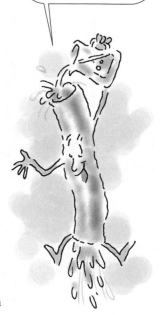

When capillary blood pressure and plasma albumin levels remain normal, the amounts of water moving into and out of a vessel are equal.

Fluid gains and losses

In a healthy body, fluid gains match fluid losses to maintain proper physiologic functioning. The skin, lungs, and kidneys—in fact, nearly all of the major organs—work together to maintain the balance of body fluids. To maintain fluid balance, the amount of fluid gained throughout the day must equal the amount lost. (See *How the body gains and loses fluid*.)

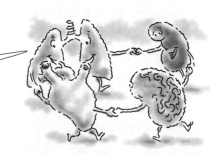

Nearly all of us major body systems work together to maintain the balance of body fluids.

How the body gains and loses fluid

Each day the body takes in fluid from the GI tract (in foods and liquids as well as from metabolism) and loses fluid through the skin, lungs, intestines (faeces) and urinary tract (urine). This illustration shows the primary sites involved in fluid gains and losses as well as the average amount of normal daily fluid intake and output.

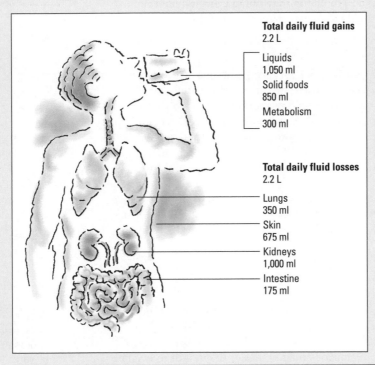

Total daily fluid gains
2.2 L

Liquids
1,050 ml

Solid foods
850 ml

Metabolism
300 ml

Total daily fluid losses
2.2 L

Lungs
350 ml

Skin
675 ml

Kidneys
1,000 ml

Intestine
175 ml

Gains

Fluid gains come mostly from drinking water and other beverages. The body also gains fluid from solid foods and the metabolism of carbohydrates, proteins and fats.

Losses

The body loses fluid through sensible and insensible means.

Sense and sensibility

Fluid losses from urination, defecation, wounds and other means are termed *sensible* because they can be measured. Urination accounts for the largest sensible fluid loss.

Memory jogger

To remember the three ways in which normal water loss occurs, think **PEE:**

Perspiration—through the skin

Exhalation—from the lungs

Elimination—through urine and faeces.

A certain amount of water must be present in urine to transport out of the body the products of metabolism that the body doesn't need. This amount is called *obligatory* water loss because it must occur daily for health. The kidneys may also put out additional water each day, depending on activities and needs. This *optional* water loss varies with climate and physical activities.

Typically, an adult loses 150 to 200 ml/day of fluid through defecation. In severe diarrhoea, these fluid losses may exceed 5,000 ml/day.

Don't count on it

Fluid losses from the skin (through perspiration) and lungs (through expiration) are called *insensible* because they can't be measured—or, to a large extent, even seen. Losses from fluid evaporation through the skin are fairly constant but depend on the body surface area. For instance, an infant has a greater body surface area than an adult, relative to their respective weights. As a result, infants typically lose more water through their skin than adults. Changes in humidity also affect the amount of fluid lost through the skin.

Likewise, respiratory rate and depth affect the amount of fluid lost through the lungs. Tachypnea causes more water to be lost; bradypnea, less. Fever increases insensible fluid losses through both the skin and lungs.

Thirst

Thirst, the conscious desire for water, is the primary regulator of fluid intake. Thirst occurs as a result of even small fluid losses. Losing body fluids or eating salty foods leads to an increase in the osmolarity (osmotic pressure) of ECF. This increase causes the mucous membranes of the mouth to become dry, in turn stimulating the thirst centre in the hypothalamus.

The brain then directs motor neurons to satisfy thirst, causing the person to drink enough fluid to restore ECF levels to normal. The ingested fluid is absorbed from the intestine into the bloodstream, where it moves freely between fluid compartments. This movement leads to a rise in the amount of fluid in the body and a drop in the concentration of solutes, thus balancing fluid levels throughout the body.

Sources of fluid

Liquids are the only water sources that meet the body's fluid needs. However, solid foods and metabolic water also contribute to total fluid intake. Solid foods supply about 700 to 1,000 ml of water daily in an average diet. By weight, solid foods range from 0% water (vegetable oil) to 95% water (lettuce). The metabolism of carbohydrates, fats and proteins yields roughly 250 ml of water daily.

> Liquids are the only water sources that meet the body's fluid needs, so advise your adults to drink 8 to 12 glasses of water per day!

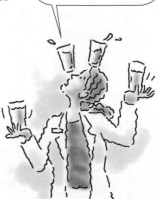

Fluids in health promotion

Many people don't drink enough fluids, which puts them at risk for chronic mild dehydration. Physical effects of dehydration include:
- increased risk of kidney stones
- reduced physical performance, such as difficulty concentrating, headache, irritability, sleepiness, dizziness and loss of balance.

Under normal circumstances, water is the best fluid to consume. Tap water is available virtually everywhere at no cost; bottled water costs relatively little and may taste better than tap water. What's more, water has no calories, fat, caffeine or cholesterol. Other good beverage choices are low-fat milk and 100% fruit juices, both of which contain essential nutrients.

Although carbonated drinks provide fluid, they also deliver empty calories along with high sugar content (unless they're diet drinks). Caffeinated beverages and alcohol actually increase fluid loss by causing frequent urination. (See *Promoting fluid intake*.)

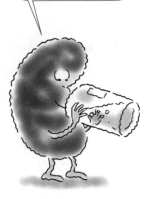

Not everybody must get stoned! Tell your patients to drink up because dehydration increases the risk of kidney stones.

NutriTips

Promoting fluid intake

To help ensure adequate fluid intake, provide the following suggestions to patients:

- Keep bottled water at your desk so you can take sips throughout the day.
- Choose liquids that taste good. If you prefer cold water, refrigerate the water bottle or a glass.
- If you do not like the taste of your water, consider installing a water filter or buy bottled water.
- Drink before you get thirsty. If you wait until you're thirsty, you'll need to drink even more fluid.
- Drink a glass of water before each meal. Water helps inhibit your appetite, so you eat less.
- Include water as part of your meal. That way, drinking water won't seem like an extra chore that calls for planning.
- Try sparkling water with a touch of lime or lemon. Sparkling water is calorie free and full of bubbles!
- Eat plenty of fruits and vegetables, which are high in water content. 150 ml of fruit juice equals one serving from the fruit group.
- Pack bottled water with your lunch to help you stay away from high-calorie soft drinks.
- Avoid alcohol and caffeinated beverages, which lead to fluid loss from frequent urination.
- Drink low-fat milk. It provides essential nutrients, such as fluids, vitamin D, calcium and protein.
- Drink extra fluids before, during and after exercise. Drink at least two glasses of fluid up to 2 hours before a competitive event, and at least one glass of water or a sports drink 5 to 10 minutes before a workout. During strenuous exercise, drink a glass of water every 15 to 20 minutes.

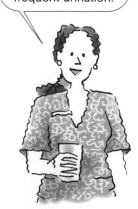

When possible, suggest that your patient wet his or her whistle with water! Drinking alcoholic beverages, such as wine, and caffeinated beverages, such as coffee and tea, can actually increase fluid loss by causing frequent urination.

Water requirement

To maintain fluid balance, a person's daily fluid intake should equal fluid output. On average, an adult loses about 1,450 to 2,800 ml of water daily from sensible and insensible losses. Roughly speaking, an adult needs 1 to 1.5 ml of water per calorie consumed. So someone who consumes 2,000 calories daily needs a total fluid intake of 2,000 to 3,000 ml. Of this intake, at least 60% should be consumed as water, with the remainder obtained from foods and metabolism. (See *Fluid balance in infants*.)

A bit more, a tad less

Despite these guidelines, actual water requirements vary greatly among individuals—and in the same individual as circumstances change. For instance the body's water requirement increases with:
- high ambient temperature—as the temperature of the surrounding environment rises, the body loses water to help maintain a normal temperature. This loss necessitates increased water intake.
- increased activity level—strenuous physical activity causes a person to lose more water through sweating and to need more water for the increased metabolic work involved in the physical activity. As a result, the water requirement rises.
- functional losses—any disease process that interferes with normal functioning of the body can affect fluid requirements. For instance, prolonged diarrhoea or vomiting may cause loss of large amounts of water, increasing the fluid need.
- different diets—if you eat a high-fibre diet, your water requirement increases because fibre absorbs water in the GI tract. A high-sodium or high-protein diet also increases the need for fluid.

Fluid imbalances

Most of the time, the body adequately compensates for minor fluid imbalances. If it can't, however, any of several problems may result. These include dehydration (fluid volume deficit), hypervolaemia (fluid volume excess) and water intoxication.

Dehydration

The body loses water all the time. A person responds to the thirst reflex by drinking fluids and eating foods that contain water. However, if water isn't adequately replaced, the body's cells can lose water. This loss causes dehydration, or fluid volume deficit. Dehydration refers to a fluid loss of 1% or more of body weight.

Signs and symptoms of dehydration include:
- dizziness
- irritability
- delirium
- extreme thirst
- dry skin and mucous membranes

Memory jogger

Remember that individuals may need a **TADD** more or less water, depending on these four factors:

Temperature

Activity

Disease

Diet.

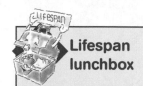

Lifespan lunchbox

Fluid balance in infants

Term infants, 0 to 6 months, need 150 ml/kg/day, and those aged 7 to 12 months need approximately 120 ml/kg/day, because of their large body water content (about 70% to 75% of total weight). Also, a relatively large amount of their total body water is located outside the cells, so body water is more easily lost than in adults.

- poor skin turgor
- increased heart rate
- falling blood pressure
- decreased urine output
- seizures and coma (in severe dehydration).

Laboratory values may include a serum sodium level above 145 mmol/L (145 mEq/L) and serum osmolality above 303 mOsm/kg (303 mmol/kg).

Treatment of dehydration involves determining its cause (such as diarrhoea and decreased fluid intake) and replacing lost fluids—orally or I.V. Most patients receive hypotonic, low-sodium fluids, such as dextrose and saline in water. (See *Dehydration in elderly people*.)

Hypervolaemia

Hypervolaemia refers to an excess of isotonic fluid (water and sodium) in the ECF. The body has mechanisms to compensate for hypervolaemia. If these fail, however, signs and symptoms develop.

Hypervolaemia can occur if a person consumes more fluid than needed, if fluid output is impaired or if too much sodium is retained. Conditions that may lead to hypervolaemia include kidney failure, cirrhosis, heart failure and steroid therapy.

Depending on the severity of hypervolaemia, signs and symptoms may include:

- oedema
- distended neck and hand veins
- heart failure
- initially, rising blood pressure and cardiac output; later, falling values.

Laboratory tests may reveal a normal serum sodium level and serum osmolality less than 280 mOsm/kg (280 mmol/kg).

Treatment involves determining the cause and treating the underlying condition. Typically, patients require fluid and sodium restrictions and diuretic therapy.

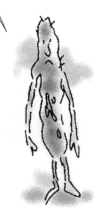

Don't hang me out to dry! Cells like me can become dehydrated if fluid balance isn't maintained.

Lifespan lunchbox

Dehydration in elderly people

Elderly people in care homes or hospitals are at particularly high risk for dehydration because of their diminished thirst perception and physical, cognitive, speech, mobility and visual impairments.

Poor skin turgor may be an unreliable sign of hydration in older people because of the reduction in the amount of subcutaneous tissue that occurs with age. Check turgor by pinching the subcutaneous tissue at the forehead or over the xiphoid process and watching for a quick return to baseline.

Water intoxication

Water intoxication occurs when excess fluid moves from the ECF to the ICF. Excessive low-sodium fluid in the ECF is hypotonic to cells; cells are hypertonic to the fluid. As a result, fluids shift into the cells, which have comparatively less fluid and more solutes. That fluid shift occurs to balance the concentrations of fluid between the two spaces.

Water intoxication may occur in a patient with the syndrome of inappropriate antidiuretic hormone, which can result from central nervous system or pulmonary disorders, head trauma, tumours or the use of certain drugs. Other causes of water intoxication include:
- rapid infusion of hypotonic solutions
- psychogenic polydipsia (a psychological disturbance in which a person drinks large amounts of fluid that aren't needed).

Quick quiz

1. Fluid gains come mostly from:
   A. Solid foods
   B. Carbohydrates
   C. Proteins
   D. Drinking water

Answer: D. Fluid gains come mostly from drinking water and other beverages.

2. Which type of fluid transport requires no energy?
   A. Active transport
   B. Diffusion
   C. Pinocytosis
   D. Sodium–potassium pump

Answer: B. Diffusion is a form of passive transport because no energy is required.

3. Dehydration may cause:
   A. Euphoria
   B. Delirium
   C. High blood pressure
   D. Anuria

Answer: B. Delirium is a possible sign of dehydration.

4. Which of the following mechanisms is the primary regulator of fluid intake?
   A. Serum potassium level
   B. Ratio of fat to skeletal muscle
   C. Thirst
   D. Active transport

Answer: C. Thirst is the primary regulator of fluid intake. Even a small fluid loss makes you thirsty and causes the osmotic pressure of ECF to rise. As a result, the mucous membranes of the mouth become dry, which stimulates thirst.

5. Which of the following factors is a source of insensible fluid loss?
A. Skin
B. Kidneys
C. GI tract
D. Wounds

Answer: A. Fluid losses from the skin and lungs are called *insensible losses* because they can't be measured or seen. Fluid losses from urination, defecation and wounds are called *sensible losses* because they can be measured.

Scoring

★★★   If you answered all five questions correctly, celebrate! The information in this chapter diffused quite easily into your system.

★★   If you answered four questions correctly, way to go! You must have learned by osmosis.

★   If you answered fewer than four questions correctly, hang in there! Give the chapter another read, and maybe you'll absorb more of the information.

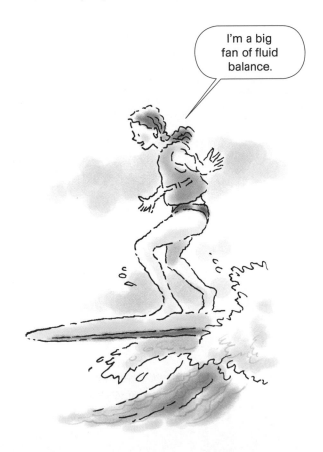

Part II

Assessment

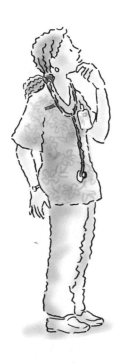

8 Assessing nutritional status

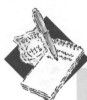

Just the facts

Assessing nutritional status is an important part of patient care. In this chapter, you'll learn:

♦ clinical uses of nutritional screening guidelines

♦ components of a comprehensive nutritional assessment

♦ physical findings that pertain to nutritional status

♦ laboratory studies used to detect poor nutrition.

Evaluating nutritional status

A healthy, balanced diet should be the goal for every individual. This goal is met when nutrient supply, or intake, meets the demand, or requirement. An imbalance occurs when there's overnutrition (supply exceeds demand) or undernutrition (demand exceeds supply).

Seeking status symbols

A patient's nutritional status is evaluated by examining information about him or her from several sources. Nutritional screening, along with the patient's medical history, physical examination findings and laboratory results, can be used to detect potential imbalances. The sources used depend on the patient and setting. A comprehensive nutritional assessment may then be conducted, by a dietitian, to set goals and determine interventions to correct actual or potential imbalances.

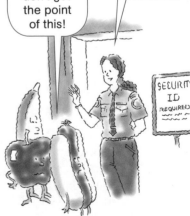

Nutritional screening is an effective way to evaluate nutritional status.

I just don't get the point of this!

Enacting a plan

Based on the information gathered in the comprehensive nutritional assessment, the patient may require restrictions in diet, such as a reduction in calories, fat, saturated fat, cholesterol, sodium or other nutrients. Other diet plans involve therapeutic correction of imbalances, such as by increasing or decreasing certain minerals or vitamins.

Nutritional screening

Nutritional screening examines certain variables to determine the risk of nutritional problems in specific populations. A screening may target pregnant women, the elderly or those with certain disorders (such as cardiac disorders) to detect deficiencies or potential imbalances. A qualified health care professional or other appropriately trained person may perform the screening on an individual who may or may not be in the target population. Routine screening should occur during the initial history and physical assessment. There are many different nutritional screening tools available, including a range of computer-based software. The tool used should be the one recommended by local policy and protocols.

Making value judgments

The most commonly examined values are:
- height and weight history
- unintentional weight loss (more than 5% in 30 days or 10% in 180 days)
- laboratory values
- skin integrity
- appetite
- diet
- present illness or diagnosis
- medical history
- functional status
- advanced age (age 80 and older).

Malnutrition Universal Screening Tool (MUST)

MUST is a common tool used in the UK and has been developed by the British Association for Parenteral and Enteral Nutrition (BAPEN). MUST is a five-step screening tool to identify adults who are malnourished or at risk of malnutrition. It is for use in hospitals, community and other care settings and can be used by all care workers. It includes management guidelines and can be used to develop a care plan. (See *How to use MUST*.)

How to use MUST

MUST is a handy screening tool for evaluating nutritional status. It provides useful information about the patient's body mass index (BMI), weight loss and acute illness. It is a simple five-stage process that includes management guidelines. Stages 1–3 enable the user to score the patient. The higher the score, the greater the risk of malnutrition.

The five MUST steps

Step 1
BMI score

BMI kg/m	Score
>20 (>30 Obese)	= 0
18.5–20	= 1

Step 2
Weight loss score
Unplanned weight loss in past 3–6 months

%	Score
<5	= 0
5–10	= 1
>10	= 2

Step 3
If a patient is acutely ill **and** there has been or is likely to be no nutritional intake for

%	Score
>5 days	= 2

Step 4
Overall risk of malnutrition
Add scores together to calculate the overall risk of malnutrition
Score 0, low-risk; Score 1, medium risk; Score 2 or more, high risk

Step 5
Management guidelines

0
Low risk
Routine clinical care
Repeat screening
Hospital—weekly
Care homes—monthly
Community—annually
For special groups, e.g. those 75 years or older.

1
Medium risk
Observe
Document dietary intake for 3 days if subject in hospital or care home
If improvement or adequate intake—little concern
If no improvement—clinical concern—follow local policy
Repeat screening
Hospital—weekly
Care home—at least monthly
Community—at least every 2–3 months

2 or more
High risk
Treat
Refer to dietitian or Nutritional Support Team according to local protocol or policy.

Improve and increase overall nutritional intake
Monitor and review care plan
Hospital—weekly
Care home—monthly
Community—monthly
Unless detrimental or no benefit is expected from nutritional support, e.g. imminent death

All risk categories
Treat underlying condition and provide help and advice on food choices, eating and drinking when necessary
Record malnutrition risk category
Record the need for special diets and follow local policy

Obesity
Record the presence of obesity. For those with underlying conditions, these are generally controlled before the treatment of obesity.

The 'Malnutrition Universal Screening Tool' (MUST) is reproduced here with the kind permission of BAPEN (British Association for Parenteral and Enteral Nutrition). The 'MUST' was developed by the Malnutrition Advisory Group (MAG) of BAPEN and was first produced in November 2003.

For further information on 'MUST', see www.bapen.org.uk.

Risk assessment

When the screening is complete, a level of risk of nutritional problems is assigned. Those individuals at higher risk should be given a comprehensive nutritional assessment by a registered dietitian, whereas those at lower to moderate risk should be periodically re-evaluated. Local policy will guide you as to when you need to make the referral to the dietitian.

Comprehensive nutritional assessment

When the nutritional screening has identified a person at risk, a comprehensive nutritional assessment is conducted to examine additional factors and better determine the degree of malnutrition. Using this assessment, a baseline nutritional status is determined and effective nutritional care is planned. Because of the extensive training required and the need for accuracy, a registered dietitian is usually responsible for conducting this assessment.

> I sentence those at high risk for poor nutrition to a comprehensive nutritional assessment.

Crunching the numbers

The comprehensive nutritional assessment is commonly performed on moderate- to high-risk patients with some degree of protein-calorie malnutrition. Major parameters examined include:
- medical history
- physical examination findings
- laboratory test results.

Multiple criteria must be examined to provide an accurate evaluation of the individual's nutritional status. No single criterion can be used to evaluate an individual, and it may not be necessary to gather all possible information for every patient. The decision to consider information is left to the dietitian's professional judgement.

Medical history

A medical history is usually gathered from the patient's medical record or through an interview with the patient.

Current and past health history

Current and past health history is important as it relates to nutritional status and affects nutrient supply or demand. Findings that may affect nutritional status negatively include:
- chewing and swallowing problems resulting from ill-fitting dentures, missing teeth or mechanical problems, such as obstruction, inflammation or oedema
- neurologic problems, such as dysphagia, Parkinson's disease, stroke or traumatic brain injury
- anorexia or loss of appetite
- cognitive impairments
- paralysis or physical disabilities that may impair the ability to feed oneself.

Excessive nutrient intake

Conditions may also be found in the patient's history that may result in excessive nutrient intake. Examples of these conditions include bulimia nervosa and obesity.

GI disorders

Other problems can also impair digestion and absorption, resulting in altered nutritional status. Check the patient's health history for inflammatory, obstructive or functional disorders of the GI tract, such as:

- lactose intolerance
- cystic fibrosis
- pancreatic disorders
- inflammatory bowel diseases
- minimal function in the small intestine due to a disorder, such as pseudo-obstruction or surgical excision (short-gut syndrome)
- radiation enteritis
- liver disorders.

Altered metabolism

Nutrition may also be affected by conditions known to accelerate metabolism. These conditions include:

- pregnancy
- fever
- sepsis
- pressure ulcers
- cancer
- acquired immunodeficiency syndrome
- major surgery
- trauma
- burns.

Some conditions, such as diabetes mellitus, hormonal imbalances and starvation, alter nutrient metabolism. In addition, diarrhoea and malabsorption syndromes, such as coeliac disease, cause increased nutrient excretion. Other conditions, such as renal insufficiency, impair nutrient excretion.

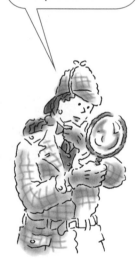

Knowing if a health problem exists helps to detect potential nutritional problems.

Detection is the key

It is important to identify any pre existing condition, in the history, that might affect nutritional status. The condition's impact on nutritional status depends on its severity and how long the patient has been afflicted. (See *Tips for detecting nutritional problems*, page 110.)

Intake information

Nutritional intake information helps you assess what and how much your patient eats. This information can help identify problems in nutritional status and behaviours that need improvement.

Survey says...

Observing what the individual eats provides an objective measurement of the kinds and amount of foods consumed. Of course, close observation is rarely possible. A questionnaire geared to nutritional problems can help fill this information gap. You may have access to computer-based programmes

Tips for detecting nutritional problems

Nutritional problems may stem from physical conditions, drugs, diet or lifestyle factors. The lists below will help you determine if your patient is at risk for a nutritional problem.

Physical condition

- Chronic illnesses (diabetes or neurologic, cardiac or thyroid problems)
- Family history of diabetes or heart disease
- Draining wounds or fistulas
- Obesity or a weight gain of 10% above the normal body weight
- Unplanned weight loss of 10% below the normal body weight
- History of or recent GI disturbances
- Anorexia or bulimia
- Depression or anxiety
- Severe trauma
- Recent chemotherapy or radiation therapy
- Physical limitation (paresis or paralysis)
- Recent major surgery
- Pregnancy, especially teen or multiple birth

Drugs and diet

- Fad diets
- Steroid, diuretic or antacid use
- Mouth, tooth or denture problems
- Excessive alcohol intake
- Strict vegetarian diet
- Liquid diet or nothing by mouth for more than 3 days
- Polypharmacy (taking more than one prescribed medication or over-the-counter medications)

Lifestyle

- Lack of support from family and friends
- Financial problems
- Isolation or homebound status

that can help in the assessment process. Open-ended questions are more useful than closed, 'yes-or-no' questions for obtaining accurate information. Important areas for questioning include:

- number of meals and snacks eaten in a 24-hour period
- unusual food habits
- time of the day most of the calories are consumed
- skipped meals
- meals eaten away from home
- number of fruits and vegetables eaten daily
- number of servings (and types) of starchy foods such as bread or grains eaten daily
- frequency of eating red meat, poultry and fish including type and amount
- frequency of meatless meals consumed
- number of hours of television watched daily
- types and amount of dairy products consumed daily
- frequency of eating desserts and sweets
- types and amount of beverages (including alcohol) consumed
- food allergies or intolerances
- dietary, vitamin and mineral supplements and why they're taken
- medications, including over-the-counter products and herbal supplements.

Diet history tools

More formal tools for taking a diet history have been developed. The 24-hour food recall and the food frequency record are tools that examine what, how much and how often a person typically eats to determine nutritional status. These may be difficult to use if the individual has a poor memory or is confused.

24-hour food recall

A quick and easy method of evaluating an individual's intake is through the 24-hour food recall. In order to complete this tool, the person must be able to recount all the types and amounts of foods and beverages consumed during a 24-hour period.

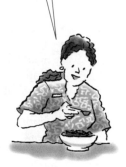

If I recall, I ate cereal for breakfast yesterday, too.

Working around the clock

The time period may be the past 24 hours or a typical 24-hour period. To help the person identify portion sizes, food models or pictures of typical portions can be used. Specific details may be necessary in some recall situations, such as food preparation (for example frying versus dry roasting meat). Open-ended questions also reveal more information than typical 'yes-or-no' questions. Once obtained, the recall information is then evaluated to see if nutritional needs are being met.

Food frequency record

The food frequency record is a checklist of particular foods that helps determine what's consumed and how often. The checklist may list the foods in one column, and the person marks off in other columns how often he or she eats the foods. The choices may include how often the food is consumed (such as per day, per week or per month) or if the food is eaten frequently, seldom or never. The checklist typically doesn't include the serving size, and it may include only specific foods or nutrients suspected of being deficient or excessive in the diet.

Getting into groups

Another method of gathering information for the food frequency record is to use the eatwell plate food groups to develop a questionnaire. This can help an individual to recall the foods they are eating, as they record the type of food consumed and how often.

Two are better than one

Either checklist provides a more complete dietary picture when used in conjunction with the 24-hour recall. When deficiencies or excesses are identified, goals may be developed to address nutritional and educational needs.

Psychosocial factors

Other factors could be uncovered during the history that may influence the patient's nutritional habits, including:

- illiteracy
- language barriers
- knowledge of nutrition and food safety
- cultural or religious influences
- social isolation
- limited or low income
- inadequate cooking resources, such as major appliances or kitchen access
- limited access to transportation
- physical inactivity or illness
- use of tobacco or recreational drugs
- limited community resources. (See *Understanding cultural and economic influences*.)

Teach according to each patient's needs

You should incorporate the patient's individual psychosocial factors into his or her teaching plan, as appropriate. For example if you identify that your patient can't read or doesn't read well, giving him or her a picture guide on which foods are appropriate and which should be avoided may be more helpful to the patient than written words alone.

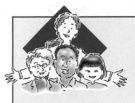

Bridging the gap

Understanding cultural and economic influences

What people eat may depend on various cultural and economic influences. Understanding these influences will give you more insight into the person's nutritional status. Consider these points:

- Socioeconomic status may affect the person's ability to purchase healthful foods in quantities needed to maintain proper health. Low socioeconomic status can lead to nutritional problems, especially for the elderly, small children and pregnant women. Many young people may be struggling with their finances if they are at university or in low-paid employment.
- Work schedule affects the amount and type of food a person eats, especially if they work full-time at night.
- Religion can restrict food choices. For example many Jews and Muslims don't eat pork products, and many Catholics avoid meat on Ash Wednesday and Fridays during Lent.

Physical findings

Physical examinations help determine your patient's health status and identify illness. Physical factors discovered during the comprehensive nutritional assessment may be related to an alteration in nutritional status and malnutrition. However, such findings as height and weight reflect chronic changes in nutritional status rather than acute processes.

Height

Measure height using a fixed measuring stick with the individual standing as straight as possible, without shoes, against a wall. Adaptations may be needed if the patient can't stand or cooperate. (See *Overcoming height measurement problems* and *Growth spurts and diminishing height*, page 114.)

Weight

Measure the person's weight using a class III-approved weighing scale (standing or sitting), or if the person has difficulty moving, approved hoists can be used. Some specialist health care units may also have scales integrated into the bed for recording the weight of bed-bound or unconscious patients. The information gathered is more helpful if weight is measured on the same scale at the same time of day (typically before breakfast and after voiding), in the same amount of clothing and without shoes. (See *Nutrition and infant growth rate*, page 114.)

Overcoming height measurement problems

A person confined to a wheelchair or one who can't stand straight because of scoliosis poses a challenge in measuring accurate height. An approximate measurement of height can be obtained by measuring the ulna length.

Point to Point
Measure between the point of the elbow (olecranon process) and the midpoint of the prominent bone on the wrist (styloid process)—nondominant side.

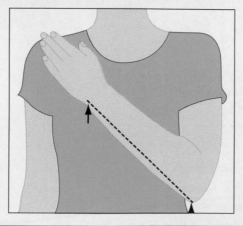

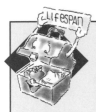

Lifespan lunchbox

Growth spurts and diminishing height

When measuring height, note the growth of children as well as diminishing height in older adults. Growth of children should be recorded on UK-WHO growth charts developed by the Royal College of Paediatrics and Child Health. Diminishing height in older adults may be related to osteoporotic changes and should be investigated.

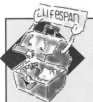

Lifespan lunchbox

Nutrition and infant growth rate

The rate of growth in infants is an indicator of nutritional status. Infants who are breastfed have satisfactory but slower rates of growth than infants who are formula-fed. However, by age 12 to 16 months, breastfed infants weigh approximately the same as infants who are formula-fed. Undernourished or sick infants with slow growth rates typically reach normal weight percentiles by age 2 years.

Body mass index

BMI measures weight in relationship to height. It can be calculated using kilograms and centimetres. (See *Calculating BMI.*) BMI can also be estimated without doing any calculations. (See *Determining BMI.*)

Using BMI to evaluate body weight requires little skill. The major disadvantage of using BMI is that it works on the assumption that excess weight is a result of excess fat. It doesn't account for other reasons such as oedema and large muscle mass.

Interpretation station

BMI is interpreted as follows:
- An underweight person has a BMI of less than 18.5 kg/m^2.
- A person whose weight is normal for his height has a BMI of 18.5 to 24.9 kg/m^2.

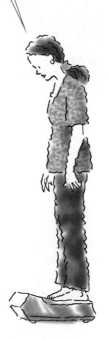

When weighing your patient, remember: same scale, same time of day, same amount of clothing and no shoes!

Calculating BMI

Use the formula below to calculate your patient's BMI.

$$BMI = \frac{\text{weight in kilograms}}{(\text{height in metres}) \times (\text{height in metres})}$$

There is a handy **BMI** calculator available online at www.NHS.uk/LiveWell.

Determining BMI

BMI measures weight in relation to height. The BMI ranges shown here are for adults. They aren't exact ranges for healthy or unhealthy weights; however, they show that health risks increase at higher levels of overweight and obesity. A very muscular person may fall in the obese range. To use the graph below, find your patient's weight along the bottom and then go straight up until you come to the line that matches his or her height. The shaded area indicates whether your patient is healthy, overweight or obese.

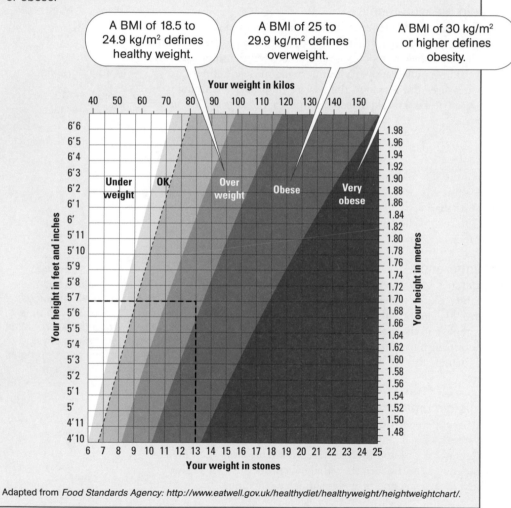

Adapted from *Food Standards Agency: http://www.eatwell.gov.uk/healthydiet/healthyweight/heightweightchart/.*

- An overweight person has a BMI of 25.0 to 29.9 kg/m².
- A person in obesity class 1 has a BMI of 30.0 to 34.9 kg/m²; in obesity class 2, a BMI of 35.0 to 39.9 kg/m²; and morbid obesity, 40.0 kg/m² or greater.

All measures other than normal place the patient at a higher health risk, and nutritional needs should be assessed accordingly.

Body composition measurements

Measurements of body composition include the triceps skinfold measurement, the midarm circumference and the midarm muscle circumference. These measurements provide quantitative information about body composition made up of fat or muscle tissue. Measurements may be compared with reference standards or may be used to evaluate changes. If measurements are less than 90% of the reference value, nutritional intervention is indicated.

Triceps skinfold measurements

Triceps skinfold measures subcutaneous fat stores and is an index of total body fat. To measure the skinfold, the individual's arm hangs freely and a fold of skin located slightly above midpoint is grasped between the thumb and the forefinger. As the skin is pulled away from underlying muscle, calipers are applied and the measurement is read to the nearest millimetre. Training is needed to complete triceps skinfold measurements. (See *Taking anthropometric arm measurements*.)

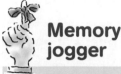

Memory jogger

To remember the three placements to take body composition measurements, think **T**otally **M**ade of **M**uscle, **M**an:

Triceps skinfold

Midarm circumference

Midarm **M**uscle circumference.

Take three

Three readings of the skinfold measurement are taken. These readings may be from the same site or other appropriate sites (bicep, thigh, calf, subscapular or suprailiac skinfolds). The readings are then added together and divided by 3 to record the average. For men, 11.3 mm is 90% of standard; for women, 14.9 mm.

Midarm circumference

Midarm circumference measures muscle mass and subcutaneous fat. To obtain this value, ask the patient to flex the forearm of his or her nondominant arm 90 degrees. Measure the distance between the acromion process of the scapula and the olecranon process of the ulna and mark the midpoint. Let the arm hang loose and measure around the arm at the midpoint. Hold the tape firmly—but not too tightly—and record to the nearest millimetre.

Midarm muscle circumference

Midarm muscle circumference provides an index of muscle mass and indicates somatic protein stores. Calculate this value by multiplying the triceps skinfold measurement by 3.14 and then subtract this value from the midarm circumference measurement. Record the value in centimetres. This value is minimally affected by oedema and provides a quick estimation.

Appearance

Physical examination of the individual may reveal signs of malnutrition related to a nutritional deficiency. However, signs may also be due to other conditions or disorders and can't be considered indicative, but only suggestive of a nutritional deficiency. In addition, remember that physical signs and

Some lab values such as levels of glucose and Hb can detect nutritional problems before physical signs and symptoms appear.

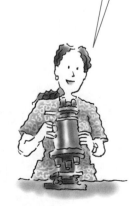

Taking anthropometric arm measurements

Follow the steps below to determine triceps skinfold thickness, midarm circumference and midarm muscle circumference.

Triceps skinfold thickness

1. Find the midpoint circumference of the arm by placing the tape measure halfway between the axilla and the elbow. Grasp the patient's skin with your thumb and forefinger, about 1 cm above the midpoint, as illustrated below.
2. Place calipers at the midpoint and squeeze for 3 seconds.
3. Record the measurement to the nearest millimetre.
4. Take two more readings and use the average.

Midarm circumference and midarm muscle circumference

1. Measure the midarm circumference at the midpoint, as illustrated below. Record the measurement in centimetres.
2. Calculate the midarm muscle circumference by multiplying the triceps skinfold thickness (measured in millimetres) by 3.14.
3. Subtract this number from the midarm circumference.

Recording the measurements

Record all three measurements as a percentage of the standard measurements (see chart below), using this formula:

$$\frac{\text{Actual measurement}}{\text{Standard measurement}} \times 100\%$$

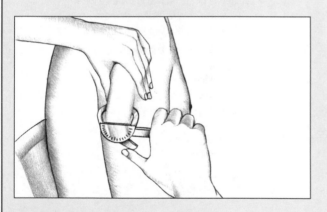

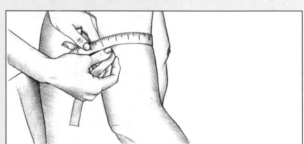

After taking and recording the measurements, consult the chart at the right to determine your patient's caloric status. A measurement less than 90% of the standard indicates caloric deprivation. A measurement over 90% indicates adequate or more-than-adequate energy reserves.

Measurement	Standard	90%
Triceps skinfold thickness	Men: 12.5 mm Women: 16.5 mm	Men: 11.3 mm Women: 14.9 mm
Midarm circumference	Men: 29.3 cm Women: 28.5 cm	Men: 26.4 cm Women: 25.7 cm
Midarm muscle circumference	Men: 25.3 cm Women: 23.3 cm	Men: 22.8 cm Women: 20.9 cm

symptoms may vary among populations because of genetic and environmental differences. (See *Evaluating nutritional disorders*.)

Laboratory data

Laboratory tests are not used routinely to assess nutritional status but can be of use in health care settings when nutritional status has been compromised by ill-health. Most of the tests provide protein-calorie information, with serum albumin used most commonly to screen for nutritional problems. Tests are done to help determine the adequacy of protein stores. Some tests measure

Evaluating nutritional disorders

This chart can help you interpret your nutritional assessment findings. Body systems are listed below with signs or symptoms and the implications for each.

Body system or region	Sign or symptom	Implications
General	• Weakness and fatigue • Weight loss	• Anaemia or electrolyte imbalance • Decreased calorie intake, increased calorie use or inadequate nutrient intake or absorption
Skin, hair and nails	• Dry, flaky skin • Dry skin with poor turgor • Rough, scaly skin with bumps • Petechiae or ecchymoses • Sore that won't heal • Thinning, dry hair • Spoon-shaped, brittle or ridged nails	• Vitamin A, vitamin B complex or linoleic acid deficiency • Dehydration • Vitamin A deficiency • Vitamin C or K deficiency • Protein, vitamin C or zinc deficiency • Protein deficiency • Iron deficiency
Eyes	• Night blindness; corneal swelling, softening or dryness; Bitot's spots (grey triangular patches on the conjunctiva) • Red conjunctiva	• Vitamin A deficiency • Riboflavin deficiency
Throat and mouth	• Cracks at the corner of the mouth • Magenta tongue • Beefy, red tongue • Soft, spongy bleeding gums • Swollen neck (goitre)	• Riboflavin or niacin deficiency • Riboflavin deficiency • Vitamin B_{12} deficiency • Vitamin C deficiency • Iodine deficiency
Cardiovascular	• Oedema • Tachycardia, hypotension	• Protein deficiency • Fluid volume deficit
GI	• Ascites	• Protein deficiency
Musculoskeletal	• Bone pain and bow leg • Muscle wasting	• Vitamin D or calcium deficiency • Protein, carbohydrate and fat deficiency
Neurologic	• Altered mental status • Paraesthesia	• Dehydration and thiamine or vitamin B_{12} deficiency • Vitamin B_{12}, pyridoxine or thiamine deficiency

by-products of protein catabolism (such as creatinine), and others measure products of protein anabolism (such as albumin level, transferrin level, haemoglobin (Hb) level, haematocrit (HCT), prealbumin, retinol-binding protein and total lymphocyte count). Other tests such as blood sugar or HbA1c can assess how well glycaemic control has been achieved in individuals managing their diabetes. Blood sugar alone can indicate a stress response.

Albumin

The serum albumin level test assesses protein levels in the body. Albumin makes up more than 50% of total proteins in blood and affects the cardiovascular system because it helps maintain osmotic pressure. Keep in mind that albumin production requires functioning liver cells and an adequate supply of amino acids, the building blocks of proteins.

Bum albumin levels

The serum albumin level decreases with serious protein deficiency and loss of blood protein due to burns, chronic malnutrition, liver or renal disease, heart failure, major surgery, infections or cancer. It also decreases as CRPC reactive protein (CRP) increases as a marker of stress and inflammation. It is of limited value in assessing nutritional status but useful when considering other clinical results to determine the extent of the disease process/illness.

Creatinine height index

The creatinine height index involves a 24-hour urine collection to measure urinary excretion of creatinine. It helps define body protein mass and evaluate protein depletion. Test results are interpreted using a formula that compares results with ideal height standards.

Creatin' creatinine confusion

Creatinine values decrease with age because of a normal decrease in lean muscle mass. The test is of limited value because results are greatly altered by age, amount of exercise, stress, menstruation and the presence of severe illness. Increased values may indicate decreased protein stores.

Transferrin

Transferrin is a 'carrier' protein that transports iron. The molecule is synthesised mainly in the liver. Transferrin levels decrease along with protein levels and indicate depletion of protein stores. The serum transferrin level reflects the patient's current protein status more accurately than albumin because of its shorter half-life. A normal transferrin value is greater than 200 mg/dl (SI, 2 g/L).

Trackin' transferrin

Decreased transferrin values may also indicate inadequate protein production due to liver damage, protein loss from renal disease, acute or chronic infection or cancer. Elevated levels may indicate severe iron deficiency.

Haemoglobin

Haemoglobin (Hb) is the main component of red blood cells (RBCs), which transport oxygen. Its formation requires an adequate supply of protein in the form of amino acids. Hb values help assess the blood's oxygen-carrying capacity and are useful in diagnosing anaemia, protein deficiency and hydration status.

Globin trekker

Decreased Hb suggests iron deficiency anaemia, protein deficiency, excessive blood loss or overhydration. Increased Hb suggests dehydration or polycythaemia. Normal Hb values vary with age and type of blood sample tested. The following values reflect normal Hb concentrations (in grams per decilitre):

- neonates—17 to 22 g/dl (SI, 170 to 220 g/L)
- 1 week—14.5 to 24.5 g/dl (SI, 145 to 245 g/L)
- 1 month—12.5 to 20.5 g/dl (SI, 125 to 205 g/L)
- 3 months—10.7 to 17.3 g/dl (SI, 107 to 173 g/L)
- 10 years—10.3 to 14.9 g/dl (SI, 103 to 149 g/L)
- adult males—14 to 17.4 g/dl (SI, 140 to 174 g/L)
- adult females—12 to 16 g/dl (SI, 120 to 160 g/L).

Haematocrit

The haematocrit (HCT) level reflects the proportion of blood occupied by the RBCs. This test for haematocrit helps diagnose anaemia and dehydration.

Don't omit haematocrit

Decreased values suggest iron deficiency anaemia or excessive fluid intake or blood loss. Increased values suggest severe dehydration or polycythaemia. Normal HCT values reflect age, sex, sample type and the laboratory performing the test. The following ranges represent normal HCT values, as a percentage, for different age groups:

- neonates—55% to 68% (SI, 0.55 to 0.68%)
- 1 week—44% to 64% (SI, 0.44 to 0.64%)
- 1 month—39% to 59% (SI, 0.39 to 0.59%)
- 3 months—35% to 49% (SI, 0.35 to 0.49%)
- 10 years—32% to 42% (SI, 0.32 to 0.42%)
- adult males—42% to 52% (SI, 0.42 to 0.52%)
- adult females—36% to 48% (SI, 0.36 to 0.48%).

Prealbumin

The prealbumin test is also more sensitive than the albumin test because of its short half-life (2 days). Levels of prealbumin are less affected by liver disease and hydration status than albumin; however, it's also more expensive to perform and therefore not routinely carried out by most clinical laboratories. The normal prealbumin value is 19 to 38 mg/dl (SI, 190 to 380 mg/L).

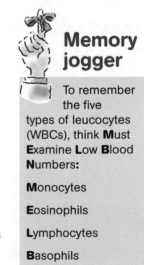

Memory jogger

To remember the five types of leucocytes (WBCs), think **M**ust **E**xamine **L**ow **B**lood **N**umbers:

Monocytes

Eosinophils

Lymphocytes

Basophils

Neutrophils.

Retinol-binding protein

Measurement of retinol-binding protein can help you detect an acute change in a patient's nutritional status. This protein responds quickly to nutritional repletion due to a small body pool and short half-life (10 to 12 hours). A normal retinol-binding protein value is SI, 1.43 to 2.86 mmol/L (2.6 to 7.7 mg/dl).

Total lymphocyte count

A lymphocyte (leucocyte) is a white blood cell (WBC), the main cell responsible for fighting infection. Leucocytes are responsible for destroying organisms as well as for phagocytosis, which promotes cellular repair. Normal WBC counts range from 4,000 to 10,000 cells/mm^3 (SI, 4 to 10 $\times$ 10^9 L). The WBC count is useful for diagnosing the severity of a disease.

There are five types of leucocytes:

 neutrophils, which fight pyogenic infections

 eosinophils, which fight allergic disorders and parasitic infections

 basophils, which fight parasitic infections

 lymphocytes, which fight viral infections

 monocytes, which fight severe infections.

The WBC differential will provide specific information about which type of WBC is being affected and is a diagnostically useful test.

Malnutrition decreases the total number of lymphocytes, impairing the body's ability to fight infection. The total lymphocyte count is used in evaluating the health of the immune system and assists in evaluation of protein stores. The total lymphocyte count may also be affected by many medical conditions, so the value is limited.

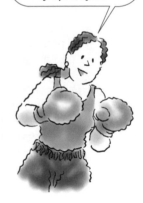

Malnutrition takes the fight out of the immune system by decreasing the number of lymphocytes.

Totalling it up

Decreased lymphocyte values may indicate malnutrition when no other cause is apparent and may point to infection, leukaemia or tissue necrosis.

Other measures of poor nutrition

In addition to the patient's medical history, physical findings and laboratory test results, you can use other criteria to detect nutritional deficiencies, including immunocompetence and bone integrity. These are not routinely completed but are ways in which nutritional status can be assessed.

Cutaneous hypersensitivity reactions

Immunocompetence may be evaluated by placing small quantities of recall antigens (*Candida*, mumps or purified protein derivative of tuberculin)

Lifespan lunchbox

Delayed hypersensitivity reactions

Age can cause delayed cutaneous hypersensitivity reactions, making the test less helpful for determining protein status. Elderly patients may have altered laboratory values because of:

- hydration status
- chronic diseases
- organ function changes
- drug regimen.

under the skin. Normally, a positive reaction occurs in 24 to 48 hours with a red area of 5 mm or more. However, in the individual with malnutrition, a delayed reaction, a reaction to only one antigen or no reaction at all (anergy) may occur. (See *Delayed hypersensitivity reactions*.)

X-rays

X-rays can be used to determine bone integrity and, especially in older women, to detect possible osteoporosis. A bone mineral density test is a specialised x-ray (DEXA scan often referred to as a DXA scan) that detects the amount of change in a bone. (Bones with higher mineral density allow fewer x-rays to pass through.) The beam detects the intensity and shows the doctor how dense the bones are. A bone scan, another type of x-ray, takes a picture of the bone and identifies fractures, tumours or inflammation. It's also sensitive enough to recognise structural changes. X-rays and other investigations such as CT scans may also be used to evaluate the GI tract for integrity and diagnose disorders that may cause malnutrition. The specific x-rays performed will be influenced by the patient's symptoms and diagnosis. Multiple tests may be necessary before a definitive diagnosis is made.

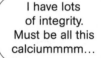

I have lots of integrity. Must be all this calciummmm…

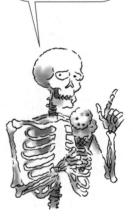

Quick quiz

1. You should measure a patient's midarm circumference whenever you:
   A. conduct a basic nutritional assessment.
   B. want to confirm an abnormal protein level.
   C. want to obtain information about body composition.
   D. determine a person's weight.

   Answer: C. Midarm circumference is one of three measurements used to provide information about the percentage of fat or muscle tissue in the body.

2. To identify individuals at moderate or high risk for nutritional problems, you can obtain information quickly by using which of the following tools?
    A.   Comprehensive nutritional assessment
    B.   Laboratory data
    C.   Physical examination
    D.   Nutritional screening

Answer: D. Screening uses a minimal amount of information to identify people at risk. Those identified as being at risk will need a comprehensive nutritional assessment.

3. Which of the following measures helps classify a person as underweight, normal or obese?
    A.   Body mass index
    B.   Triceps skinfold
    C.   Midarm circumference
    D.   Midarm muscle circumference

Answer: A. Body mass index uses the patient's height and weight to obtain a value that's useful for determining nutritional status.

4. The serum albumin test assesses:
    A.   protein levels in the body
    B.   the ratio of protein to albumin
    C.   how well the liver metabolises proteins
    D.   amino acid levels.

Answer: A. The serum albumin test assesses protein levels in the body.

Scoring

☆☆☆   If you answered all four questions correctly, wow! You've achieved star status in nutritional assessment.

☆☆   If you answered three questions correctly, you've been screened for great things! Your evaluation shows no imbalances when it comes to comprehension.

☆   If you answered fewer than three questions correctly, don't worry! If you're still feeling starved for information, go back and review this chapter.

9 Nutrition across the lifespan

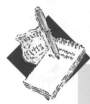

Just the facts

This chapter discusses the ways in which nutritional needs and considerations change throughout life. In this chapter, you'll learn:

♦ stages of growth and development throughout life

♦ nutritional needs unique to each stage of life

♦ nutritional problems common in each stage of life.

A look at nutrition across the lifespan

Nutrition plays a major role throughout each stage of the life cycle. From pregnancy and infancy to the older adult years, each stage of life has specific nutrition requirements to keep the body functioning at its best.

Nutrition during pregnancy

Maternal diet and nutritional status directly impact the course of pregnancy and the foetus. Malnutrition that occurs in the early months of pregnancy can affect the embryo's ability to survive; poor nutrition during the latter half of pregnancy can affect foetal growth.

Physiologic changes

Pregnancy produces various physiologic changes that influence the mother's nutritional needs and how nutrients are used in her body. These changes include alterations in metabolism, GI function and weight.

Nutrient metabolism

A pregnant woman's nutrient metabolism changes to adjust to the growing foetus:

• Carbohydrate and fat metabolism are altered during pregnancy to provide glucose to the foetus. Maternal fat stores increase during the first half of pregnancy as fat becomes the primary maternal fuel source. During the second half of pregnancy, these stores are used by the mother's body for energy, allowing glucose to be used as an energy source for the foetus.

• Protein metabolism is increased for growth of maternal and foetal tissues.

GI function

Nausea and vomiting are common symptoms of pregnancy in the first trimester. These GI alterations may be related to hypoglycaemia (low blood glucose level), decreased gastric motility, relaxation of the cardiac sphincter or anxiety. During the later stages of pregnancy some women may suffer from gastro-oesophageal reflux.

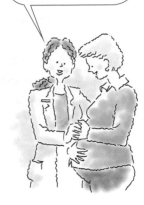

An expectant mother's body undergoes many changes that influence her nutrition needs.

Smoothing things out

During pregnancy, production of the hormone progesterone is increased, causing relaxation of smooth-muscle cells. This action helps the uterus expand to accommodate the growing foetus and slows GI motility, allowing for increased nutrient absorption.

Feeling the burn

As pregnancy progresses, the displacement of the stomach and the intestines caused by the enlarging uterus may contribute to heartburn and constipation. Some women also experience taste and odour changes and some become thirsty frequently.

Weight gain

Growth of the foetus, the placenta, maternal blood volume, maternal fat stores and tissues all contribute to weight gain during pregnancy. A women will normally be weighed at her first antenatal booking appointment in order to calculate her body mass index (BMI). She will not normally be weighed again unless there are concerns about her weight or obvious weight loss.

Fluid factors

A woman's body gains a large amount of water during pregnancy—total body water can increase by 7 to 10 L. This fluid weight gain accounts for a large percentage of weight gain at term. Up to 75% of women experience oedema. Minor oedema may be considered normal as long as the mother

Pregnancy weight gain recommendations

Here are recommendations for weight gain during pregnancy, based on body mass index (BMI).

Prepregnancy weight status	Recommended gain
Underweight (BMI less than 18.5 kg/m²)	12.7 to 18.1 kg
Normal weight (BMI 18.5 to 24.9 kg/m²)	11.3 to 15.9 kg
Overweight (BMI 25 to 29.9 kg/m²)	6.8 to 11.3 kg
Obese (BMI 30 kg/m² or more)	6.8 kg
Twin pregnancy	15.9 to 20.4 kg

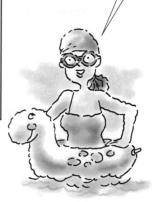

The weight a woman gains during pregnancy is primarily water—up to 7 to 10 litres!

doesn't have other complications, such as hypertension and proteinuria. In addition, blood and plasma volume increase significantly during pregnancy.

Tipping the scales towards a healthy infant

The amount of weight gained during the second and third trimesters can be a valuable indicator of foetal development. Inadequate weight gain during pregnancy increases the risk of having a low-birth-weight (LBW) infant—a baby weighing less than 2,500 g. LBW babies may be malnourished, especially if born full-term and of normal length, and have a higher incidence of postnatal complications and mortality.

Putting on pounds for pregnancy

Current weight gain recommendations are influenced by prepregnancy weight status. The higher a woman's weight is before pregnancy, the lower the amount of weight she needs to gain during pregnancy to produce a healthy-sized baby. However, young adolescents should be encouraged to achieve gains at the upper ends of the ranges to accommodate for their own growth during pregnancy. (See *Pregnancy weight gain recommendations*.)

Bad influences

It's important to remember, however, that other factors also influence birth weight; adequate maternal weight gain doesn't ensure the delivery of a healthy-birth-weight infant. These factors include:
* smoking
* alcohol intake
* maternal health status. (See *Cultural practices during pregnancy*.)

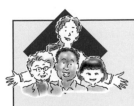

Bridging the gap

Cultural practices during pregnancy

When assessing the nutritional status of pregnant women, be sure to ask about cultural food preferences, restrictions and taboos because these practices can impact care.

- In the UK the largest ethnic minority groups, South Asians and Afro-Caribbeans, may have reduced intakes of iron or calcium containing foods. They may also have a different view about weight gain during pregnancy and are at greater risk of obesity.
- Pregnant Filipino women may avoid prunes because they believe these fruits cause a baby to be wrinkled. They may also avoid squid because it's thought to cause the umbilical cord to twist in the womb.

Nutrient needs

The requirements for many nutrients increase during pregnancy. Calorie and protein requirements increase to meet the needs of the heart's increased workload, increased energy needs for respiration, growth of maternal tissues, uterine muscles and the baby's rapid growth. Vitamins and minerals—specifically folate (folic acid), B vitamins, calcium and iron—also play critical roles in this phase of the life cycle and require specific attention.

> For the second trimester of pregnancy, we're adding 300 calories per day to your menu.

Calories

During the first trimester, energy needs are essentially the same as those in a nonpregnant woman. In the second and third trimesters, however, the increased need for energy ranges from 300 to 400 kcal/day. An additional 300 kcal/day is equal to only two extra cups of low-fat milk and one slice of bread. Because nutrient needs increase more than calorie needs, a pregnant woman's food choices need to be nutrient dense. More calories may be needed for active, large or nutritionally deficient mothers.

Protein

Recommended protein intake during pregnancy increases by only 10 to 15 g/day, to 60 g/day total. Many nonpregnant women consume more than this already and don't need to increase protein intake. Foods rich in protein include lean meat and chicken, fish (pregnant women should aim for at least two servings of fish a week, including one of oily fish), eggs and pulses (such as beans and lentils). These foods are also good sources of iron.

Carbohydrates

Pregnant women should be encouraged to consume plenty of starchy foods such as bread, pasta, rice and potatoes.

Folate

Folate also is critical during the early periconceptional period (from approximately 2 months before pregnancy to 6 weeks' gestation) to ensure healthy embryonic tissue development and prevent spina bifida and neural tube defects. The daily recommended intake of folate is 400 µg.

The *Food Standards Agency (FSA)* recommends that women of childbearing age who may become pregnant obtain adequate amounts of synthetic folic acid each day from fortified foods such as breakfast cereals or supplements in addition to eating a varied diet rich in folate.

A fortified feast

In recent years, fortification of folic acid in refined grain products, such as breads and breakfast cereals, has helped improve the folate status in women of childbearing age. Foods that contain highly usable forms of folate include oranges, orange juice and pineapple juice.

Vitamin D and calcium

Vitamin D is important for the absorption of calcium needed during pregnancy for the formation of the foetal skeleton and teeth.

All women should be informed at the booking appointment about the importance for their own and their baby's health of maintaining adequate vitamin D stores during pregnancy and whilst breastfeeding. In order to achieve this, women may choose to take 10 µg of vitamin D per day, as found in the Healthy Start multivitamin supplement. Particular care should be taken to enquire as to whether women at greatest risk are following advice to take this daily supplement. These include:
- women of South Asian, African, Caribbean or Middle Eastern family origin
- women who have limited exposure to sunlight, such as women who are predominantly housebound, or usually remain covered when outdoors
- women who eat a diet particularly low in vitamin D, such as women who consume no oily fish, eggs, meat, vitamin D-fortified margarine or breakfast cereal
- women with a prepregnancy BMI above 30 kg/m^2.

Increasing calcium one cup at a time

A diet that includes three cups of milk or calcium-fortified soy milk or two cups of calcium-fortified orange juice and one cup of milk can provide adequate calcium for the increased needs during pregnancy.

Iodine

Adequate iodine intake is essential for the production of thyroxin, the thyroid hormone responsible for controlling the increased metabolic rate that occurs during pregnancy.

Iron

Pregnant women can become deficient in iron and should be encouraged to have iron-rich foods. They should, however, avoid liver as it contains high levels of vitamin A. Consuming foods or drinks, such as orange juice, high in vitamin C can help the body to absorb iron. Tea and coffee can make it harder for the body to absorb iron so cutting down on these drinks at mealtimes can help to improve iron levels in the body.

Iron is essential to maintain the increased haemoglobin synthesis necessary for increased maternal blood volume as well as the baby's necessary prenatal iron storage.

Ironing out iron difficulties

Because iron occurs in such small amounts in food and can be difficult to be absorbed, some pregnant women may be prescribed additional iron supplements. Some of this iron is transferred to the foetus, where it's stored in the liver for use during the first 4 to 6 months of life. The remainder is used to support the mother's blood volume.

Developing a healthful diet

A daily diet that supports a healthful pregnancy can be arranged using recommendations of the *FSA* and *Eat well be well* intake patterns. For example, an easy-to-implement core food plan that meets daily pregnancy needs includes:
- milk products—such as milk, yogurt and cheese
- meat and bean group—lean meats, eggs, nuts, seeds and cooked, dry beans
- vegetables—fresh, frozen, canned or dried vegetables (consume at least five portions of fruits and vegetables)
- dark green or orange vegetables
- fruits—fresh, frozen, canned or dried fruits and fruit juices, including vitamin C-rich sources
- grains—at least half should be wholegrains
- oils—emphasise those containing omega-3 fatty acids and monounsaturated fats. But no more than one portion of oily fish each week.

Fluid challenge

It's important to drink plenty of fluids during pregnancy—10 cups per day. For many women, thirst will help meet this need without much effort.

Nutrition and breast-feeding

Nutritional needs for a woman who's breast-feeding are only slightly different from those during her pregnancy. Folate and iron needs decrease after giving birth, and energy requirements increase.

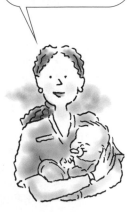

Breast-feeding requires more energy! Therefore, breast-feeding mothers can't afford to cut calories.

Fuelling milk production

While breast-feeding, a healthy woman should consume 2,300 to 2,700 kcal/day, approximately 500 kcal/day more than prepregnancy recommendations. If maternal intake is poor, which can occur when a breast-feeding woman is dieting, the nutrient content of her breast milk may become inadequate and the quantity of milk she produces may decrease.

Water hydrant

Adequate hydration encourages ample milk production, so it's important for new mothers to drink plenty of fluids—about 6 to 8 glasses each day (2 to 3 L/day). The mother should also drink one glass of fluid each time the infant nurses to ensure she's staying hydrated. Water and such beverages as fruit juices and milk are good choices to maintain adequate hydration.

Keep contaminants out!

Most substances that the mother ingests are secreted into her milk. Therefore, beverages containing alcohol and caffeine should be limited or avoided because they may be harmful to the infant. In addition, the mother should check with her health visitor or midwife before taking any medication. Some researchers believe that components of the maternal food may contribute to colic or the infant's fussiness.

Women who are pregnant or breast-feeding can reduce the risk of mercury poisoning, which can cause brain damage in the foetus and developing child, by avoiding the consumption of shark meat, swordfish and marlin. They should also limit their intake of other fish and shellfish. (See 'Nutritional concerns'.)

Nutritional concerns

During their antenatal care pregnant women should be informed of foods that may put them or their foetus at risk including:
- soft mould ripened cheeses, such as Camembert, Brie and blue-veined cheese
- pate (including vegetable pate)
- liver and liver products
- uncooked or undercooked ready-prepared meals
- uncooked or cured meat, such as salami
- raw shellfish, such as oysters
- fish containing relatively high levels of methylmercury, such as shark, swordfish and marlin, which might affect the nervous system of the foetus.

The *FSA* has also recently announced that pregnant women should limit their consumption of:
- tuna to no more than two medium size cans or one fresh tuna steak per week
- caffeine to 300 mg/day. Caffeine is present in coffee, tea and colas.

Other important nutrition-related considerations during pregnancy include use of artificial sweeteners, alcohol, caffeine and supplements; smoking and food-borne illnesses.

Artificial sweeteners

Currently, there's no evidence that consumption of artificial sweeteners, such as aspartame (NutraSweet) or sucralose (Splenda), is harmful during pregnancy. Regardless, many artificially sweetened beverages and foods are low-nutrient foods that serve as poor substitutes for more nutrient-rich foods in the diet.

Alcohol

Prenatal exposure to alcohol is the leading preventable cause of birth defects, mental retardation and developmental disorders. Alcohol can easily cross the maternal—foetal barrier and the growing foetus hasn't yet developed enzymes to break alcohol down, so it lingers in the foetus's circulation. Be sure to tell your pregnant patient to exclude alcohol-containing beverages from her diet.

Caffeine

Caffeine has long been suspected of causing negative effects in pregnant women. For example, some research suggests that high caffeine consumption during pregnancy can lead to miscarriage. It's also responsible for increasing heart rate, stimulating the central nervous system and acting as a diuretic.

Some evidence suggests that high caffeine intake may also affect the developing foetus. Caffeine passes through the placenta into foetal circulation, which stimulates foetal activity, leading to increased heart rate and blood pressure.

Coffee break

Because of the high amount of caffeine in coffee, general recommendations limit intake to about two cups per day during pregnancy, or no more than 300 mg of caffeine per day.

Smoking

Smoking has negative effects on an unborn child. Babies born to women who smoke during pregnancy commonly have low birth weights.

Supplements

Vitamin and mineral supplements may be recommended for an individual when a nutritional assessment indicates that she's deficient in a particular nutrient. (See *Supplements and pregnancy*, page 132.)

Herbal helpers?

Herbal supplement use is increasingly more common during pregnancy. In the early stages of pregnancy some women may use ginger to alleviate

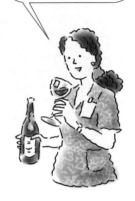

Don't toast too soon! A foetus hasn't developed the enzymes to break down alcohol. That's why it's important for mothers to avoid alcohol during pregnancy.

Supplements and pregnancy

Supplements are generally not recommended for pregnant women.

It's recommended that certain groups of women at high risk for poor dietary intake should be nutritionally assessed and the dietitian or relevant health care professional may suggest supplementation. These groups include women who:

- have poor-quality, unchangeable diets
- are pregnant with more than one baby
- smoke cigarettes
- have iron-deficiency anaemia
- abuse alcohol or use drugs.

Pregnant women should be informed that vitamin A supplementation (intake greater than 700 µg) might be teratogenic and should therefore be avoided. Pregnant women should be informed that, as liver and liver products may also contain high levels of vitamin A, consumption of these products should also be avoided.

---

nausea. However, there's little well-supported research about the safety and effectiveness of this practice and some may be detrimental to mother and baby so should be used with caution and appropriate advice from the midwife.

Food-borne illnesses

Food-borne illnesses, such as listeriosis and *Escherichia coli* infection, can be life threatening during pregnancy. Pregnant women are more susceptible to food-borne infections because of increased hormone or progesterone levels. To prevent food-borne illnesses, pregnant women should avoid raw fish, oysters and soft cheeses such as Brie, raw or undercooked meat and unpasteurised milk.

Nutrition during infancy

As humans grow, energy and nutrient requirements change to meet the body's changing needs. Tissue rebuilding and metabolic functioning go on throughout life. However, growth and activity are most rapid during infancy and childhood, resulting in increased nutritional requirements during these stages.

Growth and development

During infancy, energy, protein, vitamin and mineral requirements per kilogram of body weight are higher than at any other time during the lifespan. These high requirements are necessary to support rapid growth and development during this stage of life. An infant's birth weight doubles in the first 4 to 6 months of life and triples within the first year.

Assessing growth

The primary tool for assessing adequacy of nutrition is growth. Health care professionals chart an infant's growth (weight and length) each visit on a standardised graph, the UK-WHO growth charts, developed by the Department of Health and the Royal College of Paediatrics and Child Health. As long as the height-to-weight ratio is consistent and the infant's growth follows the curve, nutrition is most likely adequate. In addition, the infant is checked for the development of musculoskeletal milestones at an appropriate age.

Physiologic changes

During this time, important physiologic changes can be seen throughout the body, including several major body systems.

GI system

Because an infant's stomach capacity is small—approximately 90 ml at birth—and gastric emptying time is 2.5 to 3 hours, small, frequent feedings are important to meet the infant's energy needs. Digestive enzymes are produced only in small quantities at birth, which is why breast milk and formula are initially the only dietary nutrients babies consume.

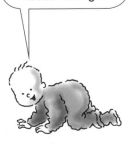

I need small, frequent meals to meet my energy needs. Off I go!

Adding to the menu

By age 3 months, secretion of digestive enzymes begins in quantities sufficient to digest some of the starches found in cereal. However, cereals and other solid foods shouldn't be added to an infant's diet until age 6 months, when lipase and bile (enzymes that help to digest fat) are produced. A full range of foods from each of the food groups should be introduced to the diet once the infant has mastered the use of spoon. If there is a family history of allergy, foods may be introduced one at a time in order to gauge infant preferences and observe for food allergies and intolerances.

Renal system

The ability of the kidneys to concentrate urine develops rapidly during the first 6 weeks. Before that, however, the infant is highly susceptible to dehydration, especially if he's being fed formula that's overly concentrated.

Neuromuscular system

An important factor in obtaining enough nutrients for small infants is their ability to ingest them. At birth, the infant relies on the sucking reflex and only gradually develops muscle control of the tongue, jaw, head and neck. Eventually, developing fine motor control allows the infant to chew and drink and to grasp food so that he can feed himself. By age 9 months, the infant can bring the thumb and first finger together to grasp objects, such as small pieces of food, a cup or a spoon.

Nutrient needs

Infants need calories to grow. Encouraging infants to eat a balanced diet using foods from all the food groups is important.

Fat free? No need!

There's no specific recommended amount of fat for infants and restriction isn't recommended. For infants up to age 2, at least 40% of calories consumed should be from fat. Protein and fat requirements are met by human milk or formula.

Fluid figures

Once eating solid foods infants need about 500 ml of fluid daily. Infants typically consume enough breast milk or formula to supply this amount. However, during periods of illness—for example, diarrhoea, vomiting or fever—or exposure to sun, additional fluids may be needed.

ABCs of supplementation

Formula and breast milk provide most of the necessary vitamins and minerals needed by the growing infant. However, supplementation is recommended for certain nutrients:
• Vitamin K is routinely given by injection to all infants at birth to supply the vitamin until the infant's intestinal tract can synthesise it on its own.
• Children between the age of 6 months and 5 years may need vitamins A, C and D. Supplements may not be needed if the child is a good eater and has a varied diet. Advice can be sought from the health visitor or General Practitioner (GP).
• Because the body's iron stores are generally depleted by age 6 months, it's recommended that infants are encouraged to eat a varied diet containing iron-rich foods like meat and green leafy vegetables. Solid foods such as iron-fortified cereals may be used to help meet these iron needs. Infants who consume a vegan or vegetarian diet may be advised to have additional iron supplements. The health visitor or GP will advise on this.

Nutrient intake

Human milk consumed through breast-feeding is considered optimal for infants. Even so, not all mothers can or choose to breastfeed. Medical conditions, cultural background, anxiety, drug abuse and various other factors can prevent a woman from breast-feeding. Rarely, some infants can't take in enough breast milk through breast-feeding to meet nutritional needs. Although breast milk is usually the best food for premature infants, some breast milk may be insufficient in calcium, protein and essential vitamins. In these cases, bottle-feeding with infant formula is an acceptable alternative or may be used to supplement breast-feeding. (See *Tips for preparing formula*.)

Breast-feeding

Breast-feeding is widely supported in the medical community. The *FSA* and the Department of Health recommend breast-feeding exclusively for the first 4 to 6 months and then in combination with infant foods until age 1. (See *Advantages of breast-feeding*.)

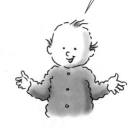

Talk about baby fat! Up to age 2, I'm supposed to consume at least 40% of my daily calories from fat.

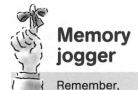

Memory jogger

Remember, **K**ids need their **ACD**:

Vitamin **K**

Vitamin **A**

Vitamin **C**

Vitamin **D**

NutriTips

Tips for preparing formula

Here are a few tips for properly preparing infant formula:

- Wash your hands before preparing formula.
- Boil water for 1 to 2 minutes, and then let it cool.
- Wash utensils in warm, soapy water and rinse them well to ensure that they're safe to use. Also, keep separate utensils for preparation.
- Avoid using microwave ovens because they fail to sanitise utensils and cause uneven heating, which increases the risk of burns.
- Always follow the manufacturer's guidelines when preparing a formula feed.
- Always add the powder to the water when mixing a feed.
- Discard a prepared bottle of formula after it has been offered to the infant or has sat at room temperature for more than 1 hour.

Advantages of breast-feeding

It's a well-known fact that breast-feeding is best for an infant. Here are five reasons why.

1. Passive immunity
Human milk provides passive immunity to the infant. Colostrum is the first fluid secreted from the breast (occurs almost immediately) and provides immune factor and protein to the neonate. Many components of breast milk protect against infection—it contains antibodies (especially immunoglobulin A) and white blood cells that protect the infant from some forms of infection. Breast-fed babies also experience fewer allergies and intolerances.

2. Easily digestible
Breast milk provides essential nutrients in an easily digestible form for the neonate. It contains lipase, which breaks down dietary fat, making it easily available to the infant's system.

3. Brain booster
The lipids in breast milk are high in linoleic acid and cholesterol, which are needed for brain development. Breast milk also contains docosahexaenoic acid (an omega-3 fatty acid that's important for brain and eye development).

4. Low protein content
Cow's milk contains proportionally higher concentrations of electrolytes and protein than are needed by human infants. It must be cleared by the immature kidneys and thus isn't recommended until after a baby is at least 12 months old.

5. Convenience and price
Breast-feeding saves the time and money that must be spent to buy and prepare formula.

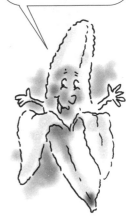

Pleased to meetcha! It's okay to introduce solid finger foods such as bananas to infants aged between 7 and 9 months.

Formula feeding

Formula feedings can provide adequate nutrition in cases where the mother shouldn't or can't breastfeed her infant. Infant formulas are constituted to provide the proper variety and amount of carbohydrates, protein, fats and micronutrients needed for healthy growth and development. UK legislation regulates the composition, labelling and inspection of infant formula to ensure infant safety.

Women are strongly urged to use commercially prepared formulas rather than homemade formulas made with cow's milk because cow's milk:
- doesn't meet all of an infant's nutritional needs
- can be difficult to digest
- can strain the infant's renal system.

Unlocking the secret formula

Most formulas are based on cow's milk, although preparations based on casein hydrosylate are available for infants who can't tolerate cow's milk-based preparations. There are also special formulas for infants with diseases, such as phenylketonuria and other metabolic diseases. Formula comes in powder form, concentrated liquid and ready-to-feed forms. Ready-to-feed formulas are convenient and prevent problems based on incorrect dilution and preparation but are more expensive. Special care should be used so that formula isn't improperly mixed and stored, which can be hazardous to the infant.

Introducing solid foods

Introducing solid foods to an infant's diet depends on such factors as nutritional need for iron, physiologic capability to digest starch and physical ability to chew and swallow. Breast milk or iron-fortified formula satisfies all of an infant's nutritional requirements until age 6 months. Signs that an infant is ready to try solid foods and eat from a spoon include the ability to sit with some support and move the head to participate in the feeding process as well as reaching and grabbing for food. (See *Solid foods and infant age*.)

Teaching points

Be sure to stress these points about feeding and nutrition to the parents of an infant:
- Be observant for behaviours that indicate feeding preferences. Turning the head away, biting and chewing followed by swallowing all indicate preferences and satiety. If the infant rejects a food initially, don't force him to eat it. Offer the food again later. It can take up to 15 tastes to get an infant to accept a solid food.
- Keep the baby in the upright feeding position.
- Let the baby decide how much to eat. Don't try to make him eat more to finish the serving or portion.
- Initially, offer iron-fortified rice cereal. Avoid wheat-based cereals until age 6 months because of the increased risk of allergic reaction.
- If there is a strong family history of food allergy introduce new foods one at a time, waiting 5 to 7 days between foods, to assess for allergy or intolerance.

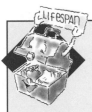

Lifespan lunchbox

Solid foods and infant age

This table gives an overview of solid foods that are appropriate for a developing infant.

Age	Type of food	Rationale
6 months	Rice cereal mixed with formula or breast milk; mashed vegetables and fruits	Less likely than wheat to cause an allergic reaction (offer vegetables first because they may be more readily accepted)
7 to 9 months	Finger foods (bananas, crackers); pureed and mashed foods	Promote self-feeding
10 to 12 months	Minced meats, cheese, yogurt, pudding; mashed egg; bite-size cooked food	Provide important source of iron, add variety to the diet and decrease the risk of choking (although the infant chews well, be careful to avoid foods likely to cause choking)
12+ months	Foods from the adult table Cow's milk can be offered as a drink	Add variety to the diet (chop or mash according to the infant's ability to chew foods)

- Offer mashed fruit (bananas, pears) or vegetables (parsnip, potato, yam)
- Avoid honey. These products may contain the harmful bacteria *Clostridium botulinum*, which can lead to botulism. Botulism can be fatal in children younger than age 1 year.
- Do not add salt or sugar to the food.

Nutritional concerns

Some nutritional concerns for the infant include iron deficiency anaemia, dental health, diarrhoea, constipation and food allergies. Some infants may suffer from colic and this can be distressing for the mother and infant.

Iron deficiency anaemia

When older infants consume few solid foods rich in iron, they're at risk for developing iron deficiency anaemia. By age 6 months, the iron stores in the liver are depleted and the infant must rely on ingestion and absorption to provide the iron necessary for tissue building.

Initially, iron-fortified cereals are recommended. Later, red-meat products can be consumed as tolerated (usually pureed) to meet iron requirements. Iron supplements are available for infants who are diagnosed with iron deficiency anaemia.

Dental health

Fluoride and dental caries are two potential nutrition-related problems that can compromise dental health. Fluoride is incorporated into forming teeth, including those in early stages of development. Most infants who live in areas where fluoridated water is available don't require an additional source of fluoride.

The bottle can let a baby down

Dental caries are a potential problem if an infant is put to bed with a bottle. An infant can fall asleep with formula in its mouth, which leads to the development of caries. Fruit juices can also contribute to dental caries.

Colic

Repeated crying episodes that don't respond to feeding, holding or nappy changes are characteristic of infants with colic. The infant is generally unhappy and fussy and cries a lot. About 10% to 20% of infants suffer from colic, which is thought to be due to swallowing air (for bottle-fed babies, when nipple holes are too large or too small) or to a reaction to gas-producing foods. (See *Tips for reducing colic*.)

Diarrhoea

Noninfectious diarrhoea, which may result from overfeeding and food intolerances, can put an infant at risk for dehydration.

Because an infant's body is 75% water, fluid loss due to diarrhoea can quickly cause dehydration. A careful diet history commonly uncovers the cause of diarrhoea.

Although it isn't uncommon, diarrhoea can be dangerous and parents should notify the infant's health care provider if diarrhoea persists beyond 12 hours or if it's accompanied by fever or vomiting.

Battling dehydration

If an infant develops diarrhoea, rehydration drinks which are special electrolyte-replacement formulas, may be recommended to help with rehydration in the

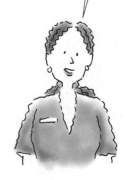

Diarrhoea puts infants at high risk for dehydration.

NutriTips

Tips for reducing colic

Colic usually resolves by about age 3 months and isn't associated with later dysfunction or disease. Here are several ways to reduce the discomfort caused by colic:

- Change the diet for mothers who are breastfeeding. Avoid onions, cow's milk, chocolate, broccoli, cauliflower and brussels sprouts.
- Change the routine. Try different positions during feeding. Also try using warm water, holding, rocking and using a pacifier.

short term. Babies who are breast-fed should continue to feed from the breast. Formula is commonly withheld temporarily. The infant should receive 150 ml/kg of the electrolyte solution. After about 12 hours, if diarrhoea has stopped, formula can be offered with additional feeds or rehydrate solutions.

Constipation

Constipation is rare in breast-fed infants. However, it's occasionally a problem for formula-fed infants. In many cases, it's a result of inadequate carbohydrate intake or consumption of overly concentrated formula. The parents should be instructed to follow the manufacturer's guidelines in mixing the formula and, for older infants, add fibre to the diet by feeding fresh fruits and vegetables as indicated.

Food allergies

Foods that commonly pose allergy risks include milk, eggs and wheat. If there is a strong family history of food allergies it's important to introduce solid foods to the diet slowly to assess for allergy or intolerance. If a reaction occurs after the introduction of a food, the response should be noted for further evaluation. If a similar reaction occurs the second time the food is consumed, the food should be eliminated from the diet. It's important to discuss suspected allergies with health visitor or GP.

Nutritional considerations for premature infants

Babies who are born prematurely (gestational age less than 37 weeks) require special nutritional care. Each premature infant has different needs, depending on its weight and length of gestation. Breast milk is especially beneficial in easing digestion for premature infants.

Other nutritional concerns in premature infants include:
- increased caloric and nutrient requirements
- lack of enzymes that enable digestion and absorption
- neuromuscular immaturity
- small gastric capacity
- risk of dehydration due to immature kidney function and proportionally high body-surface area
- risk of hypoglycaemia due to immature liver function, hypothermia or respiratory distress syndrome
- vitamin E deficiency due to inability to digest and absorb fats.

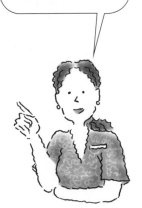

Breast milk can help ease digestion in premature infants.

Tired out

Many premature infants also have a hard time feeding long enough and efficiently enough to take in adequate amounts of breast milk. For this reason, breast milk can be expressed, saved and fed to the infant through a nasogastric tube or bottle.

Rapid response

Breast milk may be supplemented with such nutrients as calcium, phosphorus, sodium and protein, which are necessary to supplement a premature infant's rapid growth.

Nutrition during childhood

As children grow, energy and nutrient needs continue to change to meet the body's changing needs.

Growth and development during childhood

Childhood growth and development can be divided into three stages:
- toddler (aged 1 to 3 years)
- preschool age (aged 3 to 5 years)
- school age (aged 5 to 10 years).

Obtaining adequate energy and nutrient requirements during each of these stages is essential to achieving full growth and development potential.

Sprouting up

Growth during childhood is steady but not as great as during infancy or adolescence. Toddlers gain about 0.2 kg and grow 1 cm in height per month, whereas preschool children gain approximately 1.8 kg to 2.3 kg and grow approximately 5.1 cm in height per year (or about 0.4 cm per month). By the time a child reaches school age, his/her weight should be about double what it was at age 1. This decreased growth rate is commonly associated with a reduced appetite and food intake in toddlers and preschool children.

Eating behaviours

Eating behaviours vary with each stage of childhood development.

Toddler

During the toddler years, exploration and a sense of individuality begin to develop. The toddler may demonstrate a change in appetite and may be easily distracted from eating. Because of these changes, it's best to offer a toddler various foods and smaller portions. In addition, a toddler shouldn't be forced to eat foods. It's also a good idea to keep nutritious foods, such as fruits, available to serve as snacks.

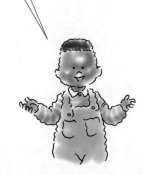

Sometimes I can be easily distracted from eating. Mom says I'm showing my individuality.

Preschool age

During the preschool-age period, parents and caregivers still have a fair amount of control over a child's food intake. Nutritional concerns focus on offering a proper selection and amount of nutrients needed by the growing child.

A preschool-age child responds best to regular mealtimes. Three meals per day aren't enough for this age group, and snacks are recommended as part of a regular eating pattern. Research indicates that snacks typically provide 20% of a child's total caloric intake and, therefore, can be a good way to provide protein, calories and nutrients to a young child. At this age, it's good to begin involving a child in meal-related activities, such as food selection and preparation.

School age

The school-age child is more independent of adults. Meeting the nutritional needs of this age group must be balanced with the child's need for decision-making and peer acceptance. A school-age child spends much of the day at school, away from parents and, in many cases, only marginally supervised at lunchtime. In addition, peers' behaviours are an increasing influence, as is exposure to different types of food and eating behaviours. A child at this age begins to make independent choices about what to eat. (See *Tips for ensuring childhood health*.)

NutriTips

Tips for ensuring childhood health

To help ensure that children take in a balanced diet and maintain a healthy lifestyle, recommend these tips to parents and caregivers:

- Schedule regular mealtimes and allow the child to participate in planning, preparation and serving as well as clean up.
- Maintain variety because it's normal for a child to prefer certain foods for a while and then suddenly refuse to eat them.
- Have nutritional snacks readily available, especially when the child gets home from school. Carrot and celery sticks and yogurt are good possibilities.
- Do not prepare special foods but encourage the child to eat family meals.
- Have the child get up early enough to be able to eat breakfast unhurriedly. Breakfast is an important meal.
- Encourage physical activity. Sports are increasingly an important and beneficial part of a young child's life. Also, keep in mind that physical activity other than sports is valuable as well and should be encouraged. Walks, bike rides and other forms of loosely organised activities can be beneficial.
- Eat with a child to model good eating habits.
- Avoid using food as a reward or bribe.
- Turn off the television during meals and avoid other distractions.

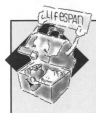

Lifespan lunchbox

Energy and protein requirements for infants, children and adolescents

This table lists the recommended dietary allowances for energy and protein needs of infants and children.

Age	Estimated energy requirement (kcal/day)*
First 6 months	515 to 645
7 to 12 months	765 to 865
1 to 3 years	Boys 1,230 Girls 1,165
4 to 6 years	Boys 1,715 Girls 1,545
7 to 10 years	Boys 1,970 Girls 1,740
11 to 14 years	1,790 to 3.308

*Actual energy requirement depends on activity level and gender.
Estimated protein requirements for infants and children

   0–12 months (12.5–14.9 g/day)
   1–3 years (14.5 g/day)
   4–10 years (19.7–28.3 g/day)

Actual protein requirements are weight dependent.

Nutrient needs

Preschool children need approximately 1,000 to 1,600 kcal/day. School-age children need between 1,200 and 2,200 kcal/day, depending on specific age, sex and activity level (sedentary, moderately active or active). Protein requirements vary by age group. (See *Energy and protein requirements for infants, children and adolescents*.)

Supplemental information

Research confirms that most normal, healthy children in the UK don't require supplementation of vitamins and minerals in their diet.

Nutritional concerns

Some things to consider when planning nutritional care for a child include caffeine consumption, irregular eating habits, overeating and obesity and lead poisoning.

Caffeine

Children may ingest caffeine in such products as chocolate, and soft drinks. The *FSA* recommends that coffee and tea are not suitable drinks for infants and children.

The facts about caffeine

Some people believe that because caffeine is a stimulant, its consumption leads to hyperactivity. However, research has disproven this assumption. Even so, although most children don't require caffeine restriction, parents should be aware of how much caffeine a child ingests daily.

Irregular eating habits

Be aware of patterns of irregular eating, such as food fads, skipped meals and overeating, when preparing nutritional care for a child. Some irregular eating habits are a major concern for this age group.

Bag the fad?

Children commonly go on food fads where they eat one particular food in preference to most others. As long as they're getting adequate amounts of nutrients, food fads aren't problematic and parents should be reassured that they are unlikely to cause their child any harm.

Physiologic anorexia may be logical

At times, some children will display a lack of interest in food, especially as growth rate fluctuates. This 'physiologic anorexia' isn't a cause for concern, as long as intake doesn't drop off too sharply and the child is behaving normally otherwise.

Don't let 'em skip out on you

Skipping meals, especially breakfast, is common in older children. The maintenance of a regular pattern for meals and snacks (within reason) is very important to help children eat regularly. Getting children up early enough before school so that they wake up fully and become hungry will help in getting them to eat breakfast.

Overeating and obesity

Overweight and obesity are growing problems in children from industrialised cultures. Obesity is defined as being 20% or more above the mean weight for children of the same height and age. The cause of the increase in childhood obesity rates is thought to be sedentary lifestyle and consumption of high-fat, starchy food in greater proportion than proteins and complex carbohydrates.

According to the *Office National Statistics (ONS)*, the incidence of weight problems among children and adolescents is significantly increasing, with as much as 20% of boys and 26% of girls aged 2 to 19 years being overweight.

Sticks and stones break bones but names hurt, too

Although the major health concern is in overweight children going on to become overweight adults with ill-health effects, obese children also undergo psychosocial stress. They're the target of teasing and disapproval, due to conceptions among adults that obesity is related to weakness and laziness, and the fact that these perceptions are passed on to children.

Not merely baby fat

The severity of childhood obesity is affected by the age of onset and the presence of factors such as parental obesity. If obesity develops after age 3, the likelihood of lasting into adulthood is greater; the same is true if the obesity is severe or if one or more parents is obese. Studies show that obese children's intake isn't significantly higher than that of nonobese children. Experts currently believe that lack of physical activity is the reason for the weight gain.

Setting a schedule for success

Prevention and treatment are based on establishing regular meal and snack times, having nutritious snacks readily available and encouraging (especially through role modelling) regular physical activity. The *FSA* recommends that children shouldn't be placed on weight reduction diets without first consulting with a professional.

According to the *FSA*, the goal for overweight children and adolescents is to reduce the rate of weight gain while allowing for normal growth and development. The guidelines recommend that children and adolescents consume foods with less calories and increase physical activity to control their weight. They should participate in at least 60 minutes of physical activity on most, if not every day of the week. Children and adolescents should consume a balanced diet that contains some fat but should avoid saturated fat, which is found in butter, hard-fat spreads, cheese, fatty meat and meat products, biscuits, pastry and cakes. The majority of fats should come from polyunsaturated and monounsaturated fats.

Lead poisoning

Children under age 6 are susceptible to lead toxicity because they have a higher rate of intestinal absorption, their neurologic tissues are still developing and they tend to put things in their mouths, increasing the risk of exposure. Lead poisoning can cause stunting of growth as well as cognitive deficits and other neurologic problems. Lead toxicity occurs more readily (and is, therefore, more common) in children with iron deficiency.

Nutrition during adolescence

Nutritional requirements during adolescence are more individualised than during other periods of life. They depend on the timing and duration of the growth spurt, which can vary from person to person and is different for males and females.

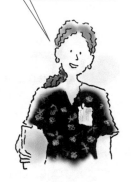

The risk of growing into an obese adult increases if a child's obesity develops after age 3.

Protein needs vary with the degree of growth and development, and requirements based on developmental age are more accurate than those based on chronological age.

Growth and development during adolescence

During adolescence, increases in lean body mass, skeletal mass and body fat that occur during puberty influence energy and nutrient needs. The growth rate is different for boys and girls and each growth rate is individualised.

Girls get a head start...

In girls, the growth spurt usually begins between ages 10 and 11, peaks at age 12 and ceases at age 15. Girls have lower caloric needs during this time because of more fat deposition (particularly to the abdomen and pelvic girdle).

...But boys bone up

In boys, the growth spurt usually begins between ages 12 and 13, peaks at age 14 and stops at age 19. Because boys experience an increase in muscle mass, bone and lean body tissue, they have higher caloric needs during this stage.

Nutrient needs

Sedentary adolescent boys require 1,800 to 2,400 kcal/day, whereas those who are moderately active require 2,000 to 2,800 kcal/day. Adolescent girls who are sedentary require 1,600 to 1,800 kcal/day, while those who are moderately active require 2,000 kcal/day. Adolescent boys who participate in sports may need up to 3,200 kcal/day while athletic adolescent girls may need up to 2,400 kcal/day. Active adolescents may need additional niacin, thiamine and riboflavin. Three servings of dairy products per day are recommended to help adolescents meet their calcium requirements of 1,300 mg/day.

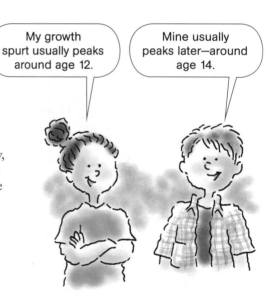

My growth spurt usually peaks around age 12.

Mine usually peaks later—around age 14.

Zinc again!

Zinc is important during adolescence for its role in sexual maturation. Males who are deficient in zinc experience growth failure and delayed sexual development. Generally, boys and girls consume adequate amounts of iron and zinc in their diets unless they follow strict vegetarian diets.

Focus on folate

Because of folate's role in deoxyribonucleic acid, ribonucleic acid and protein synthesis, poor folate status can be an issue for adolescent females who become pregnant. Inadequate intake of folate before pregnancy can increase the incidence of spina bifida and neural tube defects. Studies show that many adolescents have inadequate folate levels. However, this number may be reduced by the fortification mandates requiring that grains and cereals be enriched with folate.

More to watch for

According to the *FSA*, dietary intakes of calcium and iron may be of concern for children and adolescents. Adolescents who do not consume dairy products, cut out foods such as red meat or green leafy vegetables or rely on highly processed foods are at more risk of becoming deficient in these nutrients.

Developing a healthful diet

Many adolescents in the UK eat low-nutrient, high-calorie, high-sugar, high-fat foods. Usually, these diets fall short of meeting the requirements recommended by the *FSA*. Many adolescents, especially adolescent girls, also don't consume adequate amounts of vitamins and minerals.

Snack attack

Usually, adolescents get one-fourth to one-third of all their energy and major nutrients from snacks. In addition, soft drinks are a favourite beverage among adolescents. These drinks contain large amounts of calories in the form of sugar, which is filling and may interfere with intake of more nutritious foods. Soft drinks also commonly replace milk as the drink of choice and may hinder an adolescent from getting adequate amounts of calcium.

Although snacking seems like a nutritional problem, it can become a healthy part of the adolescent diet. Snacking habits can be slightly altered to allow the adolescent independence in choices and to help establish a healthful lifelong eating pattern. These habits can be achieved by using Eatwell recommendations to plan snacks. One good tip for improving snacking behaviour is to have nutritious foods already prepared and available. Good examples include fortified cereals, fresh fruit, cut up vegetables and high-fibre, multigrain snack bars.

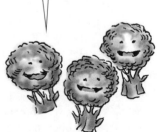

We're a cut above the rest! If you keep us around in pre-cut pieces, we make a pretty good snack!

Nutritional concerns

Some common nutritional concerns for adolescents include dieting and eating disorders, calcium deficiency, tobacco and alcohol use, hormonal contraceptive use and special diets.

Dieting and eating disorders

Because of preoccupations with appearance and peer acceptance, adolescents are notorious for fad dieting. Meals are skipped, food intake is severely restricted or whole food groups may be cut out of the diet. Dieting behaviours should be monitored because they may lead to more serious eating disorders. Dieting behaviours should be of particular concern in an adolescent who isn't overweight.

Adolescent preoccupations with eating can range from mild body shape dissatisfaction to serious eating disorders, such as anorexia nervosa and bulimia nervosa. Symptoms of eating disorders should be further investigated because inadequate nutritional intake can adversely affect growth, development and health outcomes. Keep in mind that you should be supportive and understanding of an adolescent's feelings while promoting adequate nutritional intake.

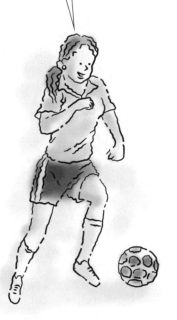

Getting enough calcium during my teen years can help me avoid osteoporosis later in life.

Calcium deficiency

Inadequate calcium intake is a common concern, especially for teenage girls, because lack of calcium during this critical time can greatly affect the development of osteoporosis later in life. It's common for teens to stop drinking milk, so suggest yogurt, cheese and calcium-fortified soya milk or orange juice to help an adolescent continue to meet their calcium requirements.

Tobacco and alcohol use

The use of tobacco, alcohol and other drugs can also impact an adolescent's nutritional health. It's important to discuss these issues with adolescents, making them aware of the adverse affects associated with these substances.

Tobacco troubles

Tobacco, which may be consumed by an adolescent who's trying to lose weight, has been associated with a range of health problems, most of which don't manifest during adolescence.

Drinking away needed nutrients

Alcohol consumption can interfere not only with the ingestion of required nutrients but also with their digestion and absorption.

Hormonal contraceptive use

It's common for adolescent girls to begin taking hormonal contraceptives—some as a form of birth control and some to decrease or regulate bleeding associated with menstruation. Hormonal contraceptives may also help with iron deficiency problems. Use of progestin-based contraceptives may be a concern for weight-conscious teens because these forms have been reported to increase appetite.

Special diets

Some adolescents, such as athletes and vegetarians, choose to follow special diets that can affect their nutritional requirements.

Athletes

An athlete's dietary intake should follow the *FSA* guidelines for healthy eating, although the athlete's increased energy needs may require him to consume the upper limit of the recommendations. Depending on the duration and intensity of his/her sport, an athlete may require 500 to 1,500 extra calories per day to meet his/her energy needs. If an athlete loses much weight, caloric intake is most likely inadequate to support growth and development and should be increased. Protein should supply 15% to 20% of total calories.

Keep an eye on iron

Iron loss during exercise puts an athlete at higher risk for developing iron deficiency anaemia. Iron status should be monitored in athletes, especially vegetarians and females who have begun menstruating.

Vegetarians

Lacto-ovo vegetarians generally aren't at great risk for inadequate intake of protein, calcium, phosphorus, zinc and other nutrients obtained from meat. However, strict vegetarians or vegans are at a risk for deficiencies if their diets aren't well planned.

Nutrition and the adult

Because growth and maturation are complete by early adulthood—approximately age 19—nutritional considerations for the adult focus more on maintaining a healthy body weight and physical fitness, avoiding excess weight gain and continuing to build strength. General calorie requirements for adults are established by the recommended dietary allowances and depend on activity levels.

According to the *Committee on Medical Aspects of Food Policy (COMA) 1991*, for adults aged 19 to 49 years, a sedentary man requires 2,500 kcal/day; a moderately active man, 2,400 to 2,800 kcal/day and an active man, 2,800 to 3,000 kcal/day. A sedentary woman in this age range requires 1,800 to 1,940 kcal/day; a moderately active woman, 2,000 to 2,200 kcal/day and an active woman, 2,200 to 2,400 kcal/day.

Fighting illnesses before they begin

Between ages 40 and 60, such chronic illnesses as heart disease, hypertension and diabetes commonly begin to develop. Establishing

Memory jogger

The *Food Standards Agency's* **ABCs** of good nutrition can help adults establish healthful eating and exercise habits. They encourage people in the UK to:

Aim for exercise every day

Build a health base (using the Eatwell recommendations)

Choose sensibly.

healthful food and exercise habits, such as reducing total fat intake, eating fruits and vegetables and maintaining a balance of food intake and physical activity to stabilise weight, can modify risk factors for developing chronic illness in later years.

Nutrition and the older adult

Life expectancy in the UK has increased dramatically over the last century. In the early 1900s, fewer than one-half of all people in the UK lived past age 65. Today, more than 55% women and 45% men in Britain are expected to do so.

Pills and ills

Older adults have special nutritional needs because their tissues and organ systems are ageing. In addition, many older adults take medications for chronic illness. More than one-third of adults over age 65 reported that they suffer from long standing or chronic illness (ONS, 2008). Nutritional health can help older adults maintain active and pleasurable lives, protect them from disease, lessen the severity of disease and hasten recovery.

Development and change

Older adults experience an array of changes that can affect their nutritional health. Some changes are directly related to the body whereas others are associated with external influences.

Physiologic changes

Even after a person reaches adulthood at age 20, the body continues to change. These changes may include gradual loss of lean body mass and gain of adipose tissue. Some changes can be offset, however, through strength training and aerobic exercise.

GI system changes

Several GI problems that affect nutritional status can arise for older adults:
• Loss of dentition, periodontal disease and jawbone deterioration can cause problems with chewing.
• Saliva production is decreased, commonly as an adverse effect of medications, and may cause difficulty swallowing.
• Secretion of gastric digestive enzymes falls off, making it more difficult to digest certain foods. Poor lactase secretion, for example, makes it difficult to digest milk products.
• Absorption of nutrients decreases as blood supply to the intestine decreases and gastric mucosa degenerates.
• Intestinal motility slows, and constipation can become a problem.

Metabolic changes

As adipose tissue replaces lean body mass, the metabolic rate slows. Glucose metabolism can be problematic in older adults, manifesting as glucose intolerance.

Central nervous system (CNS) changes

Common CNS problems that can prevent an older adult from eating a balanced diet include tremors, slowed reaction time, short-term memory loss, cognitive deterioration (from such diseases as Alzheimer's disease) and depression.

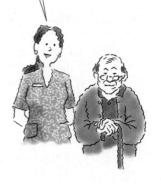

A multitude of physiologic changes can affect the nutritional intake of older adults.

Renal system changes

As blood flow decreases and new renal tissue fails to generate, the ability to clear nitrogenous and other waste products from the body is impaired. In addition, loss of sphincter tone can contribute to urinary incontinence in many older adults. Males may also experience prostate dysfunction.

Sensory changes

All sense organs lose some function as people age, and some people are more severely affected than others:
- Hearing loss begins to develop at about age 30.
- Loss of visual acuity, especially in low-light settings, begins at approximately age 40.
- Sense of smell or olfactory function decreases.
- Taste changes due to olfactory function loss, visual acuity loss and loss of taste buds and saliva. Sweet and salty tastes are the first to be lost, followed by bitter and sour.
- The sense of thirst is less acute, leaving older adults at risk for dehydration. Dehydration can manifest in older adults as confusion or lethargy.

Economic and social changes

The focus on physiologic function during nutritional assessment may lead to other factors—such as economic and social changes—being overlooked.

Spare changes

Many older adults live on fixed incomes, and approximately 20% of adults older than age 65 live in poverty. Economic hardships can limit a person's ability to eat a well-balanced diet. In many cases, meat and dairy products are cut out of the diet because of their cost. However, these foods are important to the health of older adults because they provide protein and various other nutrients, such as iron, B vitamins and zinc.

Isolating the problem

Some older adults experience social isolation due to lack of mobility, loss of sensory acuity and other functional limitations. In addition, coping with the loss of friends and lack of interest in eating can also add to isolation, leading to poor eating habits and severely affecting nutritional intake. This situation is compounded in elderly patients in nursing homes or residential care, who experience inadequate diets due to quality of food, food preferences, illnesses and taste alterations.

Nutrient needs

The *FSA guidelines* include recommendations for the older adult. Calorie requirements diminish and nutrient requirements may stay the same or increase with age.

Calories

Calorie needs diminish as the human body ages and lean muscle mass decreases. Exact calorie requirements in an older adult depend on degree of mobility, illness, overall health and level of fitness.

According to COMA, for adults 51 years of age and older, a sedentary man requires 2,000 to 2,200 kcal/day, a moderately active man requires 2,200 to 2,400 kcal/day and an active man requires 2,400 to 2,800 kcal/day. A sedentary woman in this age range requires 1,600 kcal/day, a moderately active woman requires 1,800 kcal day and an active woman requires 2,000 to 2,200 kcal/day.

Protein

Currently, the recommendation for daily protein intake for an older adult is the same as that for other adults: 0.75 g/kg of body weight or 53 g/day for males and 40 g/day for females. Impaired GI tract function and medications, however, can lead to decreased absorption of amino acids and micronutrients, leading to increased intake requirements. Some studies suggest that up to 1.1 g/kg/day may be necessary to maintain nitrogen balance.

Iron

Although the physiologic requirement for iron is lessened in older adults, decreased absorption of iron due to antacid interference, decreased stomach acid secretion, blood loss from disease (such as GI ulcers) or medications (such as aspirin), and the inability to ingest adequate amounts of iron-rich foods put some older adults at risk for iron deficiency. Leading sources of iron in the UK diet include ready-to-eat cereals and beef.

Calcium

The RNI of calcium is 700 mg for adults aged 51 and older. Low calcium intake has been linked to colon cancer and hypertension. In many cases in

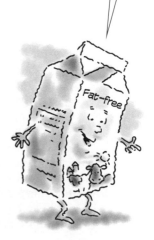

Low calcium intake has been linked to colon cancer and hypertension.

this population, the reference nutrient intake (RNI) for calcium isn't achieved and supplements are recommended.

Magnesium

Magnesium is needed for bone and tooth formation, nerve activity, glucose utilisation and synthesis of fat and proteins. A high percentage of adults aged 70 and older don't meet the RNI for magnesium (300 mg/day for men, 270 mg/day for women). Magnesium can be an issue for older adults, not only because of low intake from food but also because of malabsorption due to GI disorders, chronic alcoholism and diabetes. Signs of deficiency include personality changes (such as irritability and aggressiveness), vertigo, muscle spasms, weakness and seizures.

Maxing out magnesium levels

Magnesium is also overconsumed by some elderly patients. Many medications used by older adults, such as magnesium-based antacids and cathartics, may lead to magnesium overdose. Signs of magnesium toxicity include diarrhoea, dehydration and impaired nerve activity.

Vitamin D

Vitamin D levels are also subject to age-associated changes. The skin's decreased ability to synthesise vitamin D in older adults may be compounded by their limited exposure to sunlight due to use of sunscreen or limited mobility. In addition, medications commonly used by older adults may also interfere with vitamin D metabolism. Fortified foods such as milk are the main sources of vitamin D; however, older adults tend to consume less milk and other vitamin D sources, such as fortified cereals, eggs, liver, salmon and tuna. The *FSA* recommends that older adults should consider taking 10 µg of vitamin D supplements a day if they are not able to consume adequate dietary amounts.

Older people who rarely get outdoors (as well as women who always cover up their skin when they're outside) are at a higher risk of being short of vitamin D and so are also advised to take 10 µg of vitamin D supplements a day.

B vitamins

As the body gets older, it uses vitamin B_{12} less efficiently. Vitamin B_{12} deficiency can occur due to lack of intrinsic factor secretion, which is required for vitamin B_{12} absorption. Another cause is inadequate secretion of gastric acid, which can impair the ability to break down foods and make B_{12} available for absorption. B_{12} is better absorbed in synthetic form and can be found in fortified foods, such as cereals and soy products. Some older people may require regular injections of vitamin B_{12}, cobalamin, if they are unable to absorb vitamin B_{12} from their diet.

Risk factors for poor nutrition

Researchers estimate that as many as two-thirds of older adults are at risk for nutritional deficits. The populations at the greatest risk are those with limited education, those who live alone and those with limited incomes.

Older adults who have limited mobility due to chronic disease are at increased risk for malnutrition as well, especially those in care or residential homes. Only about 6% of the community elderly population suffers from malnutrition. However, the risk is much higher after admittance to a health care setting.

Teaching points

Because of the high prevalence of nutrition-related problems among this age group, it's important to stress these points to your elderly patient:
• Concentrate on variety and pleasure. If calories are a concern, try to moderate portion size rather than cutting foods out altogether. Follow the *FSA guidance* paying special attention to protein intake.
• Choose high-fibre foods. Whole grain breads, breakfast cereals and dried peas or beans are good choices. Fresh fruits and vegetables are also high in fibre and should be encouraged. Be aware, however, that many older adults can't tolerate or chew raw fruits and vegetables. In this case, cooked fruits and vegetables can be substituted but shouldn't be overcooked.
• Drink six to eight 250 ml glasses of water per day. It is important that even if older people have urinary incontinence that they continue to drink plenty of fluids. Older people who are taking diuretic medication should also be advised not to restrict their fluid intake unless advised to by their general practitioner, dietitian or hospital doctor.
• While not generally necessary individuals should take supplements as recommended. General recommendations are to take vitamin and mineral supplements that contain no more than 100% of RNIs. There's no conclusive, scientific evidence that herbal supplements have beneficial effects on the health of older adults.

Nutritional screening for the older adult

It's important to accurately assess the nutritional status of the older adult to reduce the risk of disease and promote health. BAPEN recommend the use of the MUST screening tool. (See the section on MUST in Chapter 8.) Here are some additional guidelines:
• Physical assessment of height and weight can be challenging in older adults, especially those who are bedridden or obese. Using mid upper arm circumference instead will provide an estimate of the body mass index.
• An adequate diet history can also be difficult to obtain unless family and friends are available to give additional information.

• A thorough diet history is important for understanding social and economic limitations (such as access to a food market), in addition to cognitive ones.
• The patient should be asked specifically about unintentional weight gain or loss in the previous 6 months.
• Ongoing height and weight measurements are important for noting trends. Dentition should be assessed regularly as well.
• Blood tests for haemoglobin, haematocrit, serum lipids and glucose are important. An especially valuable parameter for assessment of protein status is serum albumin, which should be 3.5% or higher. Urinalysis for glucose, ketones, protein and occult blood is important to assess kidney function and glucose metabolism.

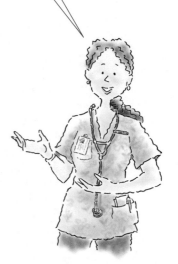

Don't mistake the lethargy and confusion that can result from dehydration with 'normal' ageing in the older adult.

Nutritional concerns

The consequences of poor nutrition are especially severe for older adults. Primary nutritional concerns for elderly patients include dehydration and decreased immunity.

Dehydration

Dehydration can cause lethargy and confusion, which are commonly overlooked as effects of the 'normal' ageing process.

Decreased immunity

Inadequate protein intake can make older adults more susceptible to infectious diseases and exacerbations of chronic diseases as well as pressure ulcers and other wounds.

Quick quiz

1. What vitamin is essential in a pregnant woman's diet to prevent neural tube defects?
    A. Vitamin E
    B. Folic acid
    C. Vitamin C
    D. Iodine
Answer: B. Folic acid ensures healthy embryonic development.

2. Infants have trouble with cow's milk-based formulas because:
    A. cow's milk has inadequate amounts of lactose.
    B. cow's milk has small amounts of protein.
    C. infants can't digest milk protein from cows.
    D. the taste of the formula is sour.
Answer: C. Cow's milk protein is hard for an infant to digest because the intestinal tract isn't mature.

3. What vitamin is absorbed less efficiently by older adults?
    A. Vitamin B$_{12}$
    B. Vitamin E
    C. Vitamin A
    D. Vitamin C

Answer: A. Older adults have decreased secretion of intrinsic factor, which is necessary for vitamin B$_{12}$ to be absorbed in the intestinal tract.

Scoring

☆☆☆   If you answered all three questions correctly, take centre stage! You should receive a lifespan achievement award!

☆☆   If you answered two questions correctly, you've hardly been upstaged. In fact, you're developing nicely into your role of nutrition-know-it-all!

☆   If you answered fewer than two questions correctly, don't get stage fright! Look over the chapter again and you're sure to become a star of stages of nutrition!

Part III

Clinical nutrition

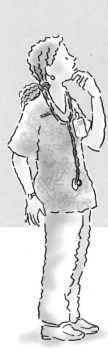

10 Feeding patients

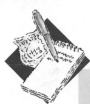

Just the facts

Knowing how to feed patients is an important part of their nutritional care. In this chapter, you'll learn:

♦ purposes, advantages and disadvantages of oral supplemental feedings, enteral nutrition and parenteral nutrition

♦ tubes used for enteral feedings

♦ components of oral supplements and enteral and parenteral nutrition formulas

♦ enteral and parenteral nutrition monitoring

♦ complications of enteral and parenteral nutrition.

A look at patient feeding methods

Ideally, a patient meets his or her nutritional needs by chewing and swallowing—in other words, through normal oral intake. However, ensuring adequate nutritional intake is more difficult if your patient is unconscious or acutely ill, can't chew or swallow, is too weak or confused to eat or needs extra nutrients to speed healing.

A patient who can't or won't consume an adequate oral diet needs an alternative feeding method. Depending on his or her condition, he or she may require oral supplemental feedings, enteral nutrition (tube feedings) or parenteral nutrition.

It's okay to be choosy

When choosing the optimal feeding method, one principle holds sway: If the gut works, use it. Whenever possible, a patient should eat orally and independently. If he or she can't take in enough nutrients through a healthy balanced diet to maintain adequate nutrition, first consider giving oral supplements. If he or she is unable or unwilling to take oral supplements, provide enteral nutrition. Consider parenteral nutrition as a last resort—to be used only when oral supplements and enteral feedings are out of the question.

Oral supplemental feeding: Sip feeds

Oral supplemental feedings (primarily beverages) may be given between or with meals if your patient can't meet his or her nutritional requirements through normal oral intake. They're also used extensively to wean patients from enteral or parenteral nutrition therapy.

Oral supplements come in several categories—milk-based drinks, prepared liquid supplements, specially prepared foods and modular products. Commercially available formulas differ in calories, protein source, osmolality, lactose content and cost. The choice of supplement depends on such factors as the condition of the patient's GI tract, the degree of digestion required and the patient's nutritional needs.

Taster's choice

Such oral supplements as Build up, Complan, Fresubin and Ensure are easy to consume and well accepted by most patients. Because they leave the stomach quickly, they can be used as between-meal snacks. Each brand tastes different. A patient who doesn't like one brand may accept another.

Milk-based supplements

Milk-based supplements may be made from scratch, prepared with powdered commercial mixes such as Complan or Build up or bought as commercially prepared products. They provide significant proteins and calories, have an acceptable taste and are relatively cheap. However, they aren't appropriate for patients who need complete nutritional support or who have lactose intolerance.

Commercially prepared liquid supplements

Commercially prepared liquid supplements vary in composition, taste and cost. Besides convenience, they offer consistent quality and a range of flavour choices. Standard commercial supplements are low in residue and contain no lactose. Typically, they provide 1 to 1.5 cal/ml, with 14% to 16% of total calories coming from protein. Examples include Fresubin, Jevity and Ensure. Depending on the brand, one serving (250 ml) of a commercially prepared supplement provides about 240 to 250 cal and 3.8 to 10 g of protein.

Commercial supplements should be used only after the patient's nutritional requirements have been thoroughly evaluated.

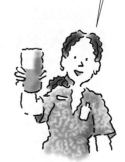

Oral supplemental feeding—most of which come in liquid form—can help your patient meet his or her nutritional needs.

Variations from the form

Many commercial supplements come in variations of the standard formula, including high-protein, high-calorie, light and added-fibre versions. Ensure and Jevity offer high-protein, high-calorie and added-fibre supplements. Ensure also offers a light version, which contains less fat and fewer calories than standard supplements.

Commercially prepared supplemental foods

As an alternative to liquid supplements, manufacturers have introduced puddings, bars and other food products that provide a concentrated source of calories and protein. Ensure Pudding, for instance, provides 170 cal and 4 g of protein.

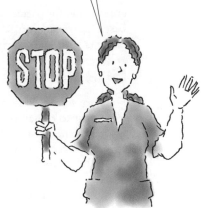

Commercial supplements should be used only after the patient's nutritional requirements have been thoroughly evaluated.

Modular supplements

Modular supplements boost nutrient intake without increasing intake volume. They contain a single nutrient—either carbohydrate (for example hydrolysed cornstarch), protein (such as whey protein) or fat (such as medium-chain triglycerides)—for use in a special situation. For instance a patient with chronic renal failure who needs to gain calories without increasing protein intake may receive carbohydrate-fortified mashed potatoes.

Modular supplements (only under the instructions of a dietitian) may be added to foods, other types of oral supplements or tube (enteral) feedings. They include products such as:
- Polycal, Maxijul and Caloreen (carbohydrate modules)
- Vitapro (protein module)
- Calogen and Liquigen (fat modules).

Be aware, however, that modular supplements are subject to calculation errors, may lead to nutrient imbalances if added to tube feeding and may become contaminated by bacteria. Also, they cost more than standard formulas.

Elemental formulas

Elemental formulas are available in liquid or powder form and contain partially digested nutrients that are useful for the patient with impaired digestion or absorption. These formulas contain little lactose and residue and can be ingested or given through a tube. An example includes Elemental 028 (SHS). A semi-elemental feed is one that contains a mixture of whole and partially digested nutrients: an example is Peptisorb.

Elemental formulas are expensive and should be used only for patients with limited GI function or metabolic disorders. Also, they're less palatable than commercially prepared supplements, so some patients may reject them.

Disease-specific supplements

Specialised formulas are tailored for patients with certain diseases or disorders. A specialised formula may have:
- decreased carbohydrate content for patients with respiratory disease
- increased branched chain amino acids for patients with liver disease
- decreased protein content for patients with kidney disease
- added fibre for patients with constipation.

Most commercial complete liquid sip feeds are lactose free and are suitable for patients with lactase deficiency. Elemental formulas based on free amino acids and monosaccharides are suitable for patients with malabsorption.

Special considerations

Here are some additional points about supplemental feeds that are important to remember:
- Supplements should be used only when medically indicated and on the advice of a registered dietitian.
- An intact (polymeric), rather than a predigested nutrient, supplement should be used if the patient has a functioning GI tract and needs all of the essential nutrients in a specific volume. Intact formulas are made from whole complete proteins or protein isolates. Because they contain complex protein, carbohydrate and fat molecules, they require normal digestion and absorption. Dozens of commercially prepared intact formulas are available.
- A complete nutritional supplement should always be used if the formula is the patient's sole nutritional source. Complete supplements include Ensure, Fortisip and Fresubin.
- Patients with water restrictions, such as those with syndrome of inappropriate antidiuretic hormone, can receive increased calories with formulas that provide 1.5 to 2 cal/ml.
- Nutrient-dense formulas are hyperosmolar and may cause diarrhoea.
- Oral supplements should be given between meals and at least 1 hour before the next meal.
- To minimise taste fatigue, serve oral supplements cold and offer various flavours. Most commercial brands have a range of sweet and savoury flavours. The most common to be prescribed are vanilla, strawberry and chocolate.

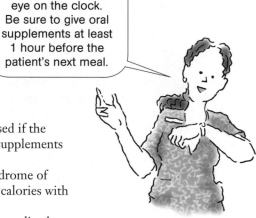

Keep your eye on the clock. Be sure to give oral supplements at least 1 hour before the patient's next meal.

Enteral nutrition

Enteral nutrition (also called tube feeding) delivers a liquid feed through a tube placed in the patient's stomach (gastric feeding) or intestine (duodenal or jejunal feeding). Enteral nutrition therapy preserves the health of the GI mucosa and stimulates lymphoid tissue in the GI tract. It's less likely than parenteral nutrition to cause infection or fluid and electrolyte imbalance, and it's cheaper.

For patients with normal digestion, nutrients in tube feedings should be provided intact rather than predigested. Because intact nutrients force the body to produce all the secretions and enzymes needed for digestion, they preserve normal functioning of the gut.

Gastric enteral nutrition typically is indicated for:
• patients who can't eat normally because of dysphagia, oral or oesophageal obstruction, or injury
• patients who are unconscious or intubated
• patients who are recovering from GI tract surgery and can't ingest food orally or who are unable to meet their full requirements through oral intake.

Duodenal or jejunal enteral feedings decrease the risk of aspiration because the formula bypasses the pylorus. (See *Indications for enteral nutrition*.)

Feeding tubes

The type and placement of a feeding tube for enteral nutrition depends on:
• anticipated duration of enteral feedings
• condition of the patient's GI tract
• patient's overall condition
• patient's aspiration risk.

Location explanation

A feeding tube is identified by where it enters the body and where its tip is placed. A tube may be placed:
• through the mouth, with its tip resting in the stomach (orogastric tube), jejunum (orojejunal tube) or duodenum (oroduodenal tube)
• through the nose, with its tip resting in the stomach (nasogastric [NG] tube), jejunum (nasojejunal [NJ] tube) or duodenum (nasoduodenal tube)
• through a surgical opening, with its tip resting in the stomach (gastrostomy tube) or small intestine (jejunostomy tube).

Surgical solutions

A percutaneous endoscopic gastrostomy (PEG) tube is placed through the abdomen into the stomach without the need for laparotomy or general anaesthesia. It's held in place with a button.

For jejunal access, a percutaneous endoscopic jejunostomy (PEJ) tube may be placed. This tube commonly has two ports—a gastric port used to decompress gastric secretions and a jejunal port used for feedings.

Indications for enteral nutrition

Enteral nutrition may be used for a patient with:

• dysphagia (difficulty swallowing)
• coma
• mechanical ventilation.

Enteral nutrition may also be used for a patient in a hypermetabolic state, which may result from burns, sepsis, multiple trauma and cancer. For a patient in this state, nutritional needs can't be met with oral diet alone.

(For indications and contraindications for PEG and PEJ tubes, see *Percutaneous feeding tubes*.)

Tube selection

Follow these guidelines for proper tube selection:

- NG tubes typically are used in patients who have satisfactory stomach emptying and are expected to need enteral feedings for at least 30 days, or if the duration of enteral feedings hasn't been determined.
- NJ tubes may be used for patients with impaired stomach emptying, pancreatitis or a high risk of aspiration.
- Nasoduodenal tubes are used for patients with impaired stomach emptying or a high risk of aspiration.
- Orogastric, oroduodenal and orojejunal tubes can be used in critically ill patients to minimise the risk of sinusitis.

Other tube features

Feeding tubes are classified by length, diameter and presence or absence of a weighted tip. The outer diameter is measured in French sizes. Each French size unit equals 0.33 mm. Although a tube with a smaller diameter promotes patient comfort, it's more likely to clog. PEG tubes, with their larger diameters, are less likely to clog. All feeding tubes need to be flushed often to prevent clogging.

Enteral feeding formulas

In enteral feeding formulas, osmolality (the number of particles in solution, expressed as milliosmols per kilogram [mOsm/kg]) is determined by the concentration of sugars, amino acids and electrolytes. Isotonic formulas have roughly the same osmolality as blood—about 300 mOsm/kg.

Most patients tolerate formulas that are isotonic or mildly hypertonic (with a slightly higher osmolality than blood). Formulas that are more hypertonic are poorly tolerated—especially when delivered at full strength into the intestine. The high osmolality draws water into the intestine to dilute the particle concentration, causing nausea, abdominal cramping and diarrhoea.

Content with the contents

Formula residue consists of fibre (carbohydrates not digested in the GI tract), undigested food, intestinal secretions, bacterial cell bodies and cells shed from the intestinal lining. Enteral formulas vary in their residue content. Most standard intact formulas are low in residue, although some have added fibre.

Fibre may help normalise bowel function in patients with diarrhoea or constipation. With long-term tube feedings, adding fibre to the formula may help maintain GI integrity. However, formulas that contain fibre may cause gas and bloating in some patients. They're usually inappropriate as initial feedings in patients who have been on bowel rest, have certain GI disorders or have undergone GI surgery.

Percutaneous feeding tubes

A percutaneous endoscopic gastrostomy (PEG) or percutaneous endoscopic jejunostomy (PEJ) tube is used to deliver enteral nutrition to a patient who:

- needs long-term tube feedings (more than 4 weeks)
- requires gastric decompression
- has a swallowing dysfunction
- has mental status problems that prevent oral intake
- has a tracheoeso-phageal fistula.

These tubes are contraindicated for patients with:

- GI obstructions
- haemodynamic instability
- coagulation disorders
- no stomach
- scarring from pre-vious abdominal surgery.

Types of enteral feeding formulas

More than 80 types of enteral feeding formulas are available. They range from inexpensive standard formulas to costly disease-specific ones. Dietitians will advise and recommend the most appropriate enteral feed.

Standard formulas

Standard formulas provide about 1 kcal/ml and have a moderate protein content.

Calorie-dense formulas

Calorie-dense formulas range from 1.2 to 2 kcal/ml. Those used for patients with renal failure are low in potassium, phosphorus and magnesium; they also require less volume. Other calorie-dense formulas are simply high in calories as they have a higher protein content per 100 ml of feed.

Fibre-containing formulas

Fibre-containing formulas usually provide 10 to 15 g of fibre per 1,000 cal. The fibre source may be mostly insoluble fibre or a mixture of soluble and insoluble fibre. These formulas help to prevent constipation and solidify loose stools. To prevent faecal impaction, the patient must be adequately hydrated.

High-protein formulas

High-protein formulas are given to patients with high-protein needs—for example those with major wounds, critical illnesses or burns; those recovering from surgery or trauma; and overweight or elderly patients who have high-protein needs relative to their calorie needs.

Elemental formulas

Elemental (hydrolyzed) formulas contain partially digested nutrients, including proteins in the form of amino acids, or amino acids along with peptides. Used for patients with impaired digestion or absorption, these formulas provide 1 to 1.5 kcal/ml, with 8% to 17% of total calories coming from protein.

Disease-specific formulas

Disease-specific formulas are tailored to meet the nutritional needs of patients with specific medical problems. These are used only when advised by a dietitian or nutrition team as their benefits compared with standard formulas are not well supported by clinical research.
• Diabetic formulas contain fibre and relatively low amounts of carbohydrates. Useful for patients with hard-to-control blood glucose levels, they're effective among patients in long-term care facilities. However, their effectiveness in acute-care patients hasn't been established.
• Renal formulas are dense in calories; low in potassium, magnesium and phosphorus; moderately low in protein and low in fat-soluble vitamins.
• Pulmonary formulas are dense in calories, high in fat and relatively low in carbohydrates.

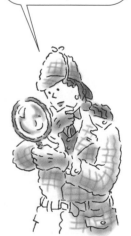

It's elemental, my dear Watson. Because elemental formulas contain partially digested nutrients, they aid digestion and absorption.

• Immune-enhancing formulas may contain extra arginine, omega-3 fatty acids, nucleic acids and glutamine. They're sometimes used in hospitals in an attempt to reduce infectious complications. However, experts haven't determined which patient populations benefit from these formulas.

Modular formulas

Modular formulas are used when the patient's nutritional needs can't be met with other available formulas. They provide supplemental proteins, carbohydrates, lipids and fibre. A modular formula can be added to a tube feeding or infused through the tube between feedings.

Administering enteral nutrition

Enteral feedings may be given continuously or on a cyclic or nocturnal schedule.

Never a dull moment

Recommended when the formula is delivered directly into the patient's small intestine, *continuous* feedings are administered 24 h/day by gravity drip or infusion pump. The rate is increased gradually to allow the patient's GI tract to adjust to the formula. To prevent clogging, the tube should be flushed every 4 to 6 hours. To prevent contamination, the formula bag should hang no longer than 4 hours, unless it's packaged in a sterilised delivery system when it can be used for 24 hours before being changed.

Night-time is the right time

Overnight feeding usually delivers a feed over 8 to 14 hours. The feed may be infused over a longer period to allow gradual transition to nocturnal feedings—for instance if the patient can't tolerate rapid increases in the hourly feeding rate.

Overnight feedings give the patient increased daytime mobility. They're also used during the transition to an oral diet to supply part of the patient's caloric needs. As oral intake improves, the volume of tube feedings can be reduced until the patient's oral intake is sufficient to discontinue tube feedings. Also, if the patient's caloric needs can't be met during the daytime alone, the patient may benefit from extra calories delivered during night-time feedings, such as in the patient with cystic fibrosis.

Gastric feeding

Generally, gastric feeding can be given via syringe, infusion pump or intermittent gravity drip. Infusion pumps are the most common method of administering a feed.

Bolus feedings

Bolus feedings provide a 4- to 6-hour volume of solution over 20 to 30 minutes. They're given by syringe into tubing that leads to the stomach.

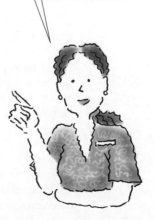

The adverse effects of bolus feedings aren't bogus! Bolus feedings may cause abdominal discomfort, cramping and nausea.

Bolus feedings may cause abdominal discomfort, cramping and nausea. However, some community patients prefer this method, especially if they work or go to school. To prevent contamination or clogging, the tube should be flushed with water after each bolus feeding.

Intermittent feeding

NG feeding can be given by gravity or through feeding pumps. Jejunal or duodenal feedings are given by infusion pump because of the gastric emptying rate.

Typically, the patient receives four to six feedings daily of up to 500 ml per feeding. The infusion rate and volume per feeding are based on patient tolerance and requirements. Flush the feeding tube with sterile or cooled boiled water before and after each feeding to prevent clogging.

Initiating feeding

Tube placement must be verified, usually by examining x-rays or pH indicator strip, before feeding begins. To check tube placement, remove the cap or plug from the feeding tube and attach a syringe. Gently aspirate gastric secretions. Examine the aspirate and place a small amount on the pH test strip. Proper placement of the tube is likely if the aspirate has a typical gastric fluid appearance (grassy-green, clear and colourless with mucous shreds or brown) and the pH is 5 or less. To help prevent aspiration during feeding, elevate the patient's head at least 30 degrees during feeding and for at least 30 minutes afterwards.

Tube feedings don't need to be diluted. Give additional fluids as flushes to maintain tube patency before and after each feed.

When giving an isotonic formula, follow NHS Trust Protocol or nutrition care plan devised with the dietitian. Normally the feed will start at full strength, infusing at a rate of 30 to 50 ml/h. Increase the rate by 25 ml/h every 12 to 24 hours, until the desired rate is achieved. Use a much slower infusion rate if the patient is malnourished, under severe stress or receiving intestinal feedings. After patient tolerance is established, increase the rate gradually.

Flushing the tube

To help ensure patency, flush the feeding tube with 20 to 30 ml of water at least every 4 hours, before and after each feed, before and after administering medications through the tube, before and after bolus and intermittent feedings and after checking gastric residual volumes. Administering medications through fine bore feeding tubes should be avoided. If, however, medications are required, the pharmacy can advise of the appropriate preparation for administration via a feeding tube. The pharmacy department can also advise about alternative medications and routes of administration. If a feeding tube becomes blocked, special preparations containing pancreatic enzyme solution may be used to flush feeding tubes.

When administering enteral nutrition to your patients, be aware of indications of low tolerance, including high gastric residual content, diarrhoea, nausea, vomiting and abdominal distension.

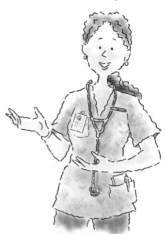

Monitoring tolerance

When monitoring your patient's tolerance of enteral feeding, evaluate the factors listed here.

High gastric residual content

If your patient is receiving gastric feedings, assess gastric emptying by aspirating and measuring residual gastric contents after 4 hours of feeding. In most situations you should reinstill any aspirate obtained. Be aware, however, that experts disagree on the need for measuring residual gastric contents and what constitutes a high gastric residual content. Local policy and protocols will provide guidance on the need for measuring the gastric residual. Research suggests that in patients with residual volumes under 500 ml, tube feeding shouldn't be stopped unless the patient is prone to aspiration, such as the sedated patient. Each patient's clinical situation and risks should be evaluated when determining whether to stop a tube feed. Interventions such as elevating the head of the bed, assessing the abdomen for distension and providing duodenal or jejunal feeding may reduce the risk of aspiration.

Diarrhoea

If your patient develops diarrhoea (more than three liquid stools per day), perform a thorough assessment to determine the cause. Review the patient's medications for those with laxative effects—including those sweetened with sorbitol, antibiotics, laxatives, magnesium and electrolyte supplements.

It isn't difficile, or is it?

If medications are ruled out as the cause of diarrhoea, a stool specimen tested for *Clostridium difficile*. If the stool tests positive for this organism, avoid giving anti-diarrhoeal medications (such as paregoric, Lomotil and Imodium), which slow intestinal peristalsis and prolong intestinal transit time. Instead seek advice and follow locol protocol. Diarrhoea can be reduced by providing a pectin- or fibre-containing medication, such as Fybogel or Normacol.

Regardless if *C. difficile* is confirmed or not, consult the dietitian who will advise on adding fibre to the tube feeding—either by changing to a fibre-containing formula or by mixing a modular fibre supplement with water and infusing it through the feeding tube several times daily.

Since administering cold tube feedings may lead to diarrhoea, check the temperature of the tube feeding. Allow the feeding solution to warm to room temperature before administration. Avoid giving cold feeds straight from the refrigerator. Reducing the flow rate or volume of the feeding may also help resolve diarrhoea. Before changing the flow rate of the feed, seek the advice of the registered dietitian. Be sure to practise good hand washing when preparing feedings and handling tube feeding equipment. If these measures don't relieve diarrhoea, consult the doctor and dietitian about a prescription for anti-diarrhoeal medication.

I don't mean to be difficile. It's just who I am.

Nausea

A patient who experiences nausea during tube feeding may need to switch to a formula with a higher caloric density to reduce feeding volume. Discuss with the registered dietitian before adjusting the flow rate of the feed. If this doesn't help, consider giving a prokinetic agent such as Maxolon. Prokinetic agents increase upper GI tract motility and relax the pyloric sphincter and duodenal bulb, thus shortening GI transit time.

Vomiting

If the patient vomits during a tube feeding, stop the feeding immediately. Then perform a thorough assessment to evaluate:
- adequacy of gastric emptying (check gastric residual contents)
- proper tube tip location
- possible bowel obstruction, ileus or constipation.

In re-establishing the feed, discuss with the dietitian, nutritonal team or relevant health care professional who may advise you to reduce the infusion rate, adjust the formula or switch formulas—for example from one that contains fibre to one that doesn't. If enteral feeding is not recommenced, make sure a nutritional plan is in place to ensure that the patient's nutritional needs are met.

Emptying promises

If your patient has impaired gastric emptying, the doctor may prescribe a prokinetic agent. If the problem persists, the patient may need to have a feeding tube placed in the small bowel, antiemetic medications or further evaluation to determine the cause of vomiting. If the patient has diabetic gastroparesis, a normal blood glucose level must be maintained.

Abdominal distension

Check for abdominal distension during every shift, measuring from one iliac crest to the other. An increase greater than 8 cm from the baseline measurement is the cause for concern.

Changing the equipment

For patients in hospitals or nursing home settings, tubing and formula bags should be changed every 12 to 24 hours or according to local policy and procedure. For the community patient, tubing and bags can be changed less frequently—for example every 24 hours, according to local policy.

Safe keeping

Make sure that the date, time the feed is commenced and signature of person commencing the feed is identified according to local protocol. To avoid contamination, use clean technique when setting up and administering tube feeds. Discard unused refrigerated tube feedings after 24 hours. In an open system, hang only 4 hours of tube feeding at a time. Change a closed system (one that uses ready-to-hang containers) every 24 hours according to the manufacturer's guidelines.

Complications

Enteral nutrition can lead to various complications, including aspiration, GI problems and metabolic imbalances.

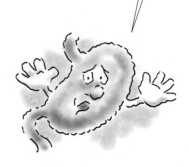

Oh no! Enteral feedings can cause me to become crampy and bloated.

Aspiration pneumonia

One of the most serious complications of tube feedings, aspiration pneumonia, can occur whether the patient receives feedings in the stomach or intestine. To help prevent aspiration, elevate the head of the bed at least 30 degrees during feedings and for about 30 minutes afterwards. Discontinue feedings at least 30 minutes before treatments that require the patient's head to be lowered. If an endotracheal tube is in place, keep the cuff inflated during feedings.

GI problems

Enteral feedings can lead to such GI problems as diarrhoea, abdominal cramps, bloating or gas. To help prevent these problems, warm the formula to room temperature before administration.

Metabolic problems

Enteral feedings can lead to fluid imbalances, such as dehydration or overhydration. Assess the patient's fluid and electrolyte status and serum glucose levels before feedings begin and throughout enteral tube feeding. Keep an accurate fluid balance chart.

Clogged feeding tube

Causes of a clogged feeding tube include:
- failure to flush the tube adequately after medication delivery or before and after each feed
- withholding of tube feedings
- use of calorie-dense formulas
- use of a small-diameter feeding tube
- use of gravity drip (the roller clamp may allow residual formula to cling to the wall of the tube, creating build-up)
- delivery of inappropriate medications and other products via the enteral tube
- gastric residual (gastric acid mixes with formula in the tube and causes coagulation)
- stopping or slowing the feeding without adequate flushing (which lowers gastric pH, reducing gastric acid dilution of the formula and possibly causing backflow of excess formula into the tube).

To help prevent clogging, flush the tube with sterile or cooled boiled water after giving medication, whenever a tube feeding is withheld, and at least every 4 hours.

The logistics of unclogging

Flushing the tube with water usually dislodges a clog. If that doesn't work, an enzyme mixture can be prescribed to declog the tube. Research doesn't support the use of cola or cranberry juice to unclog feeding tubes. Pancreatic enzyme solution may be used to keep tubes patent in patients at risk for clogged tubes.

Home enteral nutrition

If your patient will receive enteral nutrition at home, teach him or her and the family how to use an infusion control device to maintain accuracy. Provide instructions on proper use and care of the syringe or bag and tubing, care of the tube and insertion site and formula storage. The specialist nutrition nurse, if available, can assist in this.

Instruct the patient to discard any formula not used within 24 hours. Tell him or her to use a new bag daily. Teach family members which signs and symptoms to report to the doctor or home care nurse as well as measures to take in an emergency.

Parenteral nutrition

Parenteral nutrition is the administration of predigested nutrients directly into the bloodstream through an I.V. line. Used for patients who can't receive nutrients through the GI tract, parenteral nutrition enables body cells to function despite the patient's inability to eat, digest or absorb food. (See *Indications for parenteral nutrition*.)

The patient's diagnosis, history and prognosis determine the need for parenteral nutrition. Generally, parenteral nutrition isn't indicated for patients with a normally functioning GI tract or for well-nourished patients whose GI tracts will resume normal function within 10 days. Also, it may be inappropriate for patients with a poor prognosis or when the risks outweigh the benefits.

To use or not to use...

In many hospitals, nutrition support teams participate in the decision to use—or not use—parenteral nutrition. These teams will include registered dietitians, doctors, nurses and pharmacists. If the patient is extremely ill, it is important that family members are included in any discussions about parenteral nutrition.

Drawbacks

Like any invasive procedure, parenteral nutrition poses certain risks, including catheter-related infection, hyperglycaemia (high blood

---

Indications for parenteral nutrition

Generally, parenteral nutrition is prescribed for a patient who can't absorb nutrients through the GI tract for more than 10 days. Common conditions that may make parenteral nutrition necessary include:

- GI trauma
- pancreatitis
- short-bowel syndrome
- ileus
- inflammatory bowel disease
- intractable vomiting and diarrhoea
- GI tract cancer
- GI haemorrhage
- GI obstruction
- paralytic ileus
- GI fistula (high-output [more than 500 ml/day] enterocutaneous fistula)
- severe malabsorption
- severe radiation enteritis.

glucose level) and hypokalaemia (low blood potassium level). Such complications can be minimised with careful monitoring of the catheter site, infusion rate and laboratory test results.

Another disadvantage of parenteral nutrition is the need for vascular access. If poor vasculature rules out peripheral access, central access may be necessary, perhaps requiring surgical intervention.

Show me the money

Parenteral nutrition is also expensive—about 10 times as expensive as enteral nutrition for the solutions alone. Therefore, it's used only when necessary.

Types of parenteral nutrition

Parenteral nutrition may be given through a central or peripheral I.V. line. The administration routes depend on what level of parenteral nutrition is required.

Total parenteral nutrition

A patient who needs parenteral nutrition for more than 5 days usually requires total parenteral nutrition (TPN). TPN provides total caloric needs. It's delivered through a central line, typically placed in the subclavian vein with its tip resting in the superior vena cava. Central lines can also be inserted via a peripheral vein, peripherally inserted central catheter (PICC). This large central vein can tolerate the concentrated, hypertonic solutions that supply full nutritional support. Alternatives are the internal jugular and femoral veins.

Indications for TPN include:
• poor tolerance of long-term enteral feedings
• chronic vomiting or diarrhoea
• GI disorders that prevent or severely reduce absorption, such as bowel obstruction, Crohn's disease, short-bowel syndrome and bowel fistulas.

Peripheral parenteral nutrition

Peripheral parenteral nutrition (PPN) delivers nutrients through a short catheter inserted into a peripheral vein. It meets basic nutritional needs without the risks involved with central venous access. PPN may be used for:
• administration of parenteral nutrition via a peripheral catheter, which should be considered for patients who are likely to need short-term parenteral nutrition (less than 14 days) who have no need for central access for other reasons
• patients who can't absorb enteral feedings
• patients who are receiving oral or enteral feedings and need to supplement low-calorie intake.

Generally, PPN provides fewer nonprotein calories than TPN because it uses lower dextrose concentrations. PPN must infuse a much larger fluid

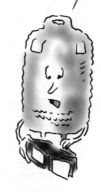

In addition to putting your patient at risk for catheter infection, hyperglycaemia and hypokalaemia, parenteral nutrition can lead to empty wallet syndrome. Parenteral solutions cost 10 times more than enteral ones.

volume to deliver the same number of calories as TPN. Therefore, most patients who require parenteral nutrition support receive TPN rather than PPN. (See *Nutrition by many other names. . .*)

Catheters used for parenteral nutrition

The type of catheter used depends mainly on how long the patient is expected to require parenteral nutrition and whether or she will receive a central or peripheral infusion. PPN is administered through a peripheral vein. TPN is administered using one of the methods listed here. Parenteral nutrition must be delivered via a dedicated lumen that is used for nothing else.

For short-term use

For short-term TPN, a stiff, triple-lumen catheter is typically used. Generally, the I.V. line is inserted percutaneously into the jugular or subclavian vein—usually at the bedside, with a nurse assisting. Strict sterile technique is essential to prevent infection. The catheter tip rests in the vena cava or right atrial area. The line can also be inserted using a PICC—a PICC line.

For long-term use

A longer silicone central catheter, such as a Hickman or Groshong catheter, is used for long-term TPN. The catheter is tunnelled to allow separation of the vein entry site from the skin exit site, thus lowering the infection risk. The catheter tip rests in the vena cava.

Take your PICC

A PICC may be used if the patient will need parenteral nutrition for several weeks to several months. PICCs are associated with fewer insertion complications and infections than lines inserted directly into a central vein.

Inserted via the basilic, median antecubital, cubital or cephalic vein, the PICC is threaded to the superior vena cava or subclavian vein or to a noncentral site such as the axillary vein. Many hospitals will have trained nurses who are responsible for the management of PICCs.

Parenteral nutrition solutions

The type of parenteral solution that should be administered depends on the patient's condition and metabolic needs and whether it will be given through a peripheral or central line. The solution usually contains proteins, carbohydrates, electrolytes, vitamins and trace minerals. A lipid emulsion provides the necessary fat.

Nutrition by many other names...

Parenteral feeding is known by various names.

- Total parenteral nutrition (TPN)—delivers total caloric needs through a central vein
- Parenteral nutrition (PN)—is administered through a central vein
- Peripheral parenteral nutrition (PPN)—delivers basic caloric needs through a peripheral vein.

Parenteral solutions may contain the following elements, each offering a particular benefit:
- dextrose—in parenteral nutrition solutions, most of the calories that can help maintain nitrogen balance come from dextrose. The number of nonprotein calories needed to maintain nitrogen balance depends on the severity of the patient's illness. Dextrose provides 3.4 kcal/g.
- amino acids—amino acids supply enough protein to replace essential amino acids, maintain protein stores and prevent protein loss from muscle tissue. Commercial amino acid solutions range in concentration from 3% to 15%.
- fats—a concentrated energy source, fats prevent or correct fatty acid deficiencies. They're available in several concentrations and can provide 30% to 50% of daily calories. Lipids can be infused separately (as a lipid emulsion) or mixed with the carbohydrate and protein.
- electrolytes and minerals—the amount of electrolytes and minerals added to the solution is based on the evaluation of the patient's serum chemistry profile and metabolic needs.
- vitamins—to ensure normal body functions and optimal nutrient use, the patient needs daily vitamins. A commercially available mixture of fat- and water-soluble vitamins should be added to the solution. Parenteral nutrition formulas should contain vitamins A, D, C, E, K and B_{12}; thiamin; riboflavin; pyridoxine; niacin; pantothenic acid; folic acid and biotin.
- trace elements—trace elements promote normal metabolism. Most commercial solutions contain zinc, copper, chromium, selenium and manganese. Some peripheral nutrition formulas also contain sodium, potassium, chloride, acetate, phosphorus, magnesium and calcium.
- water—the amount of water added to a parenteral nutrition solution depends on the patient's fluid requirements and electrolyte balance.
- other components—depending on the patient's condition, the doctor may order such additives as insulin or heparin. Iron isn't routinely included because of the risk of anaphylactic reactions. However, iron dextran may be added after a test dose is given to determine patient tolerance. Medications other than insulin or heparin also aren't generally added because of the risk of incompatibilities between the nutrients and medications.

> Parenteral nutrition formulas should contain all four of us—and some of our buddies, too!

TPN solutions

TPN solutions are hypertonic, with an osmolarity of 1,800 to 2,600 mOsm/L. Electrolytes, minerals, vitamins, micronutrients and water are added to the base solution to satisfy daily requirements. Lipids may be given as a separate solution or as an admixture with dextrose and amino acids. (See *ABCs of TPN*.)

Maintaining glucose balance

Glucose balance is extremely important in a patient receiving TPN. Adults use 0.8 to 1 g of glucose per kg of body weight per hour. That means a patient can tolerate a constant I.V. infusion of hyperosmolar (highly concentrated)

ABCs of TPN

To determine the appropriate dosage and administration of total parenteral nutrition (TPN), the doctor collaborates with the dietitian and pharmacist. Basic components of TPN include:

- dextrose
- amino acids
- lipids (may be given separately or mixed in a 3-in-1 solution)
- sterile water
- vitamins
- mineral and trace elements.

glucose without the need to add insulin to the solution. As the concentrated glucose solution infuses, a pancreatic beta-cell response causes serum insulin levels to rise.

Slow and steady

To allow the pancreas to establish and maintain the necessary increased insulin production, start with a slow infusion rate and increase the rate gradually as ordered. Abruptly stopping the infusion may cause rebound hypoglycaemia.

PPN solutions

PPN solutions usually consist of dextrose 5% in water to dextrose 10% in water ($D_{10}W$) and 2.75% to 4.25% crystalline amino acids. Alternatively, PPN solutions may be slightly hypertonic, such as $D_{10}W$, with an osmolarity no greater than 600 mOsm/L.

Lipid emulsions

Lipid emulsions prevent and treat essential fatty acid deficiency and provide a major source of energy. In an oral diet, lipid or fat intake should provide 20% to 35% of calories. In parenteral nutrition solutions, lipids provide 9 kcal/g. I.V. lipid emulsions are oxidised for energy as needed. As a nearly isotonic emulsion, a concentration of 10% or 20% can be infused safely through a peripheral or central vein.

Administering parenteral nutrition

Parenteral nutrition may be given on a continuous or cyclic schedule. With *continuous* delivery, the patient receives the infusion over a 24-hour period. The infusion begins slowly and increases to the optimal rate, as ordered, to help prevent such complications as hyperglycaemia from a high dextrose load. Most hospital patients who receive parenteral nutrition are on a continuous delivery schedule.

Night cap

With overnight feeding, the patient receives the entire 24-hour volume of solution over a shorter period—perhaps 10, 12, 14 or 16 hours. If the patient ambulates during the day or will be discharged soon on parenteral nutrition, changing to a cyclic night-time schedule allows freer movement during the day. If the patient on a night-time schedule isn't sleeping well because of increased urination at night, a daytime schedule may be preferable. Home parenteral nutrition programs have boosted the use of cyclic parenteral nutrition.

Administering TPN

TPN solutions must be infused through a central vein, using one of these devices:
• a PICC whose tip lies in a central vein
• a central venous catheter
• an implanted vascular access device.

A patient on overnight feeding is freer to move about during the day.

Long-term therapy requires:
- a silicone central venous catheter, such as a Hickman, Broviac or Groshong catheter
- an implanted reservoir, such as an Infuse-A-Port
- an implanted vascular access device.

Solution dilution

Because TPN fluid has about six times the solute concentration of blood, peripheral I.V. administration can cause sclerosis and thrombosis. To ensure adequate dilution, the central venous catheter is inserted into the superior vena cava—a wide-bore, high-flow vein.

Inspecting the infusate

Make careful inspection of the infusate a habit. Check for clouding, floating debris and colour changes. Any of these could indicate contamination, problems with the solution integrity or a pH change. If you see anything suspicious, notify the pharmacist. Also inform the doctor that there may be a delay in hanging the solution; he or she may want to order $D_{10}W$ until a new container of TPN solution is available.

Start your infusions!

After removing the TPN solution from the refrigerator, let it warm to room temperature. (Administering chilled solution can cause discomfort, hypothermia, venous spasm and venous constriction.) Then, using an aseptic technique, begin the infusion as prescribed. Watch for swelling at the catheter insertion site. This may indicate extravasation of the TPN solution, which can cause tissue damage.

A port of last resort

Remember the parenteral nutrition infusion port is a dedicated line for feeding only; never add medication to a TPN solution container. Do not use a TPN infusion port for another infusion. To prevent infection, don't use the TPN line to piggyback or infuse blood or blood products, give a bolus injection, administer simultaneous I.V. solutions, measure central venous pressure or draw blood for laboratory tests. In unavoidable circumstances, the TPN port may be used for electrolyte replacement or insulin drips.

Administering PPN

Because PPN solutions have lower tonicity than TPN solutions, a patient receiving PPN must be able to tolerate infusion of large fluid volumes. Administer the solution through the largest peripheral vein available so the blood can dilute the solution adequately.

Well that isn't so swell

When starting the PPN infusion, watch for swelling at the peripheral insertion site. Swelling may indicate infiltration or extravasation of the solution, which can cause tissue damage.

Withdrawing blood samples

Avoid contaminating a blood sample with parenteral nutrition solution. Otherwise, blood glucose level and certain other values may be extremely high. Generally, blood should never be withdrawn from a parenteral nutrition line. If unavoidable, follow the local policy on withdrawing blood from a parenteral nutrition line.

Complications

Complications of parenteral nutrition therapy may be catheter related, metabolic or mechanical in nature. (See *Complications of parenteral nutrition.*)

Catheter-related complications

The most common catheter-related problems are catheter clogging, catheter dislodgment, cracked or broken tubing, pneumothorax and hydrothorax, and sepsis:
• clogged catheter—suspect a clogged catheter if the infusion flow rate is interrupted or if greater pressure is needed to maintain the infusion at the desired rate.
• catheter dislodgment—the most obvious sign is when the catheter comes out of the vein. You may note that the dressing is wet. With a peripheral catheter, the insertion site may be red or swollen. With a central catheter, swelling may appear around the insertion site. Catheter dislodgment may cause bleeding from the insertion site and an air embolism.
• cracked or broken tubing—if the catheter or vascular access device is damaged, infusate may leak from a cracked part of the insertion site. If the infusion tubing is damaged, the I.V. insertion site remains dry. Both situations pose the risks of bleeding, contamination and air emboli.
• pneumothorax (air in the pleural cavity) and hydrothorax (fluid in the pleural cavity)—these complications usually result from trauma to the pleurae during insertion of a central venous access device.
• sepsis—the most serious catheter-related complication, sepsis can be fatal. To prevent it, provide meticulous, consistent catheter care.

Metabolic complications

During parenteral nutrition support, rapid intracellular electrolyte shifts may occur, leading to such complications as:
• high or low blood glucose level
• hyperosmolar hyperglycaemic nonketotic syndrome

Complications of parenteral nutrition

• pneumothorax (air in the chest)
• haemothorax
• venous thrombosis (a blood clot)
• lymphatic injury
• air embolism (leakage of air into the catheter, obstructing blood flow)
• catheter embolisation (the catheter tip breaks off and obstructs blood flow)
• phlebitis (vein inflammation)
• nerve damage at the insertion site
• infection or sepsis
• hyperglycaemia
• hypertriglyceridaemia
• electrolyte imbalances, including refeeding syndrome
• liver dysfunction
• fluid overload or dehydration.

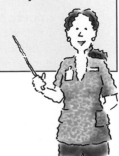

- high or low blood potassium level
- low blood magnesium, phosphate and calcium levels
- metabolic acidosis
- liver dysfunction.

Refeeding syndrome: A complication of enteral and parenteral nutrition

Although refeeding syndrome can occur in patients fed by mouth or enteral nutrition, it's most likely to occur in parenterally fed patients because the I.V. route can infuse larger amounts of nutrition. A potentially fatal complication, refeeding syndrome results from rapid and immediate refeeding of a malnourished patient, whose total body stores of potassium, magnesium and phosphorus are depleted. Accustomed to a state of near-starvation, the patient is at risk of an adverse metabolic response to the introduction of calories and protein. When parenteral nutrition begins and endogenous insulin is released, intravascular potassium, magnesium and phosphorus move into the cells. Because the body's stores of these electrolytes are already decreased, intravascular levels may become dangerously low. In fact, overaggressive parenteral nutrition has been fatal for some patients.

Any patient who has had very little food intake for more than 5 days is at risk of some refeeding problems. If you are concerned, advice should be sought from the registered dietitian and doctors and local policy adhered to.

In general, nutrition support should be commenced at 50% of nutritional need for the first 2 days before increasing to full needs if close clinical and biochemical monitoring reveals no refeeding problems.

Patients at high risk of developing refeeding syndrome include those with:
- BMI < 16 kg/m^2
- unintentional weight loss of >15% within the previous 6 to 8 months
- very little or no nutrient intake for >10 days
- low levels of potassium, phosphate or magnesium prior to any feeding.

Clinical management will include provision of thiamine and other B group of vitamins along with balanced multivitamins and trace element supplements.

Mechanical complications

Mechanical complications of parenteral nutrition therapy can be life threatening:
- air embolism—suspect this problem if the patient becomes apprehensive and develops chest pain, tachycardia, hypotension, cyanosis, seizures, loss of consciousness, cardiac arrest or a churning heart murmur.
- venous thrombosis—this complication causes pain, redness or swelling at the catheter insertion site; swelling of the arm, neck or face; malaise; fever and tachycardia.
- extravasation—suspect extravasation if swelling and pain occur around the insertion site.
- phlebitis—pain, tenderness, redness and warmth at the insertion site and along the vein path may indicate phlebitis.

Monitoring your patient

During parenteral nutrition support, monitor the results of routine laboratory tests, including serum electrolyte levels, blood urea nitrogen and arterial blood gas values. Report abnormal findings to the doctor so that appropriate changes in the nutrition solution can be made. (See *Keeping an eye on lab values*.)

In addition, check glucose levels as ordered, using glucose monitoring sticks (known as BM sticks) or serum tests. Monitor serum triglyceride levels, which should stay within the normal range during continuous TPN infusion. Typically, alanine aminotransferase, aspartate aminotransferase, alkaline phosphatase, cholesterol, triglyceride, plasma-free fatty acid and coagulation tests are performed weekly. Also, evaluate the patient for signs and symptoms of nutritional abnormalities, such as fluid and electrolyte imbalances and disturbed glucose metabolism. Some patients may need supplementary insulin throughout TPN support.

Discontinuing therapy

If your patient has been receiving PPN, it can be discontinued without weaning because the dextrose concentration is lower than in TPN. With TPN, the patient is weaned while receiving an additional form of nutrition, such as enteral feedings. If the transition to oral or tube feedings will be rapid, parenteral nutrition can be discontinued relatively quickly. Local protocol will guide you, but current recommendations are to reduce the TPN rate by 50% for 1 hour, and then discontinue TPN and check the patient's blood glucose level 1 hour later.

If the transition to oral or tube feedings is expected to be gradual (for example if the tube feeding rate will be advanced only by small amounts each day), TPN should be reduced gradually to avoid overfeeding.

Home parenteral nutrition

Patients who require prolonged or indefinite parenteral nutrition may be able to receive the therapy at home. Home parenteral nutrition reduces the need for prolonged hospitalisation and allows the patient to resume many of his normal activities.

Home parenteral nutrition is low-volume high-cost support for patients with intestinal failure, and guidance for its use is available through the two UK regional centres. Support for patients can be obtained through these centres and the contracted providers of the TPN.

It is important to meet with the patient before discharge to make sure he or she knows how to perform the administration procedure and how to handle complications. If the patient can't manage the TPN himself, a well-trained caregiver must be available to assist with setting up and maintaining the infusion system and changing catheter dressings. The patient should be monitored regularly by a clinician with expertise in parenteral nutrition support.

Keeping an eye on lab values

If your patient is receiving parenteral therapy, biochemical monitoring is important. Keep on eye on key parameters including:

- serum glucose
- serum sodium
- serum potassium
- serum chloride
- carbon dioxide
- blood urea nitrogen
- serum creatinine
- serum calcium
- serum magnesium
- serum phosphorus
- liver function
- serum triglycerides
- nitrogen balance
- routine blood glucose every 6 hours
- weight (two to three times per week)
- bone densitometry (with long-term parenteral therapy).

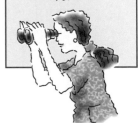

Quick quiz

1. Enteral nutrition is preferred over parenteral because:
    A. it disturbs the GI mucosa
    B. feeding tubes are easier to place than I.V. lines
    C. it's more physiologic than parenteral nutrition
    D. it costs less

Answer: C. Enteral nutrition is a more physiologic way to receive nutrition.

2. A patient receiving gastric feedings should:
    A. have his or her head elevated at least 30 degrees during the feedings
    B. have his or her head elevated for 15 minutes after the feeding
    C. remain flat in bed
    D. lie supine

Answer: A. A patient receiving a gastric feeding should have his or her head elevated at least 30 degrees during feedings and for at least 30 minutes afterwards.

3. What's the maximum amount of time that enteral solutions are permitted to hang before the bag must be replaced?
    A. 4 hours
    B. 8 hours
    C. 12 hours
    D. 24 hours

Answer: C. Don't allow enteral solutions to hang for more than 24 hours.

Scoring

⭐⭐⭐ If you answered all three questions correctly, great job! You've totally taken in the essentials of patient feeding.

⭐⭐ If you answered two questions correctly, way to go! You obviously used the correct administration route to feed yourself this information.

⭐ If you answered fewer than two questions correctly, don't worry! Take a break and then come back and try a different method of intake.

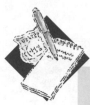

11 Obesity and eating disorders

Just the facts

Overeating and eating disorders are among the most common causes of nutritional problems. In this chapter, you'll learn:

♦ definitions for the terms overweight and obesity

♦ causes of overweight and obesity

♦ treatments for overweight and obesity

♦ signs and symptoms of anorexia nervosa and bulimia

♦ nutritional interventions used to treat eating disorders.

A look at overweight and obesity

Overweight and obesity in the UK have increased. In 2003–2004, the mean body mass index (BMI) of men and women in the UK general population was 27 kg/m² outside the healthy range 18.5 to 25 kg/m². According to the 2004 Health Survey for England, nearly a quarter of men (23.6%) and women (23.8%) were obese. In 2006 a report for the Department of Health predicted that these will increase to approximately 33% in men and 28% in women by 2010. (See *Weight changes in the ageing adult*, page 182.)

The high cost of too many calories

Excess weight substantially increases the risk of diabetes, cardiovascular disease, certain types of cancer and other diseases. Other obesity-related diseases that require identification and appropriate management include gynaecologic abnormalities, osteoarthritis, gall bladder disease and stress incontinence. The risk of death from all causes in obese people is 50% to 100% greater than in people with normal weight. In addition, the annual health care cost of obesity is approximately £7 billion.

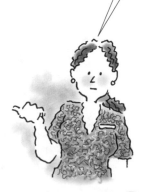

Obesity is a major contributor to preventable deaths and costs more than £7 billion in medical expenses annually.

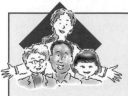

Bridging the gap

Cultural beliefs about weight

Be aware that some cultures and races consider overweight a positive characteristic. Many ethnic populations, for example, believe that carrying extra pounds is important to allow for weight loss during illness.

Lifespan lunchbox

Weight changes in the ageing adult

As a person ages, the risk for overweight or obesity increases. After age 60, the risk tends to decrease; however, sudden or profound weight changes aren't a normal result of ageing.

In addition to the risk of morbidity from obesity-related diseases, obesity can increase the morbidity of other pre-existing disorders. Overweight and obese patients with existing coronary artery disease, type 2 diabetes, stroke and sleep apnoea are at high risk for developing disease-related complications that may lead to death.

Obesity is also associated with complications during surgery, pregnancy, labour and delivery. It's a major contributor to preventable deaths, and it also leads to low self-esteem, negative self-image, hopelessness and negative social consequences, such as stereotyping, prejudice, social isolation and discrimination. (See *Cultural beliefs about weight*.)

Causes

The basic cause of obesity is an energy imbalance that results when the number of calories taken in exceeds the number of calories used for energy. A recurring imbalance leads to weight gain over time. This imbalance most commonly results from overeating or inactivity or both.

The 500 rule

An easy way to put weight gain in perspective is to recall the so-called '500 rule'. Because 0.45 kg (1 lb) of body fat equals 3,500 kcal, a person who eats 500 kcal more per day than his or her body requires will roughly gain 0.45 kg (1 lb) of body fat in 1 week (500 kcal/day × 7 days = 3,500 kcal).

Other explanations

You may notice that some people who are overweight eat only moderate amounts of food but still gain weight and that some average-weight people overeat but never gain weight. That's because there are other possible influences on fat accumulation in the body:

• A *family history* of obesity increases a person's chance of becoming obese by 25% to 30%. In addition, body fat distribution is influenced by genetics. Families also share diet and lifestyle habits that may contribute to obesity. (See *Obesity in ethnic groups*.)

Your genes may play a role in how well you fit into your jeans.

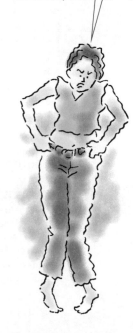

• *Environment* also strongly influences obesity. This includes such lifestyle behaviours as eating habits, diet and level of physical activity. British people tend to eat high-fat foods and put taste and convenience ahead of nutrition. Also, most people in Britain don't get enough physical activity. Only 13% of the population achieve the recommended 30 minutes of physical activity each day.

• *Nutrition* plays an important role in weight gain. Consuming low-fat foods and snacks can decrease the amount of fat in a diet but commonly increases the amount of calories consumed by increasing consumption of carbohydrates. The high fat content in high-fat foods also contributes to increased calorie consumption.

• *Psychological factors* may also influence eating habits. Many people eat in response to positive emotions, such as excitement, or negative emotions, such as boredom, sadness and anger.

• Some *illnesses* can lead to obesity or a tendency to gain weight. Examples include hypothyroidism, Cushing's syndrome, depression and certain neurological problems that can lead to overeating. Also, drugs such as steroids, antipsychotics and some antidepressants may cause weight gain. A general practitioner can tell whether underlying medical conditions are causing weight gain or making weight loss difficult.

• *Sociocultural factors*, such as race, gender, income, education and ethnicity, may also contribute to overweight and obesity.

Evaluating weight

The Department of Health issued guidance in 2008—Healthy Weight, Healthy Lives—to improve the health of the population by tackling the issue of obesity. According to these guidelines, assessment of overweight involves evaluation of three key measures: BMI, waist circumference and a patient's risk factors for diseases and conditions associated with obesity. The guidelines define overweight as having a BMI of 25 to 30 kg/m² and obesity as having a BMI of 30 kg/m² or above.

Obesity is categorised into three classes:
• BMI between 25 and 30 kg/m²—overweight
• BMI between 30 and 40 kg/m²—obese
• BMI over 40 kg/m²—morbidly obese.

A complicated relationship

The relationship between body weight and good health is more complicated than simply comparing the number on the scale to a weight range table. Weight range tables aren't appropriate to use for all individuals because not all people who have a weight in the 'healthy' range are necessarily at their healthy weight. For example some people may have more fat and less muscle. In contrast, a weight above the healthy range may be fine if your patient has more muscle than fat. (See *Calculating BMI*, page 114.)

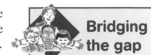

Bridging the gap

Obesity in ethnic groups

The prevalence of overweight and obesity in ethnic minorities is different than in Caucasians, especially in ethnic women. Black Caribbean and Irish men had the highest prevalence of obesity. For women, risk ratios were higher for Black African, Black Caribbean and Pakistani women. Pakistani and Bangladeshi men and women, and Black Caribbean and Black African women, were more likely to have raised waist hip ratio (WHR) and raised waist circumference than the general population.

Pear- or apple-shaped?

The illustrations below depict an apple-shaped person and a pear-shaped person. Studies indicate that where excess body fat is deposited may be a more important and reliable indicator of disease risk than the degree of total body fat.

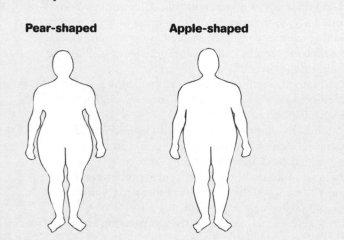

Pear-shaped   **Apple-shaped**

Weight distribution

Where your patients' body fat is may be a more important indicator of health problems than how much fat they have. People with a high distribution of fat around their waists (apple-shaped) as opposed to their hips and thighs (pear-shaped) are at greater risk for such diseases as type 2 diabetes, dyslipidaemia, hypertension and cardiovascular disease. (See *Pear- or apple-shaped?*)

Evaluating weight at the waist

To evaluate weight distribution, measure waist circumference. Locate the upper hip bone and the top of the iliac crest. Place a measuring tape in a horizontal plane around the abdomen at the level of the iliac crest. Before reading the tape measure, ensure that the tape is snug, but doesn't compress the skin, and is parallel to the floor. Measure at the end of expiration. If the measurement is greater than 88.9 cm (35 in.) for women or 102 cm (40 in.) for men with a normal BMI, your patient has a greater risk of health problems. If the BMI is 35 kg/m² or higher, waist measurement is irrelevant because disease risk is already high based on the BMI alone.

Evaluating risk factors

Determining how many health risk factors your patient has will further help you assess his or her need for weight control. The more risk factors present, the more your patient will benefit from weight loss. Risk factors include:

- personal or family history of heart disease
- male older than age 45
- postmenopausal female
- cigarette smoking
- sedentary lifestyle
- hypertension
- high low-density lipoprotein (LDL) cholesterol or low high-density lipoprotein (HDL) cholesterol
- high triglycerides
- diabetes or impaired fasting glucose.

Treatment

Treatment of obesity can be long and difficult. No single treatment method or combination of methods is guaranteed to produce weight loss or maintain weight in all people. Treatment can be directed using guidelines from the Department of Health. (See *Treatment algorithm for obesity*.)

Treatment algorithm for obesity

This algorithm can help guide your treatment of an obese patient.

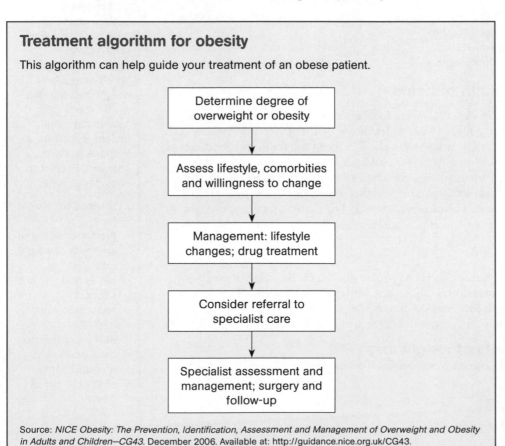

Source: *NICE Obesity: The Prevention, Identification, Assessment and Management of Overweight and Obesity in Adults and Children—CG43*. December 2006. Available at: http://guidance.nice.org.uk/CG43.

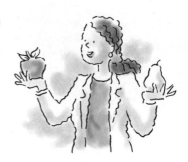

Before beginning any weight-loss therapy, it's important to determine a patient's motivation level. (See *Assessing motivation*.) Also, in 95% of cases in which weight loss occurs too rapidly, people regain the weight they have lost. Explain to your patient that slow, steady weight loss will help with long-term weight management.

Benefits of weight loss

The benefits of weight loss include:
- reduced risk of diabetes and cardiovascular disease
- reduced risk of developing hypertension
- lower triglyceride levels
- higher HDL cholesterol levels
- lower LDL and total cholesterol levels
- lower blood glucose level in nondiabetic patients and some patients with type 2 diabetes.

Goals of weight loss

The general goals of weight loss and management are to:
- reduce body weight and maintain healthy body composition (percentage of fat mass versus lean mass)
- maintain a lower body weight over the long term
- prevent further weight gain.

10% reduction = health benefits

The initial goal of weight loss is to reduce body weight by 10% at a rate of 0.45 to 1 kg (1 to 2 lb) per week with a calorie deficit of 500 to 1,000 kcal/day. Health benefits can be realised and obesity-related risk factors can be decreased with this moderate goal. After this goal is achieved, evaluation and goal setting can determine further weight loss. After 6 months of treatment, the rate of weight loss usually plateaus and the focus of treatment should turn to weight maintenance for the next 6 months. Then, after 6 months of weight maintenance, weight-loss efforts can be resumed.

Success!

The health care professional and patient must agree on weight-loss goals. Patient involvement is crucial to the treatment plan's success. In general, a successful weight loss plan yields weight regain of fewer than 3 kg in 2 years and a reduction in waist circumference of at least 4 cm.

Components of weight loss

The three components of weight-loss therapy are:

 diet therapy

 increased physical activity

 behavioural therapy.

Assessing motivation

It's important to determine the patient's motivation level before beginning weight-loss therapy. A weight-loss attempt will be more successful if the patient is motivated to make lifestyle changes. Factors to consider include:

- reasons for weight loss
- previous history of attempts at weight loss
- family and social support
- attitude towards exercise
- ability to exercise
- time availability
- understanding of the impact of obesity on disease risk
- financial considerations.

Menu maven

Serving up a weight-reducing diet

Key advice for encouraging people to lose weight

Nutrient	Recommend
Calories Thinking of food? Try:	Reduce intake only approximately 600 kcal/day from usual intake • trimming the fat off meat • choosing low-fat varieties of dairy and other products • increasing your intake of starchy foods instead of fatty ones • eating less sugary foods • increasing your intake of a variety of fruit and vegetables (aim to eat at least five portions a day)

These methods should be used for at least 6 months before pharmacotherapy is attempted. Weight-loss surgery is an option for patients with extreme obesity.

Dietary management

Diet, or nutrition, management includes instructing patients how to modify their diets to decrease caloric intake. A key element of the current recommendation is a moderated reduction in calories to achieve a slow, progressive weight loss of 0.5 to 1 kg (1 to 2 lb) per week. Calories should be reduced only to the level required to achieve the goal weight. (See *Serving up a weight-reducing diet.*)

How low to go?

For sustainable weight loss, recommend diets that have a 600 kcal/day deficit (that is 600 kcal less than the person needs to stay the same weight) or that calories are reduced by lowering the fat content (low-fat diets), in combination with expert support and intensive follow-up.

• Low-calorie diets (1,000 to 1,600 kcal/day) may also be considered, but are less likely to be nutritionally complete.

• Very low calorie diets (less than 1,000 kcal/day) may be used for a maximum of 12 weeks continuously, or intermittently with a low-calorie diet (for example for 2 to 4 days a week), if the person is obese and has reached a plateau in weight loss.

• Any diet of less than 600 kcal/day should be used only under clinical supervision.

NutriTips

Controlling caloric intake

Include these tips when teaching your patient about caloric intake:

- Consume plenty of fresh fruits and vegetables, lean meat, wholegrain and high-fibre foods, skimmed milk and low-fat dairy products.
- Eat sensible portions.
- Stick with steamed, grilled or baked foods made without cheese or high-calorie sauces.
- Use oil and vinegar or lemon instead of prepared salad dressings.
- Request milk for coffee instead of cream.
- Use non-stick cooking spray, and trim all visible fat before cooking.
- Replace high-fat ingredients with low-fat substitutes.
- Halve the amount of meat in stews and casseroles.
- Use herbs, spices and cooking wine to enhance flavour.
- When food shopping, buy smart, read labels and stick to your list.

Education is the key

Successful weight reduction is more likely to occur when the patient's food preferences are included in the menu and when dietary education is performed. (See *Controlling caloric intake*.)

When educating your patient, be sure to:
- cover the energy value of different foods as well as discuss food composition, such as fats, carbohydrates (including dietary fibre) and proteins
- encourage the reading of nutrition labels
- promote new habits of purchasing, especially a preference to low-calorie foods
- instruct on food preparation, especially the need to avoid adding high-calorie ingredients (such as fats and oils) during cooking
- warn against the overconsumption of high-calorie foods
- stress the importance of adequate water intake, reducing portion sizes and limiting alcohol consumption.

Increased physical activity

Exercise plays a critical role in the loss and maintenance of body weight. Exercise is important for increasing energy expenditure, maintaining or increasing lean body mass and promoting the loss of fat. These changes in body composition result in improved body dimensions and possibly in an increased metabolic rate.

Getting physical

Efforts to lose weight through physical activity alone generally produce an average weight loss of only 2% to 3%. Exercise affects the rate of weight

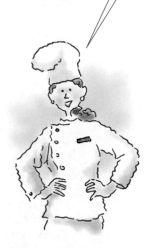

Diet doesn't mean don't eat. People should reduce calories only to the level necessary to achieve their goal weight.

loss based on the frequency and duration of the activity. Sustained physical activity is helpful in maintaining weight loss and reducing cardiovascular and type 2 diabetes risks, and may be helpful in inhibiting food intake. Even without weight loss, increasing physical activity lowers blood pressure, increases HDL cholesterol levels, improves glucose tolerance, enhances the sense of well-being, reduces tension and heightens alertness.

Slow is the way to go

For obese patients, exercise should be started slowly and increased in intensity gradually. Initial activities may simply include increasing activities of daily living, such as taking the stairs or walking at a slow pace. With time, depending on progress, the amount of weight lost and functional capacity, the patient may engage in more strenuous activities. Moderate levels of physical activity for 30 to 45 minutes, 3 to 5 days/week, should be encouraged. The long-term goal should be to accumulate at least 60 minutes of moderate-intensity exercise every day of the week.

Take a hike

Daily walking is an attractive form of physical activity, especially for obese patients. Tell your patient to start by walking 10 minutes, 3 days/week and to build to 30 to 45 minutes of more intense walking at least 5 to 7 days/week. With this regimen, an additional 100 to 200 kcal/day can be expended. A moderate amount of physical activity that burns about 150 kcal can be achieved in various ways. (See *Burning calories*.)

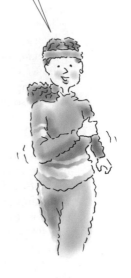

Don't move too fast! Exercise activities for obese patients should start off slow and gradually increase in intensity.

Burning calories

This chart shows the activity and duration needed to burn 160 kcal for an average 70 kg adult. Encourage the use of the online calorie calculator available from the *FSA* using the link http://www.eatwell.gov.uk/healthydiet/healthyweight/caloriecalculator/

Activity	Intensity	Duration (in minutes)
Football	Moderate	20
Walking, moderate pace (3 mph, 20 min/mile)	Moderate	37
Walking, brisk pace (4 mph, 15 min/mile)	Moderate	32
Table tennis	Moderate	32
Raking leaves	Moderate	32
Social dancing	Moderate	29
Lawn mowing (powered push mower)	Moderate	29
Jogging	Hard	20
Cricket	Medium	20
Running	Very hard	13

Reducing sedentary time, such as time spent watching television, is another way to increase activity. Patients should build physical activities into each day. For example parking farther than usual from work or shopping and walking up stairs instead of taking elevators are easy ways to increase daily physical activity.

Behaviour therapy

Behaviour therapy is a useful adjunct to planned decreases in food intake and increases in physical activity. The goal of behaviour therapy is to overcome barriers to compliance with eating and activity habits. Long-term weight reduction most likely won't succeed unless new habits are acquired. The primary assumptions of behaviour therapy are listed here:
• Changing eating and physical activity habits makes it possible to change body weight.
• Eating and physical activity behaviours are learned and can be modified.
• Environment must be changed to change patterns.

Here's the plan

Various strategies must be used for behaviour modification because no single method is superior:
• Self-monitoring of eating and physical activity—this strategy involves recording the amount and type of food, caloric value and nutrient composition of food eaten, and the frequency, intensity and type of physical activity performed each day. Recording this information allows the patient to gain insight into his or her behaviour.
• Stress management—stress triggers dysfunctional eating habits. Using coping strategies, meditation, relaxation techniques and exercise can help relieve stress.
• Stimulus control—this strategy involves identifying stimuli that encourage incidental eating and limiting those stimuli, for example by keeping high-calorie foods out of the house, limiting times and places of eating and avoiding situations in which overeating occurs.
• Problem solving—this strategy includes identifying weight-related problems and planning and implementing alternative behaviours.
• Contingency management—this strategy involves rewarding positive changes in behaviour, such as increasing exercise or reducing consumption of a specific food.
• Cognitive restructuring—cognitive restructuring involves changing self-defeating thoughts and feelings by replacing them with positive thoughts and setting of reasonable goals.
• Social support—a strong support system can help provide the emotional support needed to lose weight. Including friends and family in physical activity and diet or joining a support group can be beneficial.

Pharmacotherapy

Pharmacological treatment should be considered only after dietary, exercise and behavioural approaches have been started and evaluated. The decision to start drug treatment should be made after discussing the potential benefits and limitations including the mode of action, adverse effects and monitoring requirements, and their potential impact on the patient's motivation.

However, most studies show a rapid weight gain after the drugs are stopped. When drug therapy is effective and adverse effects are manageable, therapy can be continued for the long term; however, no one knows how long drug therapy can safely be maintained.

Because few long-term studies have been conducted on the safety and effectiveness of weight-loss medications, they should be used only by patients who are at an increased medical risk because of their weight. These patients include those with a BMI of 30 kg/m² or more and those with one of the following disorders:

- hypertension
- dyslipidaemia
- coronary artery disease
- type 2 diabetes
- sleep apnoea.

Not for everyone

Not every patient responds to drug therapy. Tests show that initial responders tend to continue to respond, while nonresponders are less likely to respond even with increases in dosage. Drug therapy should be discontinued if adverse effects are unmanageable or therapy is ineffective. The decision to add a drug to an obesity treatment programme should be made after consideration of all potential risks and benefits and only after all behavioural options have been exhausted. (See *Fat fighters*, page 192.)

Weight-loss surgery

Surgery is an option for some patients who are experiencing complications from severe and resistant obesity. Surgery should be considered if the risk of remaining obese is greater than the risk of surgery. The hospital specialist or surgeon should discuss in detail with the individual (and their family if appropriate) the potential benefits, long-term implications and risks, including complications and perioperative mortality. Long-term success of surgery depends on the patient's ability to change behaviour and commit to lifelong follow-up. About 70% of patients maintain a weight loss of 50% for 5 years. Two types of surgery are primarily used to promote weight loss: restrictive and combination malabsorptive/restrictive procedures.

Restrictive procedures

In gastric restriction, also known as *vertical banded gastroplasty* and *stomach stapling*, the size of the stomach is surgically decreased so that a patient feels full after eating a small amount of food. A vertical row of staples are inserted across the patient's stomach, decreasing the stomach's size to between 15 and 30 ml. A band decreases the opening from the upper pouch to about 1 cm, which delays gastric emptying. Over time, the pouch can stretch to hold more food. (See *Surgical weight-loss procedures*, page 193.)

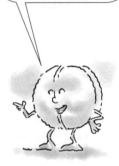

Drugs can help in the fight against fat, but make sure the adverse effects don't send your patient reeling.

Fat fighters

Two current medications used for weight loss are sibutramine and orlistat.

Sibutramine

Sibutramine (Reductil) is an appetite suppressant that works centrally by inhibiting the reuptake of norepinephrine (noradrenalin), serotonin and dopamine. The most common adverse effects are headache, insomnia, anorexia, constipation and dry mouth. It may also increase blood pressure and heart rate.

Sibutramine should be used cautiously in patients who have a history of seizures or angle-closure glaucoma. It's contraindicated in patients taking monoamine oxidase inhibitors or other centrally acting appetite suppressants and in those with anorexia nervosa. It shouldn't be given to patients with severe renal or hepatic dysfunction, coronary artery disease or a history of hypertension, heart failure, arrhythmias or stroke.

Orlistat

Orlistat (Xenical) works peripherally to inhibit pancreatic lipase and, therefore, decreases fat absorption in the GI tract. It should be used in conjunction with a reduced-calorie diet with 30% of calories from fat. Adverse reactions include headache, flatus with discharge, faecal urgency, fatty or oily stool and abdominal pain. Absorption of fat-soluble vitamins also is decreased.

National Institute for Clinical Excellence (NICE) guidance on the use of medication in the management of obesity is summarised as follows:

Orlistat

- Prescribe only as part of an overall plan for managing obesity in adults who have a BMI of:
  - $-28.0 kg/m^2$ or more with associated risk factors or
  - $-30.0 kg/m^2$ or more.
- Continue treatment for longer than 3 months only if the person has lost at least 5% of their initial body weight since starting drug treatment (less strict goals may be appropriate for people with type 2 diabetes).
- Continue for longer than 12 months (usually for weight maintenance) only after discussing potential benefits and limitations with the patient.
- Coprescribing with other drugs for weight reduction is not recommended.

Sibutramine

- Prescribe only as part of an overall plan for managing obesity in adults who have a BMI of:
  - $-27.0 kg/m^2$ or more and other obesity-related risk factors such as type 2 diabetes or dyslipidaemia or
  - $-30.0 kg/m^2$ or more.
- Prescribe only if there are adequate arrangements for monitoring both weight loss and adverse effects (specifically pulse and blood pressure).
- Continue treatment for longer than 3 months only if the person has lost at least 5% of their initial body weight since starting drug treatment (less strict goals may be appropriate for people with type 2 diabetes).
- Treatment is not recommended beyond the licensed duration of 12 months.
- Coprescribing with other drugs aimed at weight reduction is not recommended.

Inner tube

In adjustable gastric banding, a silicone rubber band is placed around the upper portion of the stomach, creating a small pouch with a narrow opening into the larger portion of the stomach. The band can be inflated or deflated

Surgical weight-loss procedures

Two types of surgical procedures promote weight loss: restrictive and combination malabsorptive/restrictive procedures.

Restrictive procedures

Adjustable gastric banding

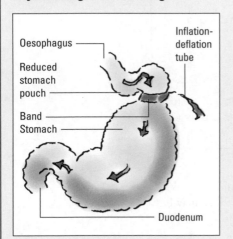

Oesophagus

Reduced stomach pouch

Band

Stomach

Inflation-deflation tube

Duodenum

Vertical banded gastroplasty

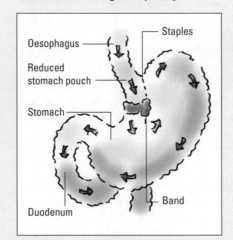

Oesophagus

Reduced stomach pouch

Stomach

Duodenum

Staples

Band

Malabsorptive procedures

Gastric bypass

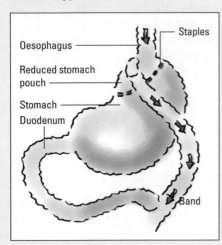

Oesophagus

Reduced stomach pouch

Stomach

Duodenum

Staples

Band

Biliopancreatic diversion

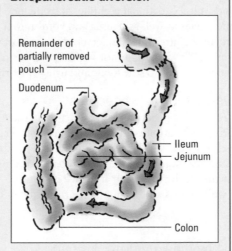

Remainder of partially removed pouch

Duodenum

Ileum
Jejunum

Colon

(continued)

Surgical weight-loss procedures (continued)

NICE guidance on surgical procedures for the management of obesity

Surgery is considered for people with severe obesity if:

- they have a BMI of 40 kg/m² or more, or between 35 and 40 kg/m², and other significant disease (for example type 2 diabetes or high blood pressure) that could be improved if they lost weight
- all appropriate nonsurgical measures have failed to achieve or maintain adequate clinically beneficial weight loss for at least 6 months
- they are receiving or will receive intensive specialist management
- they are generally fit for anaesthesia and surgery
- they commit to the need for long-term follow-up

Consider surgery as a first-line option for adults with a BMI of more than 50 kg/m² in whom surgical intervention is considered appropriate. If waiting time for the procedure is long consider orlistat or sibutramine before surgery.

---

with saline solution through a tube attached to an access port under the skin, allowing the size of stomach opening to be adjusted. This procedure may be performed laparoscopically.

Chew on these complications

Complications of gastric restriction may include bursting of the staples if too much food or liquid is consumed before the staple line heals and obstruction if food isn't chewed well. Nutritional complications include hypoalbuminaemia and vitamin deficiencies as well as nausea and vomiting. A patient undergoing restrictive gastric procedures must understand the importance of eating small meals, eating slowly, chewing food thoroughly, progressing the diet gradually from liquid to pureed foods to soft foods and using nutritional supplements.

Malabsorptive/restrictive procedures

Malabsorptive/restrictive procedures reduce stomach size as well as the number of calories and nutrients the body can absorb. Rapid dumping of food from the stomach into the small intestine limits calorie absorption, leading to weight loss. Nausea, diarrhoea and abdominal cramping may occur after this surgery, but these adverse effects improve over time. These procedures produce better weight-loss and maintenance results than gastric restriction.

Two for the road

Two types of malabsorptive/restrictive procedures are:
- gastric bypass—also known as *Roux-en-Y gastric bypass*, this procedure combines gastric restriction with a bypass of the duodenum and the first portion of the jejunum. It's the most commonly performed surgical weight-loss procedure and is recommended for long-term weight loss.

- biliopancreatic diversion—this is a more complicated surgery in which the lower part of the stomach is removed and the remaining pouch is connected to the terminal segment of the small intestine, thus bypassing the duodenum and jejunum. This surgery isn't commonly used because it can lead to nutritional deficiencies. Patients who have undergone biliopancreatic diversion must take fat-soluble vitamin (A, D, E and K) supplements. In a modified version of the procedure, a larger portion of the stomach and pyloric valve are in place, allowing control of the movement of stomach contents into the duodenum. With this variation, the patient can eat more food than following other procedures.

A look at eating disorders

Eating disorders are considered to be a psychological disorder with nutritional consequences. Eating disorders aren't a new problem; anorexia has its roots as far back as the 13th century, and bulimia dates as far back as 700 BC. Binge eating disorder was first discussed in the literature in 1959. Eating disorders usually occur before or after the onset of puberty, following a period of dieting or after other major personal stressors, such as a parent's divorce, a broken relationship or a death in the family. Dancers and gymnasts are prone to eating disorders and commonly control their eating to improve their performance.

Dancers and gymnasts are prone to eating disorders.

Added risks

Between 90% and 95% of cases of anorexia and bulimia occur in females. These eating disorders are most likely to occur between ages 12 and 13 and between ages 19 and 20. Binge eating is slightly more common in women than in men, and most people with this eating disorder are overweight or obese. Women with eating disorders also have a higher incidence of drug and alcohol abuse. People with eating disorders are more affected by depression, irritability, suicidal tendencies and passiveness, and they exhibit more health risk behaviours, such as tobacco, alcohol and marijuana use, delinquency, unprotected sex and suicide attempts.

Types of eating disorders

Three common eating disorders are anorexia nervosa, bulimia nervosa and atypical eating disorders including binge eating disorder.

Anorexia nervosa

The main characteristic of anorexia nervosa is self-imposed fasting or dieting with severe weight loss or maintenance of a weight that's 15% below the recommended weight. Other characteristics of anorexia include compulsive exercise habits and laxative or diuretic use. In most cases, an anorexic patient is overly preoccupied with food and weight and perceives themself as fat.

If left untreated, anorexia can lead to severe malnutrition, brain damage, sterility, damage to vital organs, heart failure and death.

Bulimia nervosa

Bulimia nervosa is a disorder characterised by episodes of recurrent binge–purge cycles. During binges, the patient eats large amounts of food compulsively and quickly. Weight is controlled through vomiting, emetics, laxatives, diuretics and diet pills.

The bulimic patient typically is of normal or above-normal body weight and has weight fluctuations. Because in most cases the undernutrition is less severe than that in a patient with anorexia, a bulimic patient may experience fewer medical complications. The most frequent cause of death for those with bulimia is gastric dilation and rupture.

Binge eating disorder

Binge eating disorder is a recently described condition and is listed under conditions known as atypical eating disorders. People with binge eating disorder eat very large amounts of food and feel that their eating is out of control. During a binge episode, the binge eating patient may eat faster than usual, eat until he or she feels overly full and consume vast quantities of food even if he or she's not feeling hungry. The binge eating patient may also eat alone if he or she's embarrassed about the large quantity of food being consumed. Following a binge episode, the patient may feel repulsed, depressed or guilty over his or her behaviour. Unlike the bulimic patient, the patient with binge eating disorder doesn't engage in purging, fasting or strenuous exercise after binging.

Assessment data

Assessing a patient for an eating disorder includes collecting historical data and performing a physical examination. (See also *Personal characteristics associated with eating disorders*.)

Historical data

During the health history, ask your patient about:
- current weight (it is important that weight is not made an issue and local protocol will guide you to the information required about weight and weight loss)
- complaints of fatigue, tooth sensitivity, intolerance to cold or dizziness
- abdominal complaints, such as constipation, indigestion and nausea
- regularity or absence of menses
- history or current practice of self-induced vomiting
- use of laxatives, diet pills or diuretics
- usual 24-hour food intake, including which foods are best or least tolerated
- use of vitamin, mineral and other nutritional supplements as well as over-the-counter and prescription drugs
- significant medical history as well as history of drug or alcohol abuse

Personal characteristics associated with eating disorders

Eating disorders are most common among young girls with low self-esteem but can occur at any age and are not exclusively associated with women. Other associated personal characteristics vary by disorder, as listed below.

Anorexia

- perfectionism
- concern with pleasing others
- lack of maturity
- family emphasis on high achievement
- history of bulimia

Bulimia

- difficulty controlling impulses, stress and anxiety
- pattern of hiding binge and purge cycles from family
- history of anorexia

Binge eating disorder

- tendency to eat quickly, eat until uncomfortably full, eat when not hungry and eat alone
- history of depression
- difficulty controlling impulses and stress
- difficulty expressing feelings
- family history of eating disorders

- psychosocial aspects, such as family or significant other support, emotional state and body image
- physical activity patterns.

Focusing in on food

Assess cultural, ethnic or religious influences on food intake as well as abnormal food-eating practices, such as cutting food into tiny pieces, refusing high-calorie foods, disposing of food secretly and bingeing and purging.

Physical findings

Anorexia and bulimia typically present with different signs and symptoms. Signs and symptoms of binge eating may not be as apparent.

Signs and symptoms of anorexia

Signs and symptoms of anorexia include:
- wasted appearance-weight is maintained at least 15% below that expected; in adults BMI is below 17.5 kg/m^2

- thinning hair or alopecia
- dry skin and brittle nails
- decreased heart rate or low blood pressure
- constipation
- cessation of menses—amenorrhoea
- reduced muscle mass and joint swelling
- erosion of tooth enamel.

Signs and symptoms of bulimia

Signs and symptoms of bulimia include:
- puffy cheeks due to enlarged salivary glands
- No evidence of weight loss
- evidence of self-harm
- broken blood vessels in eyes
- scars on hands (from tooth injury during self-induced vomiting).

Signs and symptoms of binge eating

Signs and symptoms of binge eating include:
- normal weight or overweight with weight fluctuations
- probability of having suffered anorexia nervosa or bulimia nervosa in the past
- fatigue
- hypertension
- joint pain.

Causes

Although eating disorders don't have an exact cause, many patients with eating disorders share common characteristics that may influence the development of the disease, including low self-esteem, feelings of helplessness and fear of becoming fat.

All in the family?

Girls who live in families that place a strong importance on physical attractiveness and weight control are at an increased risk for inappropriate eating behaviours. People who pursue professions that emphasise thinness, such as modelling or dancing, are also more likely to exhibit eating disorders.

Outcomes

Eating disorders can have serious health consequences. These consequences vary by the type of disorder.

Long-term effects of anorexia

Patients with anorexia typically have long-term health problems that result from the disorder. Malnutrition leads to irregular heart rhythms and heart failure as well as osteoporosis (due to a lack of calcium and reduced oestrogen levels). A majority of people with anorexia also experience depression, anxiety, personality disorders and substance abuse problems. About 1 in 10 women with anorexia dies of starvation, cardiac arrest or other complications.

Long-term effects of bulimia

Due to repeated purging, patients with bulimia typically have health problems associated with electrolyte imbalances and loss of potassium, such as damage to the heart muscle and an increased risk of cardiac arrest. Excessive vomiting also causes oesophageal inflammation. Patients with bulimia are also susceptible to drug addiction, obsessive–compulsive disorder, clinical depression and anxiety.

Long-term effects of binge eating disorder

The weight gain associated with binge eating disorder can produce health problems including type 2 diabetes, hypertension, high blood cholesterol levels, gall bladder disease, heart disease and certain types of cancer. Patients with binge eating may also have sleep disturbances, depression, alcohol abuse and suicidal thoughts.

Treatment

There are no universally accepted treatment plans for anorexia, bulimia or binge eating. An individualised multidisciplinary approach involving dietitians, mental health professionals and medical doctors (such as an endocrinologist) is most likely to be effective. People with anorexia nervosa requiring inpatient treatment should be admitted to a setting that can provide the skilled implementation of refeeding with careful physical monitoring (particularly in the first few days of refeeding) and in combination with psychosocial interventions. The great majority of patients with bulimia nervosa can be treated as outpatients. There is a very limited role for the inpatient treatment of bulimia nervosa. This is primarily concerned with the management of suicide risk or severe self-harm. In the absence of evidence to guide the management of atypical eating disorders (eating disorders not otherwise specified) other than binge eating disorder, it is recommended that the clinician considers following the guidance on the treatment of the eating problem that most closely resembles the individual patient's eating disorder.

Various types of therapy can be used, such as behaviour modification, family and group therapy and nutrition counselling. Antidepressants may also be helpful. Typically, eating disorders are treated on an outpatient basis; severe cases may require hospitalisation.

Nutrition therapy for patients with anorexia

The goals of nutrition therapy for the patient with anorexia are to:
- re-establish normal eating behaviours
- restore nutritional status
- maintain reasonable weight.

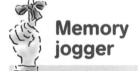

Memory jogger

To remember the goals of nutrition therapy for the patient with anorexia, think of the 3 **Rs**:

Re-establishing normal eating behaviours

Restoring nutritional status

Maintaining **R**easonable weight.

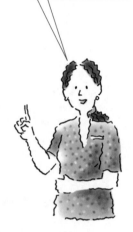

Treatment of an eating disorder includes behaviour modification, therapy and nutrition counselling.

> ### Tips for treating anorexia
>
> To help the patient with anorexia nervosa meet his or her nutritional goals, follow these tips:
>
> - To create a better response to therapy, exclude high-risk binge foods (which vary with each patient) initially but reintroduce them into the eating plan later to prevent fear of that food.
> - Provide small, frequent meals.
> - Provide one-on-one supervision during meals.
> - Whenever possible, give the patient control over food choices.
> - Only use tube feeding or total parenteral nutrition if necessary to medically stabilise the patient. Because the patient with anorexia has control issues, using enteral or parenteral nutrition unnecessarily may increase feelings of mistrust and body-image distortion and may make the individual feel a loss of control and identity.

Patient participation

Involving the patient in the planning of weight goals is imperative for patient cooperation and feelings of trust. (See *Tips for treating anorexia*.)

Keep in mind the following tips when preparing an eating plan for the anorexic patient:

- Be reasonable with calories, about 1,500 kcal/day. (Larger amounts of calories may be tolerated poorly.) In some patients, you may need to start at a lower calorie level and increase by 200 kcal/week.
- Include small, frequent meals and snacks.
- Gradually increase calories, after the patient can tolerate a full meal.
- Limit gas-producing and high-fat foods.
- Include meals based on the patient's food preferences.
- Include nutritionally dense foods to meet caloric goals.
- Include high-fibre or low-sodium foods to control constipation and fluid retention.
- Include multivitamin and mineral supplements.
- Avoid caffeine.
- Use enteral support only if necessary.

Nutrition therapy for patients with bulimia

Goals for nutrition therapy for the patient with bulimia are to:
- identify food fears
- correct food misinformation
- re-establish normal eating patterns.

Promoting compliance

A style of empathetic engagement is helpful in addressing patients with an eating disorder and has an important bearing on treatment outcomes. Although considerable attention may be necessary to address physical complications of eating disorders, these interventions need to be supported by psychological therapies. To promote patient compliance with dietary management initially, a forceful approach may be needed. Eating plans similar to those used for patients with diabetes can be used to specify meal portions, food groups and the frequency of eating. Encourage the patient with bulimia to keep a food diary, recording intake before each meal, to help control the amount he or she eats. (See *Tips for treating bulimia*.)

Meal planning for the patient with bulimia should:
- be at least 1,500 kcal/day, including snacks
- include fat, which helps delay gastric emptying and promotes satiety
- avoid large amounts of food eaten in a short amount of time
- introduce forbidden foods as appropriate.

Nutrition therapy for patients with binge eating disorder

Nutrition therapy for the patient with binge eating disorder focuses on changing unhealthy eating habits and achieving and maintaining a reasonable weight. To promote weight loss and healthy eating behaviours, nutritional interventions for the patient with binge eating disorder are similar to those for bulimia. Research is being conducted to evaluate the effectiveness of nutritional interventions. The binge eating patient who is mildly obese or not overweight doesn't need to diet since a stringent diet may aggravate binge eating.

Teaching points

Promoting self-esteem in patients with eating disorders is important for positive treatment results. This can be done by fostering decision-making, providing encouragement and support, offering choices and using a positive approach throughout all areas. Help the patient eliminate his or her preoccupation with food and avoid preaching of rules.

Syllabus

Teach your patients with an eating disorder:
- the components of a healthy diet
- appropriate food intake patterns
- the dangers of dieting, bingeing and purging
- how to recognise hunger and satiety
- how to identify food- and weight-related behaviours in themselves
- how the idealisation of thinness in our society has resulted in distorted body images and unrealistic goals for beauty.

Prevention

Prevention is accomplished by early detection and treatment.

Tips for treating bulimia

To help the patient with bulimia reach nutritional goals, encourage him or her to:

- sit down during each meal to increase awareness of eating and satiety
- eat meals slowly (at least 20 minutes) without distraction (such as television)
- use appropriate-sized utensils
- refrain from skipping meals or eating snacks.

When minor relapses occur, help the patient resume the structured eating plan immediately.

Get to them early

Because attitudes that influence the development of eating disorders develop early, prevention needs to begin early. Parents and teachers can follow these steps to help prevent the formation of eating disorders:
- Help children develop a positive self-image and sense of worth.
- Avoid pressuring children to excel beyond their capabilities.
- Recognise stressors and provide encouragement and support.
- Teach how good nutrition and exercise can keep you healthy.
- Give children the correct amount of independence, responsibility and accountability for their age group.
- Discourage dieting. If a child is overweight, discuss this with the health visitor, school nurse or general practitioner before restricting dietary intake.
- Seek professional help if a child has the signs and symptoms of an eating disorder.

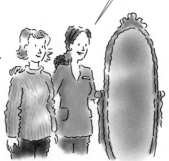

One of the most important things you can do for your patient is promote his or her self-esteem.

Quick quiz

1. Which of the following signs or symptoms doesn't indicate anorexia?
   A. Decreased heart rate and blood pressure
   B. Constipation and diarrhoea
   C. Puffy cheeks
   D. Severe weight loss, under 15% ideal body weight

Answer: C. Puffy cheeks are a sign of bulimia.

2. The need for weight loss is determined by:
   A. BMI, waist circumference and risk factors
   B. risk factors, weight and eating patterns
   C. waist circumference, weight and motivation
   D. physical activity level, BMI and risk factors

Answer: A. The need for weight loss is determined by BMI, waist circumference and risk factors.

3. The three major components of weight-loss therapy are:
   A. medications, exercise and diet therapy
   B. diet therapy, increased physical activity and behavioural therapy
   C. diet therapy, medications and surgery
   D. behavioural therapy, increased exercise and surgery

Answer: B. Diet therapy, increased physical activity and behavioural therapy are the major components of weight-loss therapy.

4. Which of the following changes is a benefit of weight loss?
   A. Lower HDL levels
   B. Higher LDL levels
   C. Increased blood pressure
   D. Reduced risk of diabetes and cardiovascular disease

Answer: D. Benefits of weight loss include higher HDL levels, decreased blood pressure and a reduced risk of diabetes and cardiovascular disease.

Scoring

☆☆☆ If you answered all four questions correctly, congratulations are in order! You've distinguished yourself when it comes to understanding eating disorders.

☆☆ If you answered three questions correctly, great! Your intake of knowledge is sure to help your brain stay properly nourished.

☆ If you answered fewer than three questions correctly, don't worry! The next chapter offers another chance to fuel up on nutritional info.

12 GI disorders

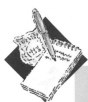

Just the facts

Nutritional support is a major component of care for patients with GI disorders. In this chapter, you'll learn:

- ♦ pathophysiology and treatment of common GI disorders
- ♦ effects of GI system malfunctions on nutritional status
- ♦ nutrition-based preventive and treatment measures for patients with common GI disorders.

A look at GI disorders

The digestive system, which is composed of the GI tract and accessory glands and organs, acts as the body's food-processing complex. It performs the critical task of supplying the essential nutrients that fuel other organs and body systems. A malfunction in the digestive system can have far-reaching metabolic effects, which can become life-threatening.

When the GI tract malfunctions, nutrition support is usually a major component of the treatment plan. That's because, in many cases, the effects of a disorder interfere with the body's ability to obtain nutrients or to use them appropriately. Therefore, nutrition support is used to control the disorder or to prevent or lessen the symptoms associated with it.

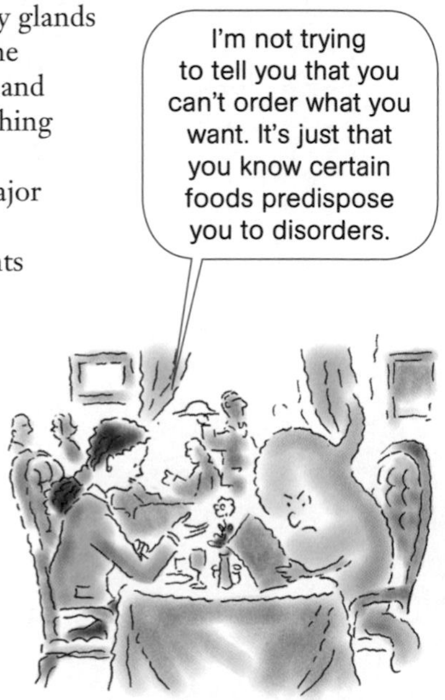
I'm not trying to tell you that you can't order what you want. It's just that you know certain foods predispose you to disorders.

Assessment

As for any disorder, a focused assessment—including a health history, a physical examination and diagnostic tests—is necessary to help confirm the presence of a GI disorder and to develop an appropriate care plan.

Health history

If you suspect your patient has a GI disorder, ask them about their major complaint. Be alert for such complaints as pain, heartburn, nausea, vomiting and a change in bowel habits—these signs and symptoms are commonly associated with GI problems. If the patient reports one of these problems, be sure to question him or her about:

- its onset, duration and severity
- measures used to treat or control it
- effectiveness of measures taken.

To determine if the patient's problem is new or recurring, ask him or her about past GI illnesses, such as ulcers, gall bladder or liver disease and GI bleeding. Also inquire about a history of surgery or trauma, especially any involving the abdomen.

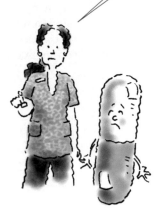

Be sure to ask your patient about recent drug use because many medications can cause adverse GI effects, such as nausea, vomiting, diarrhoea and constipation.

Current events

Follow up with questions about the patient's current health status. Be sure to inquire about medications—prescription and over the counter (including herbal preparations)—the patient is using or has used recently. Several medications, such as aspirin, sulphonamides, nonsteroidal anti-inflammatory drugs (NSAIDs) and some antihypertensive medications, can cause nausea, vomiting, diarrhoea, constipation and other GI signs and symptoms. Herbal preparations, such as ginkgo biloba and ginger, can cause stomach irritation. Also ask about the use of stool softeners, laxatives or enemas because habitual use can lead to constipation or diarrhoea.

Ask the patient if he or she's allergic to any medications or foods. Such allergies commonly cause GI problems. In addition, ask the patient about changes in appetite; difficulty chewing, eating or swallowing; and changes in bowel habits. For example has the patient noticed any changes in the colour, amount or appearance of his or her stool? Has he or she noticed any blood?

Unwanted souvenirs

Don't forget to question the patient about recent travel, especially travel to rural areas or foreign countries, because GI disorders may result from consumption of contaminated water or food.

A day in the life

Because GI function and nutrition are so closely intertwined, ask the patient to describe their typical day to provide clues about their routine activity level and eating habits. Ask them to recount what and how much they ate the previous day, how the food was cooked and who cooked it. This information not only tells you about the patient's usual intake but also gives you clues about food preferences and eating patterns as well as the patient's memory and mental status.

Family matters

Ask the patient about his or her family's health. Some GI diseases and disorders show a familial tendency or are hereditary. Disorders with a familial link include:
- ulcerative colitis
- stomach ulcers
- Crohn's disease
- coeliac disease.

Inquire about the patient's psychosocial status, including his or her occupation, home life, family and financial situation, stress level and recent life changes. Studies show that stress threatens a person's emotional and physical well-being, increasing metabolism, catabolism and the body's need for calories. Also ask about alcohol, caffeine and tobacco use as well as food consumption, exercise habits and oral hygiene.

As you proceed through the history, attempt to determine the patient's attitude and willingness to change if dietary modifications become necessary. In addition, be alert for information that might help you identify positive and negative effects that dietary interventions may have on the patient.

In conclusion...

Conclude the health history by conducting a review of body systems to gain further information for clues to the patient's problem.

Physical examination

Begin the physical examination by obtaining the patient's height and weight to calculate BMI. These findings can also be compared to a standardised height and weight table. Note any recent changes in weight.

Assessing the accessories

Increasingly, health care professionals may need to complete a physical assessment. Assess the patient's mouth, abdomen and rectum:
- Inspect the patient's mouth, noting any problems with the teeth, gums or tongue and any unusual breath odour. Then inspect the pharynx for abnormalities, lesions or exudates.
- Inspect the abdomen, noting symmetry, shape, contour and skin appearance. Check for any bulges or masses. Observe for abdominal movements and pulsations. Peristaltic waves aren't usually visible; visible rippling waves may indicate a bowel obstruction. Also, measure the patient's abdominal girth.
- Auscultate (listen using a stethoscope) the abdomen, noting the presence of bowel sounds—high-pitched, gurgling noises that occur intermittently from 5 to 34 times/min. Hyperactive sounds (loud, high-pitched, tinkling sounds that occur frequently) may be caused by diarrhoea, constipation or laxative use. Conversely, hypoactive sounds are heard infrequently and indicate diminished peristalsis.

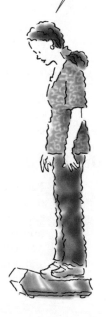

Begin your physical examination by obtaining the patient's height and weight.

- Percuss the abdomen to detect the size and location of the abdominal organs and to detect air or fluid in the abdomen, stomach or bowel. Remember that hollow organs, such as an empty stomach or bowel, should sound like a drum beating on percussion. This sound is called *tympany*. Dullness is typically heard when solid organs such as the liver are percussed. Also expect to hear dullness when the intestines are filled with faeces.
- Palpate the abdomen to determine the size, shape, position and tenderness of the major abdominal organs (including the liver) and to detect masses and fluid accumulation. Palpate all four quadrants, leaving painful and tender areas for last. After palpation, check for rebound tenderness.
- Use percussion to help estimate the size of the liver. Liver enlargement is commonly associated with such diseases as hepatitis.
- Inspect the perianal area, noting scars, fissures, discharge or haemorrhoids.
- Palpate the rectum using a lubricated, gloved finger. The rectal walls should feel soft and smooth, without masses, faecal impaction or tenderness. After palpating the rectum, test any stool adhering to the gloved finger for occult blood.

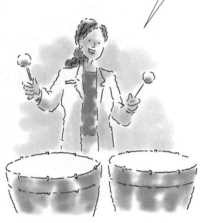

Listen to the music! The drum-beating sound of tympany is normal over a hollow organ.

Diagnostic tests

Numerous diagnostic tests may be performed for patients with GI disorders or in cases in which GI disorders are suspected. These tests may include:
- x-rays—flat plate of the abdomen, barium swallow, upper GI series, small-bowel series, barium enema and cholecystography
- ultrasound—abdominal ultrasound and ultrasound of the gall bladder
- endoscopy—upper GI endoscopy (oesophagogastroduodenoscopy), sigmoidoscopy and colonoscopy
- computed tomography scan of the abdomen
- magnetic resonance imaging of the abdomen
- GI motility studies
- stool testing—for example for occult blood, faecal urobilinogen, ova and parasites, and nitrogen.

Getting specific

In addition, specific laboratory tests are used to help diagnose GI disorders. Some of these tests can provide information about the effect of the disorder on the patient's nutrition. Common laboratory tests may include:
- haemoglobin level
- haematocrit
- serum albumin
- serum transferrin
- liver function studies
- 24-hour urine for nitrogen balance.

Dysphagia

Dysphagia, or difficulty swallowing, is one of the most common problems associated with the oesophagus. One possible cause is a mechanical obstruction, such as from a bolus of food, inflammation, a tumour, oedema or surgery of the throat. Another possible cause is interference in oesophageal motility caused by another disorder—for example a neurologic disorder such as myasthenia gravis, amyotrophic lateral sclerosis or stroke. Regardless of cause, dysphagia can severely impact the patient's nutritional intake and status as well as increase the risk of aspiration.

Pathophysiology

In preparation for swallowing, a person chews food after it's ingested. Gradually, this bolus of food is pushed towards the back of the mouth. Normally, when food reaches the back of the mouth, the receptors that surround the pharynx are stimulated and transmit impulses to the brain via the sensory portion of cranial nerves V (trigeminal) and IX (glossopharyngeal). The brain's swallowing centre is activated and relays motor impulses to the oesophagus via V, IX, X (vagus) and XII (hypoglossal). The bolus moves towards and into the oesophagus. Peristaltic movements carry the bolus through the oesophagus and to the stomach.

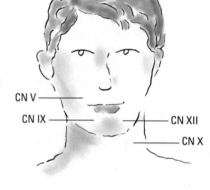

Appetite for obstruction

For the patient with dysphagia, this sequence of events becomes impaired. When a mechanical obstruction is present, although the impulses for swallowing are still at work, the obstruction physically blocks or narrows the passageway, making swallowing painful and difficult.

Obstructions can be intrinsic or extrinsic:
• *Intrinsic* obstructions originate in the oesophagus itself and can result from tumours, strictures and herniations.
• *Extrinsic* obstructions originate outside of the oesophagus, for example from a tumour or oedema due to surgery. With this type of obstruction, the lumen becomes narrowed due to pressure exerted on the oesophageal wall.

For the patient with a neural or muscular disorder, voluntary swallowing (from the time the food enters the mouth until it enters the oesophagus) and peristalsis become impaired as the upper oesophageal striated muscles malfunction. This type of dysphagia is called *functional dysphagia*.

What to look for

Patient complaints associated with dysphagia range from discomfort (feeling of something stuck in the throat) to severe acute pain on swallowing. Pain is most commonly due to distension and spasm at the site of the obstruction.

If the obstruction is in the upper oesophagus, pain typically occurs 2 to 4 seconds after swallowing. If the obstruction is in the lower oesophagus, pain commonly occurs 10 to 15 seconds after swallowing. If a tumour is present, dysphagia begins with difficulty swallowing solids, eventually progressing to difficulty swallowing semi-solid foods and liquids. If motor function is impaired, the patient reports difficulty swallowing liquids and solids.

Also be alert for these additional signs and symptoms:
- difficulty articulating words
- facial drooping
- drooling
- decreased gag reflex
- coughing or choking during or after meals
- gurgling voice
- pocketing of food in the mouth (such as in the cheeks).

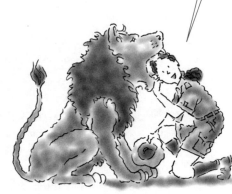

A patient with dysphagia may feel as if something is stuck in his or her throat.

Picking up the pieces

Note if a patient identifies specific foods that he or she prefers or avoids as a result of his or her discomfort. Some foods may be easier to swallow (for example thickened semi-solid foods), whereas such foods as meats may cause problems for the patient. The patient's nutritional status may suffer as a result of these self-imposed restrictions.

How it's treated

Treatment of dysphagia caused by obstruction focuses on removing or minimising the cause of the obstruction, if possible, thereby allowing a more open and free passageway for food. For example oesophageal dilatation may be performed to stretch the narrowed area of the oesophagus, or surgery may be necessary to remove a tumour or strictures. It is important to refer to a speech and language therapist (SALT) to complete a swallowing assessment and to provide therapeutic measures for dysphagia due to neurologic causes.

Dietary management

Nutrition is an important component of treatment for the patient with dysphagia because the difficulty encountered with swallowing commonly affects the types and amounts of food the patient consumes. Because the patient with dysphagia is at risk for aspiration, a SALT can recommend the types and consistency of foods that would be most appropriate and safe for the patient. (See *Dysphagia diets*, page 210.)

High-risk foods

Some foods are considered to be high risk for people with swallowing difficulties and should be avoided. They include:
- stringy, fibrous texture, e.g. pineapple, runner beans, celery and lettuce
- vegetable and fruit skins including beans, e.g. broad beans, soya beans; black-eyed peas and grapes

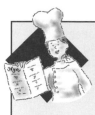

Menu maven

Dysphagia diets

Typically, a patient with dysphagia undergoes diagnostic testing to determine the underlying cause. In addition, a speech therapist is consulted to assist with a complete swallowing assessment and to provide recommendations for an appropriate diet.

Keep in mind that commercial thickeners are available for use by the patient at home.

Texture	Description of fluid texture	Fluid example
Thin fluid	Still water	Water, tea, coffee without milk, diluted squash, spirits and wine
Naturally thick fluid	Product leaves a coating on an empty glass	Full-cream milk, Complan, Build Up and commercial sip feeds
Thickened fluid	Fluid to which a commercial thickener has been added to thicken consistency • stage 1—can be drunk through a straw; leaves thin coat on the back of a spoon • stage 2—cannot be drunk through a straw; leaves a thick coat on the back of a spoon • stage 3—cannot be drunk through a straw or from a cup; needs to be taken with a spoon	Following manufacturer's guidelines, consistencies can be achieved by adding correct amounts to thin fluids
A	• smooth, pouring and uniform consistency • has been pureed and sieved to remove particles • cannot be eaten with a fork	Tinned tomato soup Thin custard
B	• smooth, pouring and uniform consistency • has been pureed and sieved to remove particles • cannot be eaten with a fork • drops rather than pours from a spoon • thicker than A	Soft whipped cream Thick custard
C	• smooth, pouring and uniform consistency • has been pureed and sieved to remove particles • can be eaten with a fork or spoon • will hold their own shape on a plate • no chewing required	Mousse Smooth fromage frais
D	• moist, with some variation in texture • has not been pureed or sieved • may be served with thick gravy or sauce • can be easily mashed • requires very little chewing	Flaked fish in thick sauce Stewed apple and thick custard
E	• dishes consisting of soft, moist food • can be broken into pieces with a fork • dishes can be made up of solids and thick sauces	Tender meat casseroles (approximately 1.5 cm diced pieces) Sponge and custard
Normal	• any foods	Includes high-risk foods

- mixed consistency foods, e.g. cereals which do not blend with milk, such as muesli, mince with thin gravy and soup with lumps
- crunchy foods, e.g. toast, flaky pastry, dry biscuits and crisps
- crumbly items, e.g. bread crusts, pie crusts, crumble and dry biscuits
- hard foods, e.g. boiled and chewy sweets and toffees, nuts and seeds
- husks, e.g. sweetcorn and granary bread.

In addition to dietary recommendations, other interventions that can help ensure adequate intake include:

- providing mouth care immediately before meals to help improve taste
- ensuring adequate rest before meals to prevent fatigue from interfering with eating
- providing small, frequent meals to prevent fatigue while maximising intake
- placing the patient in semi-Fowler's to high-Fowler's position and having them tilt their head forward to help ease swallowing
- minimising or eliminating distractions so that the patient can focus his or her full attention on eating and swallowing
- using adaptive devices as necessary, such as mugs with spouts; avoiding the use of straws (can cause more liquid to flow into the mouth than the patient can handle, increasing the risk of aspiration)
- encouraging small bites and thorough chewing if solid consistencies allowed
- offering praise and encouragement during mealtimes
- providing foods that are cool or mildly warm to stimulate the swallowing reflex
- adding flavour as necessary to stimulate salivation, helping to moisten food
- helping the patient select nutritionally dense foods.

Keep in mind that enteral feeding may be necessary if the patient still can't meet his or her nutritional requirements with these modifications.

Gastro-oesophageal reflux disease

Popularly known as *heartburn*, gastro-oesophageal reflux disease (GORD) refers to backflow of gastric contents or duodenal contents or both into the oesophagus and past the lower oesophageal sphincter (LES), without associated belching or vomiting. The reflux of gastric contents causes acute epigastric pain, usually after a meal.

Causes of GORD include:

- weakened oesophageal sphincter
- increased abdominal pressure such as with obesity or pregnancy
- hiatus hernia
- nasogastric intubation for longer than 4 days.

In addition, medications, such as morphine, diazepam, calcium channel blockers, meperidine and anticholinergic agents; food; alcohol and cigarettes may cause LES pressure to be decreased, resulting in GORD.

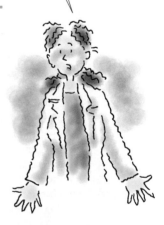

My GORD! Causes of gastro-oesophageal reflux disease include weakened oesophageal sphincter, increased abdominal pressure and hiatus hernia.

Pathophysiology

Normally, gastric contents don't back up into the oesophagus because the LES creates enough pressure around the lower end of the oesophagus to close it. Typically, the sphincter relaxes after each swallow to allow food to enter the stomach. In GORD, the sphincter doesn't remain closed—because either LES pressure is deficient or pressure within the stomach exceeds LES pressure. As a result, the normally contracted LES relaxes inappropriately and allows gastric acid or bile secretions to reflux into the lower oesophagus, where the reflux irritates and inflames the oesophageal mucosa. The high acidity of the stomach contents causes pain and irritation.

What to look for

Typically, the patient complains of burning epigastric pain that worsens with vigorous exercise, bending or lying down. Pain also may radiate to the arms and chest. The patient may report that antacids or sitting upright relieves the pain. He or she may also describe a feeling of warm fluid travelling up the throat followed by a sour or bitter taste in the mouth due to hypersecretion of saliva.

Additional signs and symptoms may include:
• odynophagia (acute pain on swallowing), possibly followed by a dull substernal ache (suggestive of severe, long-term reflux dysphagia from oesophageal spasm, stricture or oesophagitis)
• bright-red or dark-brown blood in vomitus
• chronic pain that mimics angina
• nocturnal salivation that awakens the patient with coughing, choking and a mouthful of saliva (rare).

How it's treated

Effective treatment of GORD focuses on relieving the symptoms by reducing reflux through gravity, strengthening the LES with drug therapy, neutralising gastric contents and reducing intra-abdominal pressure. The patient should be instructed to sit up during and after meals and to sleep with the head of the bed elevated. Doing this helps to reduce intra-abdominal pressure and prevent reflux.

In addition, numerous medications may be ordered, including:
• antacids to neutralise the acidic content of the stomach and minimise irritation
• histamine-2 (H_2) receptor antagonists to inhibit gastric acid secretion
• proton pump inhibitors to reduce gastric acidity.

Surgery is typically reserved for the patient who doesn't respond to treatment or develops a serious complication, such as pulmonary aspiration, haemorrhage or oesophageal obstruction or perforation. Fundoplication, which may be performed laparoscopically, involves wrapping part of the fundus around the oesophageal sphincter to strengthen the LES.

Dietary management

Nutrition is an important component of the treatment plan for patients with GORD. In mild cases, diet may reduce the symptoms enough that no other treatment is required. Typically, diet involves the use of small, frequent meals, focusing on avoiding foods that decrease LES pressure. (See *Under pressure*). If the patient is obese, a weight-reduction diet is necessary.

The patient should refrain from eating before going to bed to reduce abdominal pressure and reflux. Substances that stimulate gastric acid secretion, such as coffee, caffeine, alcohol and nicotine, should be avoided. If the patient avoids citrus products, such as orange juice, make sure he or she consumes other sources of vitamin C, such as strawberries, broccoli and other green vegetables, to prevent deficiency.

Peptic ulcer disease

A peptic ulcer is a circumscribed lesion in the mucosal membrane of the upper GI tract. Peptic ulcers can develop in the lower oesophagus, stomach, duodenum or jejunum. (See *A close look at peptic ulcers*, page 214.)

Pathophysiology

There are two major forms of peptic ulcer, both of which are chronic conditions:

 duodenal

 gastric.

Upsetting the up-side

Duodenal ulcers affect the upper part of the small intestine. This type of ulcer accounts for about 80% of peptic ulcers, occurs mostly in men between ages 20 and 50 and follows a chronic course of remission and exacerbation. Between 5% and 10% of patients with duodenal ulcers develop complications that make surgery necessary. Duodenal ulcers are small (less than 1 cm in diameter), sharply demarcated and usually deeper than gastric ulcers. These ulcers usually don't become malignant.

Mucosa corrosion

Gastric ulcers affect the stomach lining (mucosa). They're most common in men aged 50 to 60, especially those who are poor and undernourished. They commonly occur in chronic users of aspirin and alcohol. Gastric ulcers are more likely than duodenal ulcers to become malignant.

Under pressure

Various dietary substances can increase or decrease lower oesophageal sphincter (LES) pressure. Keep them in mind when planning care for the patient with gastro-oesophageal reflux disease (GORD) to reduce the symptoms of the disease.

Increase LES pressure

- protein
- carbohydrate
- nonfat milk.

Decrease LES pressure and likely to aggravate symptoms

- fat
- whole milk
- orange juice
- tomatoes
- chocolate
- nicotine
- alcohol.

A close look at peptic ulcers

This illustration shows different degrees of peptic ulceration. Lesions that don't extend below the mucosal lining (epithelium) are called erosions. Lesions of acute and chronic ulcers can extend through the epithelium and may perforate the stomach wall. Chronic ulcers also have scar tissue at the base.

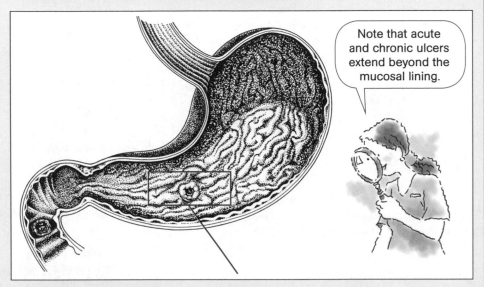

Note that acute and chronic ulcers extend beyond the mucosal lining.

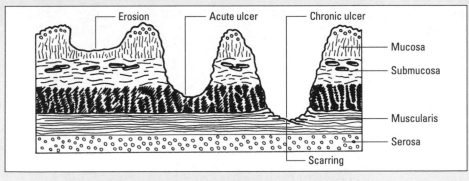

Erosion   Acute ulcer   Chronic ulcer

Mucosa

Submucosa

Muscularis

Serosa

Scarring

Everything in moderation! Chronic use of alcohol may cause gastric ulcers.

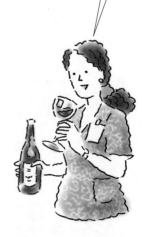

Peptic pep-squad

There are three major causes of peptic ulcers:

bacterial infection with *Helicobacter pylori* (causes 70% to 80% of peptic ulcers)

use of NSAIDs

hypersecretory states such as Zollinger–Ellison syndrome.

Researchers are still discovering the exact mechanisms of ulcer formation; however, predisposing factors include:
- type A blood (gastric ulcers)
- type O blood (duodenal ulcers)
- genetic factors
- exposure to irritants, such as alcohol and tobacco
- trauma
- stress and anxiety
- normal ageing. (See *Ageing and ulcer formation*).

Resistance breaker

In a peptic ulcer caused by *H. pylori*, acid adds to the effects of the bacterial infection. *H. pylori* releases a toxin that destroys the stomach's mucous coating, reducing the epithelium's resistance to acid digestion that causes ulcer disease.

Getting complicated

A possible complication of severe ulceration is erosion of the mucosa. This can cause GI haemorrhage, which can progress to hypovolaemic shock, perforation and obstruction. Obstruction of the pylorus may cause the stomach to distend with food and fluid, block blood flow and cause tissue damage.

Break out

The ulcer crater may extend beyond the duodenal wall into nearby structures, such as the pancreas or liver. This phenomenon, called *penetration*, is a fairly common complication of duodenal ulcers.

What to look for

A patient with a gastric ulcer may report:
- recent loss of weight and appetite
- pain, heartburn or indigestion
- feeling of abdominal fullness or distension
- pain triggered or aggravated by eating.

Painstaking problem

A patient with a duodenal ulcer may describe the pain as sharp, gnawing, burning, boring, aching or hard to define. He or she may liken it to hunger, abdominal pressure or fullness. Typically, pain occurs 90 minutes to 3 hours after eating. However, eating usually reduces the pain, so the patient may report a recent weight gain. The patient may also have pale skin from anaemia caused by blood loss.

How it's treated

Treatment of peptic ulcer disease has changed dramatically over the past few decades. Dietary changes were once the focus. However, treatment

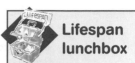

Lifespan lunchbox

Ageing and ulcer formation

In the course of ageing, the pyloric sphincter may wear down. As a result, bile can reflux into the stomach. This appears to be a common contributor to the development of gastric ulcers in the older adult.

now aims to eradicate the *H. pylori* infection. Drug therapy for this may include:

- antibiotics—tetracycline (Tetracyn), amoxicillin (Amoxil) and metronidazole (Flagyl)
- H_2-receptor antagonist—famotidine (Pepcid)
- proton pump inhibitors—omeprazole (Prilosec)
- mucosal protectors—sucralfate (Carafate).

Smoke detector

Cigarette smoking encourages ulcer formation by inhibiting pancreatic secretion of bicarbonate. It also causes acceleration of gastric acid emptying into the duodenum, which promotes mucosal breakdown.

Dietary management

Once a standard, a bland diet consumed in small, frequent meals is no longer recommended for treatment of peptic ulcer disease; research shows that this type of diet is ineffective. Instead, encourage the patient to avoid or limit the intake of foods that cause GI discomfort. Some foods that commonly are irritating include:

- alcohol
- chilli powder
- citric juices
- coffee
- cola
- hot peppers
- pepper
- tea.

In addition, advise the patient to not to eat near to bedtime to avoid dyspepsia during the night. Encourage vitamin C and protein intake to promote healing.

Dumping syndrome

Dumping syndrome occurs after certain types of gastric surgery in which part of the pyloric sphincter, or the entire pyloric sphincter, is removed or bypassed. Without proper sphincter function, food quickly passes from the stomach into the small intestine.

Pathophysiology

When the pyloric sphincter no longer functions, undigested food quickly passes into the small intestine. The presence of undigested food in the intestines raises the osmolarity (concentration of solutes) of the intestines. This increase in osmolarity causes fluid to shift from the bloodstream into the intestines, which dilutes the concentration of the intestines, leading to distension.

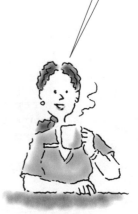

Such drinks as coffee, cola and tea are commonly irritating and should be eliminated from the diet of a patient with peptic ulcer disease.

What to look for

The following symptoms may begin about 2 weeks after surgery and typically occur within 15 to 30 minutes after eating:

- pain
- cramping
- diarrhoea
- physiologic changes brought about by the sudden fluid shift (orthostatic hypotension, tachycardia, dizziness and diaphoresis).

Delayed reaction

A secondary reaction also occurs 2 to 3 hours later. Rapid absorption of carbohydrates causes a rapid rise in blood glucose levels. In response, the body produces excessive amounts of insulin, causing a rapid decrease in blood glucose levels. The rapid decrease in blood glucose level causes:

- dizziness
- nausea
- diaphoresis.

How it's treated

Because the patient is recovering from surgery, food or fluids may be restricted until recovery. The type of surgery involved and local protocol can advise on this. Then, treatment of dumping syndrome focuses primarily on dietary advice. In addition to diet, an antispasmodic may be prescribed to delay gastric emptying.

Dietary management

Once dumping syndrome, or the potential for dumping syndrome, has been identified, the patient should be encouraged to consume small meals and limit the consumption of high-sugar foods and drinks. (See *Serving up an antidumping diet*, page 218.) Encourage the patient to consume five or more small meals per day because the stomach's capacity has been reduced. Commonly fat and protein intake is encouraged because fat is considered isotonic and protein is broken down slowly. As a result, these won't increase the osmolarity of the intestinal contents. However, fat can cause some problems following gastric resection and the registered dietitian can advise on this. Instruct the patient to avoid fluids with meals and 1 hour before or after meals. Explain the importance of lying down for 30 to 60 minutes after meals to delay gastric emptying.

Coeliac disease

Coeliac disease is a digestive disease that damages the small intestines and interferes with absorption of nutrients. People with coeliac disease can't tolerate a protein called *gluten*, which is found in wheat, rye, barley and oats.

Serving up an antidumping diet

After gastric surgery, encourage the patient to adhere to dietary restrictions to successfully combat dumping syndrome. The patient can consume:

- beverages (coffee, tea and artificially sweetened beverages)
- grains and starches (up to five servings of plain breads, crackers, rolls, unsweetened cereal, rice, pasta, corn, peas and potatoes)
- meats
- unsweetened fruit and fruit juices (up to three servings)
- vegetables (unlimited cabbage, celery, cucumbers, lettuce, and radishes; up to 2½ servings of asparagus, beets, broccoli, carrots, cauliflower, aubergines, green pepper, mushrooms, onions, tomatoes and courgette).

Encourage the patient to avoid:

- alcohol
- cereal (sweetened and those containing dried fruit)
- creamed vegetables
- desserts (cakes, biscuits, jelly and ice cream)
- fruit (dried and sweetened)
- milk and milk products (initially)
- sugar and high-sugar foods, such as honey, jam and syrup.

A gluten for punishment

Because the body's own immune system causes the damage, coeliac disease is considered an autoimmune disorder. However, it's also classified as a disease of malabsorption because nutrients aren't absorbed. Coeliac disease is also known as *coeliac sprue*, *nontropical sprue* and *gluten-induced enteropathy*.

Coeliac disease has a genetic link. Sometimes the disease is triggered or becomes active for the first time after surgery, pregnancy, childbirth, viral infection or severe emotional stress.

Pathophysiology

In coeliac disease, ingestion of gluten causes injury to the villi (tiny finger-like protrusions that line the small intestine and are responsible for nutrient absorption) in the small intestine. This leads to decreased surface area and malabsorption of most nutrients. Inflammatory enteritis may also result, leading to osmotic and secretary diarrhoea.

What to look for

Although some people have very vague signs and symptoms, the common signs and symptoms of coeliac disease include:
- recurring abdominal bloating and pain
- chronic diarrhoea
- weight loss

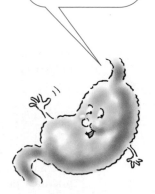

Gluten be gone! For patients with coeliac disease, following a gluten-free diet restores my villi to working order!

- pale, foul-smelling stools
- unexplained anaemia
- flatulence
- bone pain
- behaviour changes
- fatigue
- tooth discoloration.

How it's treated

Dietary intervention is key to treatment of coeliac disease.

Dietary management
The only treatment of coeliac disease is adherence to a gluten-free diet. For most people, following this diet stops symptoms, heals existing intestinal damage and prevents further damage. Improvement can occur within days of starting the diet or can take several weeks. The small intestine is usually healed, meaning the villi are intact and working, in 3 to 6 months. (It may take up to 2 years for older adults.)

Lifetime commitment

The gluten-free diet is a lifetime requirement. Eating any gluten, no matter how small the amount, can damage the intestine. This is true for anyone with coeliac disease, including those who don't have noticeable symptoms. Depending on a person's age at diagnosis, such problems as delayed growth and tooth discoloration may not improve. (See *Coeliac disease and child development*.)

A gluten-free diet requires avoiding foods that contain wheat (including spelt and triticale), rye, barley and oats. This means restrictions on most breads, pasta, cereals and many processed foods. (See *Serving up a gluten-free diet*, page 220.)

Why so glum? Gluten-free isn't so grim!

Despite these restrictions, people with coeliac disease can eat a well-balanced diet with various foods, including bread and pasta. For example instead of wheat flour, people can use potato, rice, soy or bean flour. They can obtain some gluten-free items on prescription or buy gluten-free bread, pasta and other products from supermarkets or special food companies. In addition, plain meat, fish, rice, fruits and vegetables don't contain gluten, so people with coeliac disease can eat as much of these foods as they like.

Are oats okay?

Research is currently under way to determine if patients with coeliac disease can tolerate oats. Some people with the disease can eat oats without reactions. Until studies are complete, however, encourage your patient with coeliac disease to follow his or her doctor's or dietitian's advice about eating oats.

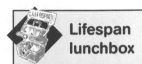

Lifespan lunchbox

Coeliac disease and child development

Some evidence suggests that whether a person was breastfed—and how long the person was breastfed—plays an important role in the development of coeliac disease. The longer a person was breastfed, the later the occurrence is of symptoms of coeliac disease and the more atypical the symptoms are. Other factors that influence coeliac disease development include the age at which a person began eating foods containing gluten and how much gluten is eaten. Gluten-containing foods should not be given to an infant before 6 months of age.

Menu maven

Serving up a gluten-free diet

Here are examples of foods that are allowed—and those that should be avoided—on a gluten-free diet. Note that this isn't a complete list. Encourage the patient and his or her family to discuss gluten-free food choices with the doctor and dietitian. Be sure to explain to your patient the importance of reading all food ingredient lists to make sure that the food doesn't include gluten.

Food groups	Servings	Foods to eat	Foods to avoid
Starch	18 units a month. 1 unit = 1 loaf bread/200 g biscuits/250 g pasta	Breads or bread products made from corn, rice, soy, arrowroot corn or potato starch, pea, potato or whole-bean flour, tapioca, cornmeal, buckwheat, millet, flax, sorghum and quinoa; hot cereals made from soy, brown and white rice; cold cereals such as puffed rice and corn; rice, rice noodles, and pasta made from allowed ingredients	Breads and baked products made with wheat, rye, triticale, barley, oats, wheat germ or bran, graham, gluten or durum flour, farina, bulgur and wheat-based semolina; cereals or pasta made from wheat, triticale, barley and oats and cereals with added malt extract and malt flavourings; most crackers
Vegetables and fruits	Five portions	All plain, fresh, frozen or canned vegetables made with allowed ingredients; all fruits and fruit juices	Creamed or breaded vegetables; canned baked beans; some French fries Some commercial fruit pie fillings and dried fruit
Milk	1,200 ml/day	All milk and milk products except those made with gluten additives; aged cheeses	Some milk drinks; flavoured or frozen yoghurt; malted milk
Meats and beans	Men more than 55 g per day Women no more than 45 g per day	All meat, poultry, fish and shellfish; eggs, dry beans, peanut butter and soybeans; cold cuts, hot dogs or sausage without fillers	Any prepared with wheat, rye, oats, barley, gluten stabilisers or fillers; self-basting turkey; some egg substitutes
Oils and sugar	Eat sparingly	Butter, margarine, salad dressings, sauces, soups and desserts made with allowed ingredients; sugar, honey, jelly, jam, plain chocolate and coconut; pure instant or ground coffee, carbonated drinks and wine.	Commercial salad dressing; prepared soups, condiments, sauces and seasonings prepared with above ingredients; hot cocoa mixes, non-dairy creamers, flavoured instant coffee, herbal teas, alcohol distilled from cereals such as gin, vodka, whiskey and beer; liquorice

What's on the menu
Here's a sample menu for a gluten-free diet.

Breakfast
- 125 ml orange juice
- 100 g rice crispies
- two slices gluten-free bread
- one egg (cooked any way)
- 200 ml milk (preferably low fat or fat free)
- 1 tsp margarine
- 1 tsp jam

Lunch
- tuna salad
- one portion salad greens with 1 tbs of fat-free dressing
- 200 ml milk
- 200 g rice pudding

Snack
- one apple

Dinner
- grilled chicken breast
- baked potato with reduced fat sour cream
- one portion steamed broccoli
- 200 ml milk
- one pear

Detection offers protection

The gluten-free diet is complicated. It requires a completely new approach to eating that affects a person's entire life. Advise a patient with coeliac disease to be extremely careful about what he or she eats in all situations, including what he or she buys for lunch at work, eats at parties and grabs from the refrigerator for a midnight snack. Eating out can also be a challenge. The person with coeliac disease needs to scrutinise the menu for foods with gluten and question the waiter or chef about possible hidden sources of gluten, such as additives, preservatives and stabilisers found in processed food. Medicines and mouthwash may also contain stabilisers. If ingredients aren't itemised, encourage the patient to check with the manufacturer. With practice, screening for gluten becomes second nature.

What if too much damage has occurred?

A very small percentage of people with coeliac disease don't improve on the gluten-free diet because the damage to the intestines is so severe that they can't heal even after eliminating gluten from the diet. There is a slight increase in the risk of bowel cancer in people who have poor compliance with dietary advice.

Lactose intolerance

Lactose intolerance refers to an inability to digest significant amounts of lactose, the predominant sugar in milk. This deficiency results from a shortage of the enzyme lactase, which is usually produced by the cells that line the small intestine.

Pathophysiology

Lactase breaks down milk sugar into simpler forms that can be absorbed into the bloodstream. When there isn't enough lactase to digest the amount of lactose consumed, the results—although not usually dangerous—may be distressing. Although not all people deficient in lactase have symptoms, those who do are considered *lactose intolerant*.

Why the lack of lactase?

Some causes of lactose intolerance are well known. For instance certain digestive diseases and injuries to the small intestine can reduce the amount of enzymes produced. In rare cases, children are born without the ability to produce lactase (primary lactase deficiency). For most people, lactase deficiency develops naturally over time. After about age 2, the body begins to produce less lactase. However, many people may not experience symptoms until they're much older. (See *Ethnicity and lactose intolerance*, page 222.)

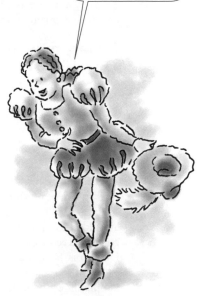

Alas! People who are lactose intolerant lack sufficient amounts of lactase, and less lactase means more metabolic mishaps.

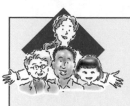

Bridging the gap

Ethnicity and lactose intolerance

In the UK, Ireland, Northern Europe and America, we think, on average, that about 5% of the adult population are lactose intolerant; however, certain ethnic and racial populations are more widely affected than others. In South America, Africa and Asia, more than 50% of the population are intolerant to lactose, which can rise to nearly 100% in some parts of Asia.

What to look for

Common signs and symptoms of lactose intolerance include:
- bloating
- flatulence
- cramps
- diarrhoea
- nausea.

These symptoms begin about 30 minutes to 2 hours after eating or drinking foods that contain lactose. The severity of symptoms varies depending on the amount of lactose each individual can tolerate.

How it's treated

Fortunately, lactose intolerance is relatively easy to treat. No treatment exists to improve the body's ability to produce lactase, but symptoms can be controlled through adjusting the diet.

Dietary management

Young children with lactase deficiency shouldn't eat any foods containing lactose. Because individuals differ in the amounts of lactose they can handle as they grow older, most older children and adults need not avoid lactose completely. Dietary control of lactose intolerance depends on each person's learning—through trial and error—about how much he or she can handle.

Limiting lactase

For those who react to very small amounts of lactose or have trouble limiting their intake of foods that contain lactose, lactase enzymes are available over the counter. One example is a liquid form that can be used with milk. A few drops are added to a pint milk, and after 24 hours in the refrigerator, the milk's lactose content is reduced by 70%. The process works faster if the milk is heated first. Doubling the amount of the liquid enzyme produces milk that's 90% lactose free.

A more recent development is a chewable lactase enzyme tablet that helps people digest solid foods that contain lactose. Three to six tablets should be taken just before a meal or snack.

Lactose-reduced milk and other products are available at many supermarkets. The milk contains all of the nutrients found in regular milk and remains fresh for about the same length of time or longer if it's super-pasteurised.

Balancing nutrition

Milk and other dairy products are a major source of nutrients in the UK diet. The most important of these nutrients is calcium. Calcium is essential for the growth and repair of bones throughout life. In the middle and later years, a shortage of calcium may lead to thin, fragile bones that break easily (a condition called *osteoporosis*). A concern, then, for both children and adults with lactose intolerance, is getting enough calcium in a diet that includes little or no milk.

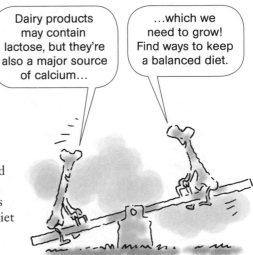

Dairy products may contain lactose, but they're also a major source of calcium…

…which we need to grow! Find ways to keep a balanced diet.

Keeping calcium on the menu

When planning meals, making sure that each day's diet includes enough calcium is important, even if the diet doesn't contain dairy products. Many non-dairy foods are high in calcium. Green vegetables, such as broccoli and kale, and fish with soft, edible bones, such as salmon and sardines, are excellent sources of calcium. (See *Sources of dietary calcium*.)

Recent research shows that yoghurt with active cultures may be a good source of calcium for patients with lactose intolerance, even though it's fairly high in lactose. Evidence shows that the bacterial cultures used in making yoghurt produce

---

Sources of dietary calcium

Here's a list of dietary sources of calcium that have little or no lactose. These items should become part of the diet of someone with lactose intolerance.

Food source	Calcium content (mg)
Broccoli (cooked), 230 g	94 to 177
Chinese cabbage (cooked), 230 g	158
Kale (cooked), 230 g	94 to 170
Turnip greens (cooked), 230 g	194 to 249
Oysters (raw), 230 g	226
Salmon with bones (canned), 89 g	167
Sardines, 89 g	371
Shrimp (canned), 89 g	98
Molasses, 2 tbsp	274
Tofu (processed with calcium salts), 89 g	225

some of the lactase enzyme required for proper digestion. Yoghurt should be given to a lactose intolerant patient only after discussions with the registered dietitian.

Although milk and foods made from milk are the only natural sources, lactose is often added to prepared foods. People with a very low tolerance for lactose need to know about the many food products that may contain lactose, even in small amounts, including:

- bread and other baked goods
- processed breakfast cereals
- instant potatoes, soups and breakfast drinks
- margarine
- lunch meats (other than kosher)
- salad dressings
- sweets and other snacks
- mixes for pancakes, biscuits and cakes.

Hidden agenda

Some products labelled non-dairy, such as powdered coffee creamer and whipped toppings, include ingredients that are derived from milk and therefore contain lactose. Encourage patients to learn to read food labels carefully, looking not only for milk and lactose among the contents but also for other ingredients that indicate that the item contains lactose, such as:

- whey
- curds
- milk by-products
- dry milk solids
- nonfat dry milk powder.

In addition, lactose is used as the base for more than 20% of prescription drugs and about 6% of over-the-counter medicines. Many types of birth control pills, for example, contain lactose, as do some tablets used to treat stomach acid and gas. However, these products typically affect only people with severe lactose intolerance.

Living with lactose intolerance

Even though lactose intolerance is widespread, it need not pose a serious threat to good health. People who have trouble digesting lactose can learn which dairy products and other foods they can eat without discomfort and which ones they should avoid. Many can enjoy milk, ice cream and other such products if they take them in small amounts or eat other food at the same time. A carefully chosen diet is the key to reducing symptoms and protecting future health.

Diverticular disease

In diverticular disease, bulging pouches (diverticula) in the GI wall push the mucosal lining through the surrounding muscle. Although the most common site for diverticula is the sigmoid colon, they may develop

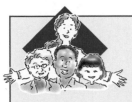

Bridging the gap

Diverticular disease around the globe

Diverticular disease is common in industrialised countries, such as the United States, England and Australia, where people tend to eat diets low in fibre. It rarely occurs in Asia and Africa, where high-fibre vegetable diets are regularly consumed. Diverticular disease initially appeared in the UK in the early 20th century, when processed foods became popular.

anywhere, from the proximal end of the pharynx to the anus. Other common sites include the duodenum, near the pancreatic border or the ampulla of Vater, and the jejunum. Diverticular disease of the stomach is rare and is usually a precursor of peptic or neoplastic disease. Diverticular disease of the ileum (Meckel's diverticulum) is the most common congenital anomaly of the GI tract.

Who and where?

Diverticular disease is common in industrialised countries, suggesting that a low-fibre diet reduces stool bulk and leads to excessive colonic motility. This consequent increased intraluminal pressure causes herniation of the mucosa. (See *Diverticular disease around the globe*.)

Diverticular disease is most prevalent in men over age 40 and people who eat low-fibre diets. More than half of adults older than age 50 have colonic diverticula.

Type two

Diverticular disease has two forms:

diverticulosis, in which diverticula are present but don't cause symptoms

diverticulitis, in which diverticula are inflamed and may cause potentially fatal obstruction, infection, perforation or haemorrhage.

Pathophysiology

The aetiology of diverticular disease hasn't been determined, but it's thought to be caused by a disordered colonic motility pattern. Diverticula probably result from high intraluminal pressure on an area of weakness in the GI wall, where blood vessels enter. Diet may be a contributing factor, because insufficient fibre reduces faecal residue, narrows the bowel lumen and leads to high intra-abdominal pressure during defecation.

In diverticulosis, the pouches formed by diverticula sometimes trap faecal material, which becomes hardened and irritates the surrounding cells. Inflammation develops, causing diverticulitis. In diverticulitis, retained undigested food and bacteria accumulate in the diverticular sac. This hard mass cuts off the blood supply to the thin walls of the sac, making them more susceptible to attack by colonic bacteria. Inflammation follows and may lead to perforation, abscess, peritonitis, obstruction or haemorrhage. Occasionally, the inflamed colon segment may adhere to the bladder or other organs and cause a fistula.

What to look for

Typically the patient with diverticulosis is asymptomatic and will remain so unless diverticulitis develops.

With mild diverticulitis, signs and symptoms include:

- moderate left lower abdominal pain
- low-grade fever
- leucocytosis.

If diverticulitis is severe, signs and symptoms include:

- abdominal rigidity
- left lower quadrant pain
- high fever
- chills
- hypotension
- microscopic or massive haemorrhage.

How it's treated

If diverticulitis develops, administer antibiotics as prescribed to combat infection and minimise inflammation. Administer analgesics as prescribed to control pain and relax smooth muscle. Give antispasmodics to control muscle spasms. Encourage the patient to exercise to increase the rate of stool passage.

If diverticulitis is refractory to medical treatment, a colon resection with removal of the involved segment may be necessary. A temporary colostomy may be needed to drain abscesses and rest the colon if diverticulitis is accompanied by perforation, peritonitis, obstruction or fistula. Blood transfusions may be necessary to treat blood loss from haemorrhage.

Dietary management

For the patient with diverticulosis, encourage fluids and a high-fibre intake that includes 25 to 30 g of fibre per day. High-fibre diets produce soft, bulky stools that move easily through the colon, decreasing pressure within the colon.

During an acute phase of diverticulitis, a low-residue diet may be recommended to reduce residue in the bowel.

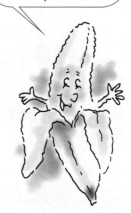

High-fibre fruits, which make good snacks for the patient with diverticulosis, include bananas, oranges and peaches.

Irritable bowel syndrome

Irritable bowel syndrome (IBS) is characterised by chronic symptoms of abdominal pain, alternating constipation and diarrhoea and abdominal distension. This disorder is common, although about 20% of patients never seek medical attention. It occurs in women twice as often as men.

Mechanisms involved in IBS include visceral hypersensitivity and altered colonic motility. IBS is generally associated with psychological stress; however, it may result from such factors as diverticular disease, ingestion of irritants (coffee, raw vegetables or fruits), laxative abuse, food poisoning and colon cancer.

Pathophysiology

Typically, the patient with IBS has a normal-appearing GI tract. However, careful examination of the colon may reveal functional irritability—an abnormality in colonic smooth-muscle function marked by excessive peristalsis and spasms, even during remission.

Contractual obligations

To understand what happens in IBS, consider how smooth muscle controls bowel function. Normally, segmental muscle contractions mix intestinal contents while peristalsis propels the contents through the GI tract. Motor activity is most propulsive in the proximal (stomach) and distal (sigmoid) portions of the intestine. Activity in the rest of the intestines is slower, permitting nutrient and water absorption.

IBS appears to reflect motor disturbances of the entire colon in response to stimuli. Some muscles of the small bowel are particularly sensitive to motor abnormalities and distension; others are particularly sensitive to certain foods and drugs. The patient may be hypersensitive to the hormones gastrin and cholecystokinin. The pain of IBS seems to be caused by abnormally strong contractions of the intestinal smooth muscle as it reacts to distension, irritants or stress.

Developing a disturbing pattern

Some patients have spasmodic intestinal contractions that set up a partial obstruction by trapping gas and stools. This causes distension, bloating, gas pain and constipation. Other patients have dramatically increased intestinal motility. Usually, eating or cholinergic stimulation triggers the small intestine's contents to rush into the large intestine, dumping watery stools and irritating mucosa. The result is diarrhoea.

If further spasms trap liquid stools, the intestinal mucosa absorbs water from the stools, leaving them dry, hard and difficult to pass. The result is a pattern of alternating diarrhoea and constipation.

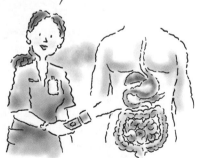

IBS pain is caused by abnormally strong contractions of the intestinal smooth muscle.

What to look for

The most commonly reported symptom is intermittent, cramping, lower abdominal pain that's relieved by defecation or passage of flatus. It usually occurs during the day and intensifies with stress or 1 to 2 hours after meals. The patient may experience alternating constipation and diarrhoea, with one being the predominant problem. Mucous passage through the rectum may also occur. Abdominal distension and bloating are common.

How it's treated

Treatment of IBS aims to relieve symptoms and includes counselling to help the patient understand the relation between stress and illness. Rest and heat applied to the abdomen are usually helpful. The use of linseed, peppermint oils and probiotics may reduce symptoms.

In addition, some medications may be used:
• 5-HT$_3$ receptor antagonist (alosetron) is a selective antagonist used for short-term treatment of women with IBS who have severe diarrhoea.
• 5-HT$_4$ receptor partial agonist (tegaserod) may be prescribed for short-term treatment of women with IBS whose primary symptom is constipation. It also relieves abdominal discomfort and bloating.
• Antidepressants have been effective, especially when diarrhoea is a predominant symptom.
• Bulk-forming agents, such as psyllium (Metamucil), are effective when constipation is the predominant symptom. In the case of laxative overuse, bowel training is sometimes recommended.
• Antispasmodics, such as propantheline or diphenoxylate with atropine sulphate, are commonly prescribed.
• A mild barbiturate, such as phenobarbital, in judicious doses is sometimes helpful as well.

Dietary management

Patients suffering from IBS should be encouraged to follow a healthy eating pattern in line with the eat well plate principles. Dietary restrictions haven't proven to be effective in treating IBS, but the patient is encouraged to be aware of foods that exacerbate symptoms. Advise the patient to chew food slowly and to eat small, frequent meals to reduce distension. Some people find a high-fibre diet effective; however, this type of diet isn't helpful for everyone. Consuming a low-fat diet has also proven beneficial for some patients.

Inflammatory bowel disease

Inflammatory bowel disease (IBD) is a chronic condition characterised by the formation of inflammatory and ulcerating lesions in the small intestine or colon. Patients commonly experience diarrhoea, fever and abdominal pain although the condition may have a relapsing/remitting pattern of occurrence.

The two major types of IBD are:
- Crohn's disease
- ulcerative colitis.

Crohn's disease details

Crohn's disease is a type of IBD that may affect any part of the GI tract from the mouth to the anus. Inflammation extends through all layers of the intestinal wall and may involve lymph nodes and supporting membranes in the area. Ulcers form as the inflammation extends into the peritoneum.

Crohn's disease is most prevalent in adults aged 20 to 40. It tends to run in families—up to 20% of patients have a positive family history.

When Crohn's disease affects only the small bowel, it's known as *regional enteritis*. When it involves the colon or affects only the colon, it's known as *Crohn's disease of the colon*. Crohn's disease of the colon is sometimes called *granulomatous colitis*; however, not all patients develop granulomas (tumour-like masses of granulation tissue).

Although it isn't necessarily all in the family, Crohn's disease sometimes occurs in identical twins, and up to 20% of affected patients have relatives who also have the disease.

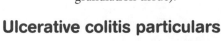

Ulcerative colitis particulars

Ulcerative colitis causes ulcerations of the mucosa in the colon. It commonly occurs as a chronic condition. As many as 1 in 1,000 people have ulcerative colitis. Peak occurrences are between ages 15 and 20 and between ages 55 and 60. It's more prevalent among women, people of Jewish ancestry and whites. (See *Inflammatory bowel disease in Jewish people*.)

Pathophysiology of Crohn's disease

Although researchers are still studying Crohn's disease, possible causes include:
- lymphatic obstruction
- infection
- allergies

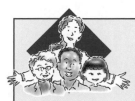

Bridging the gap

Inflammatory bowel disease in Jewish people

Crohn's disease is more common among Jewish people than in other white cultural groups. Moreover, this GI disorder is more common in Jewish men than in Jewish women. Ulcerative colitis is more common in Ashkenazi Jews than in other Jewish and non-Jewish people.

- genetic factors
- immune disorders, such as altered immunoglobulin A production and increased suppressor T-cell activity.

An inheritance you can't retire on

Genetic factors play an important role. Crohn's disease sometimes occurs in identical twins, and 10% to 20% of patients with the disease have one or more affected relatives. Researchers have identified a gene that predisposes people to the disease; however, no simple pattern of inheritance has been identified.

Groan! Crohn's

In Crohn's disease, inflammation spreads slowly and progressively. The following stages occur:
- Lymph nodes enlarge, and lymph flow in the submucosa is blocked.
- Lymphatic obstruction causes oedema, mucosal ulceration, fissures, abscesses and, sometimes, granulomas. Mucosal ulcerations are called *skipping lesions* because they aren't continuous (as in ulcerative colitis).
- Oval, elevated patches of closely packed lymph follicles—called Peyer's patches—develop on the lining of the small intestine.
- Fibrosis occurs, thickening the bowel wall and causing stenosis, or narrowing of the lumen.
- Inflammation of the serous membrane (serositis) develops, inflamed bowel loops adhere to other diseased or normal loops and diseased bowel segments become interspersed with healthy ones.
- Eventually, diseased parts of the bowel become thicker, narrower and shorter.

Getting complicated

Severe diarrhoea and corrosion of the perineal area by enzymes can cause an anal fistula, the most common complication. A perineal abscess may also develop during the active inflammatory state. Fistulas may develop to the bladder, vagina or even skin in an old scar area.

Other complications include intestinal obstruction, nutrient deficiencies caused by malabsorption of bile salts and vitamin B_{12} and poor digestion, fluid imbalances and inflammation of abdominal linings (peritonitis [rare]).

What to look for in patients with Crohn's disease

Initially, the patient experiences malaise and diarrhoea, usually with pain in the right lower quadrant or generalised abdominal pain and fever. Chronic symptoms, which are more typical of the disease, are more persistent and less severe; they include diarrhoea (four to six stools or more per day) with pain in the right lower quadrant, steatorrhea (excess fat in faeces) and marked weight loss. The patient may complain of weakness and fatigue. The patient may also present with acute inflammatory signs and symptoms that mimic appendicitis, including steady, colicky pain in the right lower quadrant; cramping; tenderness; flatulence; nausea; fever; diarrhoea; bleeding (usually mild but may be massive) and bloody stools. Joint pain and inflammation of the eyes are also common presenting complaints.

Pathophysiology of ulcerative colitis

The cause of ulcerative colitis is unknown; it may be related to an abnormal immune response in the GI tract, possibly associated with genetic factors. Lymphocytes (T cells) in people with ulcerative colitis may have cytotoxic effects on epithelial cells of the colon. Although no specific organism has been linked to ulcerative colitis, infection hasn't been ruled out. Stress doesn't cause the disorder, but it can increase the severity of an attack.

Surveying the damage

Ulcerative colitis damages the large intestine's mucosal and submucosal layers. Here's how it progresses:
• Usually, the disease originates in the rectum and lower colon. Then it spreads to the entire colon.
• The mucosa develops diffuse ulceration, with haemorrhage, congestion, oedema and exudative inflammation. Unlike Crohn's disease, ulcerations are continuous.
• Abscesses formed in the mucosa develop purulent drainage, become necrotic and ulcerate.
• Sloughing occurs, causing bloody, mucous-filled stools.

Looking closer at the colon

As ulcerative colitis progresses, the colon undergoes these changes:
• Initially, the colon's mucosal surface becomes dark, red and velvety.
• Abscesses form and coalesce into ulcers.
• Necrosis of the mucosa occurs.
• As abscesses heal, scarring and thickening may appear in the bowel's inner muscle layer.
• As granulation tissue replaces the muscle layer, the colon narrows, shortens and loses its characteristic pouches (haustral folds).

Progression of ulcerative colitis may lead to intestinal obstruction, dehydration and major fluid and electrolyte imbalances. Malabsorption is common, and chronic anaemia may result from loss of blood in the stools.

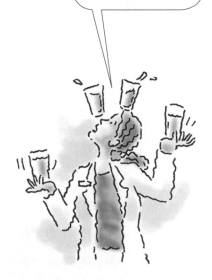

Progression of ulcerative colitis may lead to intestinal obstruction, dehydration and major fluid and electrolyte imbalances.

What to look for in patients with ulcerative colitis

The hallmark of ulcerative colitis is recurrent bloody diarrhoea—usually containing pus and mucus—alternating with symptom-free remissions. Accumulation of blood and mucous in the bowel causes cramping abdominal pain, rectal urgency and diarrhoea.

Other symptoms include:

- anorexia
- irritability
- nausea
- weakness
- weight loss
- vomiting.

How it's treated

For the patient with either type of IBD, the goals of treatment focus on reducing inflammation, relieving symptoms and preventing malnutrition. Sulfasalazine is given to treat infection and decrease inflammation. Corticosteroids are prescribed to reduce inflammation and, subsequently, diarrhoea, pain and bleeding. Immunosuppressants and immunomodulators may be given if corticosteroids fail to control the disease. Anti-diarrhoeal agents may be prescribed to relieve frequent diarrhoea in patients whose IBD is otherwise under control. Opioid analgesics may be administered to control pain and diarrhoea. I.V. therapy is administered to combat fluid losses.

Crohn's corrections

Patients with Crohn's disease may require surgery to repair bowel perforation and correct massive haemorrhage, fistulas or acute intestinal obstruction. A colectomy with ileostomy may be necessary in patients with extensive disease of the large intestine and rectum. Surgery is not surative in Crohn's disease.

Ulcerative colitis adjustments

If ulcerative colitis symptoms become unbearable or unresponsive to medications and supportive measures, the patient may require surgery to correct massive dilation of the colon. Proctocolectomy with ileostomy (to divert stool and to allow the rectal anastomosis to heal), ileoanal pull-through or pouch ileostomy (Kock pouch or continent ileostomy) may be necessary if the patient doesn't respond to drugs and supportive measures. A total colectomy in a patient with ulcerative colitis is curative.

Dietary management

Dietary management will be different depending on a number of factors such as the type of IBD, where the disease is located, previous intervention (e.g. surgery) and whether the disease is in remission or active phase. Malnutrition is a constant concern in patients with IBD, particularly Crohn's disease. Anorexia, nausea, abdominal pain and diarrhoea discourage the patient from eating. Encourage the patient to eat, and explain that eating aids healing and recovery. There are a number of dietary regimens that have been shown to be beneficial in the management of acute relapses of Crohn's disease in particular. These include the use of polymeric or elemental supplements or feeds with the exclusion of all solid foods, and the LOFLEX diet.

A diet high in protein and calories is needed to promote weight gain and healing. Calorie consumption should be sufficient to reach and maintain an acceptable body weight. Protein intake should reach 1.5 to 2 g/kg/day. If the patient's fat digestion and absorption are impaired, he or she may need to restrict fat and lactose intake. Vitamin and mineral supplements may be necessary. Vitamin B_{12} injections may be administered to the patient with Crohn's disease. Omega-3 fatty acids (fish oils) may be ordered to help make the inflammatory response less severe.

Menu matters

Encourage the patient to consume small, frequent meals, which are better tolerated than three larger meals. Also educate the patient to avoid these substances especially during the active phase and the early stages of remission:
- alcoholic beverages
- caffeinated beverages
- iced beverages
- carbonated beverages
- simple sugars
- highly spiced and fatty foods.

In some cases, patients also can't tolerate wheat and gluten, so these substances need to be avoided as well.

How low can you go?

Those who have undergone surgical procedures are also at risk for nutritional deficiencies caused by malabsorption. (See *Colostomy and ileostomy concerns*, page 234.) Many are deficient in the fat-soluble vitamins A, E and K. When portions of the ileum are resected, problems with vitamin B_{12} absorption may lead to deficiency. Patients also experience protein loss as protein-rich fluids are excreted with diarrhoea.

Deficiencies must be corrected by providing nutrients in any way that the patient can tolerate them. Nutritional supplements may be necessary. Tube feeding may be necessary if the patient is experiencing an acute exacerbation. If complete bowel rest is required due to the presence of fistulas or perforations, parenteral nutrition may be prescribed.

NutriTips

Colostomy and ileostomy concerns

Because fluid, potassium and sodium are usually absorbed in the colon, patients with colostomies and ileostomies are at risk for nutritional deficiencies. The greater the portion of the colon removed, the greater the risk of deficiencies. (Therefore, ileostomies place the patient at higher risk than colostomies.) The patient with an ileostomy is also at risk for the malabsorption of bile, fat and vitamin B_{12}, and numerous other nutrients depending on the amount of ileum available for absorption.

Dietary management

In the immediate post-operative period, the patient may be maintained on total parenteral nutrition. After healing takes place, nutrition management depends on tolerance as well as fluid and electrolyte status. A high fluid intake (8 to 10 tall glasses) is recommended to replenish fluid losses. An appropriate diet to promote healing and prevent weight loss will be recommended. The patient with an ileostomy usually requires lifelong injections of vitamin B_{12}.

Patient teaching

A patient with an ileostomy or colostomy needs to be educated about the effects of certain foods so he or she can adequately control symptoms. Use the lists below to help your patient identify the effects of certain foods.

Gas-producing foods

- apples
- asparagus
- beans
- beer
- bran
- broccoli
- cabbage
- carbonated beverages
- cauliflower
- celery
- coconut
- cream sauces
- cucumber
- eggs
- fish
- fried food
- garlic

- honey
- melon
- milk
- nuts
- onions
- prunes
- radishes
- wheat
- yeast

Foods that increase the risk of stomal blockage

- cabbage
- celery
- coconut
- sweet corn
- cucumber
- dried fruit

- green peppers
- lettuce
- mushrooms
- olives
- peas
- pickles
- pineapple
- popcorn
- seeds

Stool-thickening foods

- apple sauce
- bananas
- bread
- cheese
- creamy peanut butter
- pasta
- marshmallows

Odour-producing foods

- asparagus
- eggs
- fish
- garlic
- green pepper
- mustard
- onions
- radish
- spicy foods

Deodorising foods

- buttermilk
- cranberry juice
- parsley
- yoghurt

Diarrhoea

Diarrhoea, the abnormally frequent passage of liquid stool, is a common disorder that results in excessive loss of fluid, electrolytes and nutrients. Patients typically don't seek medical treatment; instead, they treat themselves with over-the-counter remedies. Diarrhoea can be acute (present for less than 2 weeks) or chronic (present for more than 2 weeks).

Pathophysiology

Diarrhoea can have numerous causes; however, the basic pathophysiology is the same regardless of the cause. Here's what happens:

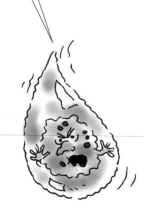

Pathogens like me can cause acute diarrhoea if your patient ingests contaminated food or water.

A substance irritates the intestinal mucosa. In response, the mucosa secretes mucous to serve as a protective barrier.

Cells secrete water and electrolytes, washing the irritating substance towards the anus.

Neuromuscular stimulation causes increased peristalsis and quickly helps rid the body of the irritating substance.

Acute

Acute diarrhoea is typically caused by pathogens or medications. When caused by pathogens, they're usually ingested through contaminated food or water. Acute infectious diarrhoea has a rapid onset after exposure to the infectious organism. Abdominal pain and fever occur when the organisms overwhelm the intestinal tract's normal defences.

Some bacteria release endotoxins that stimulate the intestinal cells to release sodium, chloride and water, worsening fluid and electrolyte loss. Some endotoxins act directly on the innervation of the GI tract, increasing peristalsis and thereby worsening fluid and electrolyte loss.

Acute diarrhoea can also be caused by medications. Some medications, such as antibiotics and NSAIDs, irritate the lining of the intestine. In response, the intestinal tract secretes mucous and fluid in an attempt to wash away the irritating substance. Some medications, such as antihypertensive agents, antiarrhythmics, bronchodilators and antineoplastics, affect the nervous system, causing increased peristaltic action.

Diarrhoea may also be caused by accidental ingestion of toxins, such as insecticides or mushrooms, or by host-transplant reactions.

Chronic

Chronic diarrhoea may result from:
• ongoing infection by such organisms as *Giardia*, *Clostridium difficile*, *Entamoeba histolytica*, *Cryptosporidium* and *Campylobacter*
• human immunodeficiency virus infection (although the specific cause is unknown)
• lactose intolerance
• adverse reaction to medications
• IBS
• IBD
• structural defects of the GI tract
• tumours.

Because chronic diarrhoea typically occurs over a long time, nutritional deficiencies are common. The impaired absorption that occurs with diarrhoea results in loss of electrolytes, minerals, vitamins, proteins and fats.

What to look for

The major manifestation associated with diarrhoea is the frequent passage of watery stool. Abdominal pain and fever are seen with acute infectious diarrhoea. In addition, dehydration and electrolyte imbalances are common.

How it's treated

Treatment of acute and chronic diarrhoea differs.

Acute actions

Before initiating treatment of acute diarrhoea, an accurate diagnosis must be made pinpointing the cause. Obtain a dietary history to determine where the patient has recently eaten. Question the patient about medical conditions that may reveal an organic cause. Also ask the patient about medications taken. A thorough physical examination and a stool culture are necessary to determine whether a pathogenic organism is present.

Anti-diarrhoeal agents, such as diphenoxylate and atropine (Lomotil), can be given to slow peristalsis; however, these agents should be avoided in patients infected by pathogens. Slowing peristalsis in these patients allows pathogen overgrowth. Patients infected by pathogens require antibiotic therapy specific to the type of organism.

I.V. therapy is initiated if fluid and electrolyte imbalance is severe. If medication is the cause, it should be discontinued and an alternative medication prescribed. If an underlying disease process is the cause, measures should be taken to treat the disorder.

Chronic corner

For chronic diarrhoea, treatment depends on the underlying cause. Stool cultures are obtained to check for and identify an infectious agent. If an infectious agent is identified, antibiotics are prescribed. If no infection is found, endoscopy may be performed to look for signs of inflammation or structural defects. A long-standing history of diarrhoea may suggest IBS.

Anti-diarrhoeal medications, such as bismuth subsalicylate (Pepto-Bismol) or loperamide (Imodium), may be given to temporarily alleviate symptoms. Stronger anti-diarrhoeal medications, such as opioid preparation, suppress peristalsis, allowing the absorption of water and electrolytes. These agents are especially effective in treating propulsive diarrhoea.

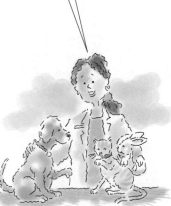

Unlike these guys, chronic diarrhoea is never 'acute' problem.

Dietary management

Nutritional support for acute diarrhoea requires no intervention other than encouraging fluid intake to replace losses. I.V. fluid therapy may be necessary depending on the severity of acute diarrhoea.

In patients with chronic diarrhoea, withhold food intake for 24 to 48 hours. Administer I.V. fluid and electrolytes to treat fluid and electrolyte imbalances. After 48 hours, encourage the patient to return to their normal diet as tolerated. Encourage the patient to consume a low-residue diet in small, frequent meals, which may be better tolerated than three large meals. (See *Serving up a low-residue diet*.)

Menu maven

Serving up a low-residue diet

A low-residue diet restricts residue and fibre. It's effective against diarrhoea because it slows transit time in the colon and reduces the frequency and volume of stool.

These foods may be included in a low-residue diet:

- meat, fish or poultry (ground or well cooked)
- eggs
- milk (up to 250 ml/day)
- fruit juices without pulp (excluding prune juice), canned fruits and ripe bananas
- vegetable juices without pulp, potatoes without skins and most well-cooked vegetables without seeds
- breads (white, refined breads; rolls; biscuits; muffins; pancakes; crackers and waffles)
- cereals (refined cereals, such as rice crispies)
- miscellaneous foods such as fruit ices, ice cream (without nuts or coconut), jelly and marshmallows.

What's on the menu

Here's a sample menu containing low-residue foods.

Breakfast	Lunch	Dinner	Snack
• apple juice • cream of rice • scrambled egg • white toast with butter and seedless jam • 200 ml milk • coffee	• tomato juice • sandwich made with white bread, turkey and mayonnaise • canned peach halves • jelly • 200 ml fruit juice (no pulp) • tea	• roasted chicken • mashed potatoes • cooked carrots • French bread with butter • rice pudding • 200 ml water • cranberry juice	• melba toast • 200 ml water

Encourage foods high in potassium, such as apricots, bananas, peaches, tomato juice, fish, potatoes and meat, to replace losses. Patients with severe diarrhoea, usually secondary to an underlying clinical condition, who don't respond to medical treatment may require elemental enteral nutrition or parenteral nutrition.

Constipation

Constipation, difficult or infrequent passage of stool, is a common complaint, especially among elderly patients. It is exacerbated by poor nutrition, low fluid intake and immobility. Individuals who complain of constipation experience prolonged periods of time between bowel movements and a sensation of incomplete evacuation after having one.

Despite what some people believe, it isn't necessary to have a bowel movement every day. Typically, people have at least three bowel movements per week.

Pathophysiology

Constipation occurs when decreased peristalsis results in prolonged transit time in the GI tract, allowing excessive fluid absorption. As a result, stool hardens, making it difficult to eliminate.

The longer stool remains in the colon, the more fluid is absorbed, making defecation more difficult and uncomfortable.

Predisposing factors include:
• sedentary lifestyle
• low-fibre diet
• dehydration
• depression
• ageing
• systemic diseases (such as multiple sclerosis, Parkinson's disease, stroke, spinal cord injury, diabetes mellitus, thyroid disease, amyloidosis, systemic lupus erythematosus and scleroderma)
• use of opioid analgesics (such as morphine)
• structural abnormalities (such as tumours, bowel obstruction, diverticulosis and anal strictures).

What to look for

Signs and symptoms of constipation include:
• prolonged period of time between bowel movements
• abdominal cramping and bloating
• firm abdomen
• straining during defecation
• small, hard faeces
• distant or muffled bowel sounds

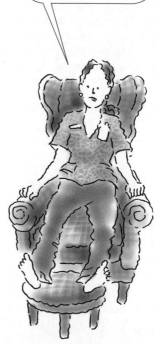

A sedentary lifestyle places patients at risk for constipation.

- backache
- headache
- decreased activity level.

How it's treated

Before treating constipation, it's important to identify the underlying cause. Obtain an accurate health history. Question the patient about unexplained weight loss, rectal bleeding or anaemia. If present, diagnostic testing and follow-up treatment is warranted. Also ask the patient about medication usage.

Encouraging elimination

Lifestyle changes are successful in relieving constipation in most cases. Encourage regular aerobic exercise, which helps maintain neuromuscular function, control appetite and enhance mood.

Explain the importance of establishing regular eating habits. Consuming food at the same time each day helps establish a regular pattern of intestinal stimulation and relaxation, which strengthens peristaltic contractions and decreases transit time through the colon. Moreover, when peristalsis becomes regular, a person can anticipate the urge to defecate and schedule around it.

Encourage the patient to increase fluid intake to at least eight 250-ml glasses per day. Drinks, such as hot coffee, tea or lemon water, help stimulate peristalsis. Inform the patient that prune juice has a laxative effect.

If diet and lifestyle changes are ineffective, fibre supplements such as Senna or Fibrogel may be necessary. As a last resort, more potent medications, such as suppositories, osmotic laxatives and stool softeners, can be used temporarily. Stimulant laxatives should be avoided if possible. Rarely, an enema may be necessary.

Dietary management

Typically a high-fibre diet is helpful in treating constipation because it increases stool bulk and speeds the passage of food through the intestines. The *FSA* recommends that adults consume a diet containing fibre daily. However, the average British adult typically consumes only one-half of the recommended amount. Adding the recommended amount of fibre to the diet isn't too difficult. (See *Serving up a high-fibre diet*, page 240.) For example a slice of white bread has 1 g of fibre, whereas a slice of multigrain bread has 3 g of fibre. Substituting multigrain bread for white bread in a sandwich increases fibre intake by 4 g. Adding bran cereal, fruits and vegetables to the diet can also greatly increase fibre intake.

Changing to a high-fibre diet may cause bloating, gas or heartburn. Therefore, it's important for a patient to initiate a high-fibre diet slowly. Include these tips when teaching the patient to help ease his or her transition:
- Gradually add small amounts of fibre to the diet by making subtle changes in eating and cooking habits. Increase the size and number of portions slowly and cut back if symptoms appear.

Menu maven

Serving up a high-fibre diet

A high-fibre diet substitutes high-fibre foods for those low in fibre. It alleviates constipation, lowers serum cholesterol levels and improves glucose tolerance in diabetics. A high-fibre diet is also helpful in preventing and treating irritable bowel syndrome and diverticular disease. Encourage the patient to consume:

- wholegrain breads and breakfast cereals
- dry peas or beans
- fresh fruits and vegetables—fruits with the skin on should be eaten whenever possible. High-fibre fruits include apples, oranges, berries, nectarines, peaches, bananas and pears. High-fibre vegetables include cabbage, greens, cauliflower, tomatoes, celery and courgette.

What's on the menu

Here's a sample menu containing high-fibre foods.

Breakfast	*Lunch*	*Dinner*	*Snack*
• prune juice	• bean soup	• roast turkey	• apple
• milk	• garden salad made	• brown rice	• milk
• multigrain toast	with lettuce, cheese,	• courgette and	• water
with butter	tomatoes, carrots,	peas	
• apple	raw broccoli	• fresh fruit salad	
• bran cereal	• wholemeal roll	• low-fat yoghurt	
• coffee	• peach	• water	
	• milk		

- Read food nutrition labels and choose foods high in fibre. Switching to high-fibre breads and cereals can significantly increase fibre intake.
- Mix high-fibre foods with other foods; for example try mixing cereals, adding fruits such as raisins or pears to salads and using apple sauce in recipes. Add lentils, pulses or beans to meat mixtures.
- Eat a meatless main dish with legumes at least once per week.
- Consume at least eight 250-ml glasses of fluid daily.

Viral hepatitis

Viral hepatitis is a common infection of the liver. In most patients, damaged liver cells eventually regenerate with little or no permanent damage. However, old age and serious underlying disorders make complications more likely.

Hepatitis may be caused by exposure to toxic substances such as carbon tetrachloride or medications that are toxic to the liver (excessive acetaminophen, for example).

Pathophysiology

Viral hepatitis is marked by liver cell destruction, tissue death (necrosis) and self-destruction of cells (autolysis). It leads to jaundice, hepatomegaly and anorexia. To date, six types of viral hepatitis have been identified: hepatitis A, B, C, D, E and G. (See *Viral hepatitis from A to G*, page 242.)

Different causes, same results

In general, the effects on the liver are usually similar among the different types of viral hepatitis. Varying degrees of liver cell injury and necrosis occur. However, the role hepatitis G plays in liver disease is unclear. This virus may cause a clinically similar systemic type of infection, affecting the liver.

What to look for

Early signs and symptoms of hepatitis infection include malaise, loss of appetite, nausea, diarrhoea and low-grade fever. As bilirubin excretion is impaired, urine becomes dark and jaundice develops. Tenderness over the right upper quadrant of the abdomen may also occur.

How it's treated

Peginterferon alfa-2a and adefovir dipivoxil have been approved for the treatment of patients with chronic hepatitis B. Interferon alpha and pegylated interferon in combination with ribavirin have been approved for the treatment of some patients with chronic hepatitis C. However, no specific drug therapy has been developed for the other forms of viral hepatitis. Treatment of viral hepatitis is mainly supportive:
- rest as needed
- I.V. hydration if vomiting is severe
- cholestyramine for severe pruritus.

Dietary management

Providing nutrients to support recovery of hepatic tissue is the goal of nutritional therapy for hepatitis. A patient who's otherwise healthy should receive a well-balanced diet. A patient who was previously malnourished should be given a high-calorie, high-protein diet. Alcohol should be avoided to prevent further hepatic damage.

Calories

Between 25 and 30 kcal/kg of body weight is recommended to meet energy needs and to avoid catabolism of protein. This intake also supports healing,

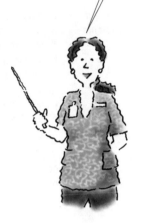

You read correctly; there's no hepatitis F. Non-hepatitis viral particles were mistakenly given this name. Now it's just a placeholder.

Viral hepatitis from A to G

This chart examines the features of each type of viral hepatitis.

Feature	Hepatitis A	Hepatitis B	Hepatitis C	Hepatitis D	Hepatitis E	Hepatitis G
Incubation	15 to 45 days	30 to 180 days	15 to 160 days	14 to 64 days	14 to 60 days	Unknown
Onset	Acute	Insidious	Insidious	Acute	Acute	Varies
Age group most affected	Children, young adults	Any age	More common in adults	Any age	Age 20 to 40	More common in adults
Signs and symptoms	Symptomatic or asymptomatic; flulike symptoms, headache, malaise, fatigue, anorexia, fever, dark urine, jaundice of skin, tender liver	Symptomatic or asymptomatic, possible arthralgia, rash, jaundice	Similar to hepatitis B; less severe with less jaundice	Similar to hepatitis B	Similar to hepatitis A (very severe in pregnant women)	Similar to hepatitis C
Transmission	Faecal–oral, sexual (especially oral–anal contact), nonpercutaneous (sexual, maternal–neonatal), percutaneous (rare)	Blood-borne; parenteral route, sexual, maternal–neonatal (virus is shed in all body fluids)	Blood-borne; parenteral route	Parenteral route (sexual, maternal–neonatal, people infected with hepatitis D also infected with hepatitis B)	Primarily faecal–oral	Exposure to blood or body fluids; parenteral route
Severity	Mild	Often severe	Moderate	Possibly severe, leading to fulminant hepatitis	Highly virulent with common progression to fulminant hepatitis and hepatic failure, especially in pregnant patients	Unknown; questionable if leads to fulminant hepatitis
Prognosis	Generally good	Worsens with age and debility	Moderate	Fair; worsens in chronic cases; can lead to chronic hepatitis D and chronic liver disease	Good unless pregnant	Unknown; results in chronic infection in 15% to 30% of adults
Progression to chronicity	None	Occasional	10% to 50% of cases	Occasional	None	Often a co-infection with hepatitis C; long-term significance associated with hepatitis C is unconfirmed

such as correcting generalised dehabilitation and fever, and rejuvenates the body's strength and endurance.

Protein

Regeneration of tissue requires adequate protein intake. Protein is also responsible for manufacturing new hepatic tissues and cells. The recommended intake of protein depends on underlying condition but should be in the range of 1 to 1.2 g/kg/day. Because protein metabolism is sometimes impaired with liver disease, resulting in toxic concentrations of ammonia, this recommendation should be adjusted to individual tolerance. Usually hepatitis isn't so severe that it significantly impairs ammonia clearance. Protein should be restricted only if ammonia levels are elevated.

Carbohydrates

The diet should provide 50% to 55% of energy from carbohydrates daily. The glucose formed from carbohydrate metabolism helps to revitalise glycogen reserves in the liver. Glucose also prevents the breakdown of protein for energy and meets the increased energy demands brought about by the disease.

Fat

A moderate amount of fat in the diet encourages the patient to eat, which is necessary because of his or her poor appetite. This fat may come from vegetable oil or milk products. The amount of fat needed should range from 30% to 35% of the daily energy intake.

Meal planning

Initially, treatment of hepatitis may require the administration of a light diet (as tolerated by the patient). As the patient's GI tolerance and appetite improve, this can be increased. Be sure to obtain the patient's food preferences to optimise food intake.

In many cases, patients with hepatitis have poor appetites. Here are some tips for encouraging intake:

- Offer smaller meals more frequently.
- Find out dietary preferences and try to offer these foods in abundance.
- Use fats (in moderation) to make food appealing.

If the patient can't eat because of persistent vomiting, parenteral nutrition may be needed.

Cirrhosis

Cirrhosis, a chronic liver disease, is characterised by widespread destruction of hepatic cells. These cells are replaced by fibrous cells in a process called *fibrotic regeneration*. When a significant proportion of hepatic tissue is irreparably damaged, the liver can no longer perform its functions.

Cirrhosis may be caused by:

- excessive alcohol ingestion
- chronic hepatitis

- bile duct disease
- exposure to toxic chemicals, such as carbon tetrachloride
- late-stage heart failure
- inherited metabolic disorders in which the body accumulates too much iron (haemochromatosis) or copper (Wilson's disease).

Cirrhosis is a common cause of death in the UK.

Pathophysiology

Cirrhosis is characterised by widespread destruction of hepatic cells; these cells are replaced by fibrous or fatty tissues. When this occurs, supporting structures are destroyed and strictures form, causing blockages of the hepatic blood flow.

There are different types of cirrhosis, each with its own aetiology. The most common types are:

- post-necrotic cirrhosis—typically a result of a complication from viral hepatitis but also can be caused by exposure to a toxin (such as arsenic or phosphorus); more prevalent in women
- portal, nutritional or alcohol-related cirrhosis—due to malnutrition and chronic alcoholism
- cardiac cirrhosis—due to prolonged venous congestion from right-sided heart failure
- biliary cirrhosis—caused by bile duct obstruction or inflammation of the bile duct
- idiopathic cirrhosis—unknown cause.

What to look for

In early stages of cirrhosis, signs and symptoms include loss of appetite, indigestion, nausea, vomiting, constipation, diarrhoea, dull abdominal aching, fatigue and jaundice. Later, signs and symptoms vary and reflect the resulting impairment of body functions and may include chronic dyspepsia, constipation, pruritus, weight loss and bleeding tendencies. (See *Complications of cirrhosis*, page 245.)

How it's treated

Cirrhotic liver tissue can't be repaired, so the first goal of treatment of cirrhosis is to reduce further destruction by removing toxins (abstaining from alcohol, for example) or other causes. In addition, treatment aims to reduce blood pressure in the portal system and provide support for those functions the body can no longer perform.

Treatment commonly includes:

- antihypertensives and diuretics to treat portal hypertension and reduce oedema
- oral antidiabetic agents to control blood glucose levels
- vitamin replacements

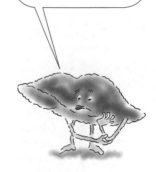

Oh dear! Damage to cirrhotic liver tissue can't be repaired, so, initially, treatment is focused on preventing further destruction.

Complications of cirrhosis

As cirrhosis progresses, impairment of other body systems and functions may occur.

Circulatory problems

Impedance of blood flow through the liver causes blood to back up into the veins that lead to the portal vein, causing portal hypertension. This has several serious consequences:

- Oesophageal varices form as blood backs up and causes the veins surrounding the oesophagus to bulge into the oesophageal lumen.
- GI bleeding develops when oesophageal varices burst and bleed into the oesophagus and stomach.
- Ascites (abdominal oedema) develops from portal hypertension as the higher pressures in the veins and low blood concentrations of protein (see below) allow diffusion of fluid from the blood into surrounding abdominal tissues; ascites causes early satiety and nausea and increases basal metabolic rate.

Metabolic problems

As the liver becomes unable to metabolise glucose, fats and proteins, additional complications may include:

- impairment of protein metabolism, resulting in low concentrations of blood proteins (such as albumin)— these proteins are needed to maintain normal osmotic pressure in the circulatory system; without them, fluid diffuses from the blood into surrounding tissues, contributing to oedema
- impairment of bile production, resulting in loss of ability to digest fats—bile is also an important excretory vehicle for bilirubin, and as bilirubin levels rise, jaundice ensues.

Coagulation problems

As cirrhosis progresses, the liver becomes unable to synthesise coagulating factors and store vitamin K, resulting in problems with blood clotting.

Vitamin deficiencies

Due to the liver's inability to create, utilise and store certain vitamins (such as vitamins A, C and K), evidence of deficiencies becomes apparent.

Anaemia

Anaemia results from the patient's poor dietary intake, impaired GI and liver function and chronic gastritis. This, in turn, affects the patient's overall ability to carry out activities of daily living.

Mental impairment

Although the exact cause of mental deterioration isn't understood, it's believed to be linked to high ammonia levels. Ammonia is a natural by-product of protein metabolism, which occurs in the liver and intestine as normal bacteria break down long-chain amino acids. With cirrhosis, ammonia levels rise because the liver no longer converts ammonia into urea to be excreted in the urine. Depletion of the vitamin B group of vitamins may also contribute to mental impairment.

Malnutrition

Due to inadequate intake, metabolism and excretion, malnutrition is a prominent feature of cirrhosis. The situation is exacerbated in cases of chronic alcohol abuse, in which the GI tract may also be dysfunctional and unable to absorb certain nutrients.

- coagulation factor replacement as needed
- electrolyte replacement (I.V. if necessary)
- blood transfusions if needed
- lactulose, an oral agent that draws ammonia into the intestine as an alternative method of excretion
- vasopressin, if necessary, to control oesophageal varices

- antibiotics to decrease intestinal bacteria and reduce ammonia production, which causes encephalopathy
- paracentesis, infusions of salt-poor albumin, and salt and fluid restrictions to control ascites
- surgical procedures, which include treatment of varices by upper endoscopy with banding or sclerosis, splenectomy, oesophagogastric resection and splenorenal or portacaval anastomosis to relieve portal hypertension.

Dietary management

Good nutritional intake is critical for the patient with cirrhosis. However, metabolism of nutrients is profoundly impaired in end-stage liver disease and difficult to achieve.

Calories

The patient with cirrhosis requires increased calories to meet the body's energy needs (35 kcal/kg dry weight). The exact requirement depends on the presence of other factors, such as active infection and ascites. Caloric intake can be enhanced by using fats, such as butter on potatoes, bread, vegetables and rice, and by using extra sugar in coffee. If steatorrhoea develops (may result from lack of bile), fats may have to be restricted.

Protein

Protein intake can be a difficult aspect of nutritional therapy for the patient with cirrhosis because the body needs additional protein for healing and tissue building, but protein metabolism can lead to high levels of ammonia in the blood. If the patient has hepatic encephalopathy current recommendations are that they should consume between 0.8 to 1.5 g/kg body weight. Most patients can tolerate up to 1.5 g/kg/day. Monitor mental status and blood ammonia levels carefully.

Fluid

Fluids should be restricted if necessary to control oedema. After oedema subsides and blood protein levels rise, fluids may be adjusted based on the patient's urine output (500 to 700 ml plus urine output per day).

Sodium

Advise your patient to avoid the addition of table salt.

Vitamins and minerals

Nearly all vitamins are depleted in people with end-stage liver disease, so daily supplements are necessary. Routine prescription of the vitamin B group of vitamins is common. Calcium, magnesium and zinc deficiencies are common.

Enteral and parenteral supplementation

At times, patients with cirrhosis can't meet their nutritional needs by oral ingestion, possibly as a result of mental impairment (encephalopathy), anorexia and vomiting or GI bleeding. In these cases, enteral or parenteral nutrition may be necessary.

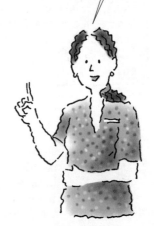

Initially, fluid and sodium should be restricted in the patient with cirrhosis to help control oedema.

Complete feeds for patients with cirrhosis include those with branched-chain amino acids, which when metabolised do not produce ammonia. These are available but are not commonly used.

Gall bladder disease

Gall bladder disease typically refers to conditions involving the formation of stones (cholelithiasis) in the gall bladder. Stone formation can give rise to several related disorders, including:
- cholecystitis (acute or chronic inflammation usually due to a stone becoming lodged in the cystic duct)
- choledocholithiasis (stones that pass out of the gall bladder and become lodged in the common bile duct)
- cholangitis (infection of the bile duct most commonly due to choledocholithiasis)
- gallstone ileus (obstruction of the small intestine by a gallstone).

Risky business

Certain risk factors predispose a person to stone formation. These include:
- high-calorie, high-cholesterol diet and associated obesity
- elevated oestrogen levels from hormonal contraceptive use, postmenopausal hormone replacement therapy or pregnancy
- use of clofibrate
- such diseases as diabetes mellitus, ileal disease, haemolytic disorders, hepatic disease and pancreatitis.

Prognosis

Prognosis is usually good with treatment; however, if infection occurs, prognosis depends on the severity of the infection and the effectiveness of antibiotic treatment. (See *Gall bladder disease in middle age*.)

Pathophysiology

Gall bladder disease and its related disorders stem from a common cause: the formation of stones (calculi). Although the exact cause of stone formation is unknown, abnormal metabolism of cholesterol and bile salts clearly plays an important role.

Welcome to the stone age

Here's what's known about gallstone formation:
- The liver continuously makes bile, which the gall bladder concentrates and stores until it's needed for fat digestion.
- Changes in the composition of bile may cause gallstone formation. Changes in the gall bladder lining's absorptive ability may also play a part.

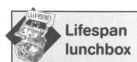

Lifespan lunchbox

Gall bladder disease in middle age

Generally, gall bladder disease occurs during middle age. In patients aged 20 to 50, occurrence is six times more common in women. After age 50, the incidence in men and women equalises. It then increases with each subsequent decade.

• Certain conditions, such as age, obesity and oestrogen imbalance, cause the liver to secrete bile that's abnormally high in cholesterol or that lacks the proper concentration of bile salts. When the gall bladder concentrates this bile, inflammation may occur. Excessive reabsorption of water and bile salts makes bile less soluble. Cholesterol, calcium and bilirubin precipitate into gallstones.

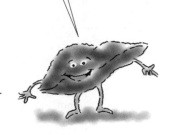

Such factors as age and obesity can cause me to excrete bile that's high in cholesterol, which can result in gallstones.

Stone cold problems

When fat enters the duodenum, the intestinal mucosa secretes cholecystokinin, which stimulates gall bladder contraction and emptying. If stones are present, one can lodge in the cystic duct. The gall bladder then contracts but can't empty, causing it to become inflamed and distended. Bacteria growth, usually *Escherichia coli*, may contribute to the inflammation. Oedema of the gall bladder obstructs bile flow, which irritates the gall bladder. Cells in the gall bladder wall may become oxygen-starved and die as the distended organ presses on vessels and impairs blood flow. The dead cells slough off, causing the gall bladder to adhere to surrounding structures.

An alternative route

Alternatively, a stone can travel to the common bile duct and become lodged. When this happens, bile can't flow into the duodenum. Bilirubin is absorbed into the blood, causing jaundice. Biliary narrowing and swelling of the tissue around the stone can also cause irritation and inflammation of the common bile duct. This inflammation can travel the biliary tree into any of the bile ducts, causing scar tissue, fluid accumulation, cirrhosis, portal hypertension and bleeding.

What to look for

Although the patient with gall bladder disease may be asymptomatic, acute cholelithiasis, acute cholecystitis and choledocholithiasis produce these classic symptoms of a gall bladder attack:
• sudden onset of severe steady or aching pain in the mid-epigastric region or the right upper quadrant, possibly radiating to the back, the right shoulder or between the shoulders or the front of the chest, which typically occurs after ingestion of a fatty meal or ingestion of a large meal after fasting for an extended time
• nausea and vomiting
• chills and low-grade fever
• jaundice (with common bile duct obstruction)
• dark-coloured urine and clay-coloured stools (with common bile duct obstruction and chronic cholecystitis).

Typically, the patient reports that milder GI symptoms preceded the acute attack. These symptoms may include indigestion, vague abdominal discomfort, belching and flatulence after eating meals or snacks rich in fat.

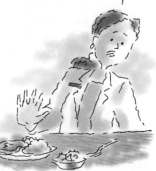

Hold the gravy! A gall bladder attack produces severe pain that typically occurs after eating a fatty meal.

How it's treated

During an acute attack, treatment focuses on administration of opioids for pain relief, antispasmodics and anticholinergic agents to relax smooth muscles and decrease ductal tone and spasm, and antiemetics to relieve nausea and vomiting. A nasogastric tube may be inserted and connected to low intermittent suction for abdominal decompression. I.V. fluids and antibiotics may be given to patients with severe acute cholecystitis.

Lithotripsy (ultrasonic shock wave therapy) may be used to break up gallstones and to allow them to pass naturally. Oral ursodeoxycholic acid may be used to dissolve the stones.

Did someone say surgery?

Surgery, usually elective, remains the most common treatment of gall bladder disease. It's commonly recommended if the patient has symptoms frequent enough to interfere with his or her regular routine, if he or she has complications or if he or she has had a previous attack of cholecystitis. Various surgical approaches may be used, including:
• cholecystectomy—removal of the inflamed gall bladder performed abdominally, laparoscopically, or percutaneously
• choledochostomy—creation of an opening into the common bile duct for drainage
• endoscopic retrograde cholangiopancreatography (ERCP)—for removal of gallstones.

Dietary management

Dietary advice for patients with gall bladder disease focuses on minimising stimulation of the gall bladder. Because fat is implicated in stimulating the gall bladder, a low-fat diet is typically suggested to reduce gall bladder stimulation and thus relieve pain. However, controversy exists about limiting fat in the diet. Several research studies demonstrate that the incidence of fat intolerance for patients with gall bladder disease is no greater than that for the general population. Therefore, dietary management is based on the individual's ability to tolerate specific foods.

If a patient is asymptomatic or has recovered from an initial attack of biliary colic, a low-fat diet is usually recommended. The amount of fat intake allowed varies, depending on the patient. (See *Serving up a low-fat diet*, page 250.)

Because of impaired bile secretion, deficiencies of fat-soluble vitamins may occur, necessitating vitamin replacement with water-soluble forms of vitamins A, D, E and K. In addition, the patient is encouraged to eat small, frequent meals to prevent future attacks.

Coffee talk

Caffeinated and decaffeinated coffee have been shown to raise levels of cholecystokinin in the blood. Remember, cholecystokinin (released when

Menu maven

Serving up a low-fat diet

When providing a low-fat diet for your patient, follow these suggestions for choosing foods:

- meat, poultry, fish, dry beans, eggs and nut group—use only lean cuts, skinless poultry and egg whites or substitutes
- milk, yoghurt and cheese group—use fat-free milk products only
- bread, cereal, rice and pasta group—use whole grains and enriched products
- fruit and vegetable groups—all fruits and vegetables are allowed as long as they aren't prepared with fat
- miscellaneous—jelly, cream crackers

The person on a low-fat diet should avoid:

- fatty or heavily marbled meats
- lunch meats
- egg yolks
- canned fish packed in oil
- fruits or vegetables prepared in butter or cream sauce
- whole, 2% or 1% milk and milk products
- breads and bread products prepared with added fat, such as muffins, cakes, doughnuts, granola-type cereals and buttered popcorn
- chocolate, toffee, fudge and most desserts
- creams and sauces.

What's on the menu

Here's a sample menu that's perfect for the low-fat diet:

Breakfast	*Lunch*	*Dinner*	*Snack*
• 68 g porridge oats (cooked) • fat-free/skimmed milk • tea • wholewheat toast with 1 tsp low-fat spread	• tuna sandwich (3 oz of tuna salad prepared with 1 tbs of light mayonnaise on two slices wholewheat bread) • tossed salad with fat-free dressing • one apple • fat-free/skimmed milk	• 3 oz grilled chicken breast • 68 g rice • peas and carrots • tea • fat-free/skimmed milk	• fruit • fat-free/skimmed milk

fat enters the duodenum) stimulates the gall bladder to contract and empty; therefore, patients with gall bladder disease who are experiencing symptoms should avoid coffee.

For acute cholecystitis

For the patient with acute cholecystitis, oral foods and fluids are typically withheld and I.V. fluid and electrolyte therapy is initiated. After 12 to 24 hours, the patient may be started on a clear liquid diet and may subsequently progress to a regular diet as tolerated.

After cholecystectomy

Controversy exists about the type of diet to follow after a cholecystectomy. Immediately after surgery, the patient should be given nothing by mouth until bowel sounds return and then progress to a regular diet as tolerated. In the post-operative period, some surgeons recommend a low-fat diet for 4 to 5 weeks, whereas others recommend a regular diet.

Quick quiz

1. Which intervention would be appropriate for a patient with GORD?
   A. Lying down immediately after eating
   B. Eating chocolate
   C. Drinking fat-free milk
   D. Eating large, infrequent meals

Answer: C. A patient with GORD should consume foods that increase LES pressure, such as fat-free milk and nonfat milk.

2. Which factor is associated with the development of peptic ulcer disease?
   A. *H. pylori* infection
   B. Poor dietary habits
   C. High-fat diet
   D. Recent weight loss

Answer: A. *H. pylori* infection, NSAID use and hypersecretory conditions are the major causes of peptic ulcer disease.

3. A patient with dumping syndrome experiences light-headedness, tachycardia and diaphoresis 15 to 30 minutes after eating. Which statement most likely explains these symptoms?
   A. Hypoglycaemia is occurring due to increased insulin secretion.
   B. There's a sudden influx of stomach contents into the small intestine.
   C. The patient has probably eaten too much too quickly.
   D. The patient has eaten too many fatty foods.

Answer: B. Dumping syndrome is a complication of gastric surgery that occurs when the pyloric sphincter is disturbed. Because the pyloric sphincter no longer functions, undigested food is quickly dumped from the stomach into the small intestine. As food digests in the jejunum, fluid shifts from the circulating blood to the jejunum. The rapid decrease in circulating blood volume causes light-headedness, tachycardia and diaphoresis.

4. Which of the following grains would be allowed on a diet specific for someone with coeliac disease?

    A. Rye
    B. Wheat
    C. Corn
    D. Barley

Answer: C. Corn is the only grain listed here that doesn't contain gluten. A person with coeliac disease needs to be on a gluten-free diet.

5. You're educating a patient with lactose intolerance about calcium-rich foods. Which of the following foods is a poor source of calcium?

    A. Sardines
    B. Yoghurt
    C. Processed breakfast cereal
    D. Kale

Answer: C. Even though some breakfast cereals are calcium fortified, most contain hidden lactose that would be unacceptable for the patient with lactose intolerance. Yoghurt, despite being a dairy product, has been shown to be acceptable to patients with lactose intolerance because of its active cultures, which produce some of the lactase enzyme required for proper digestion.

6. A patient with chronic diarrhoea is ordered to follow a low-residue diet. Which of the following foods would be an appropriate choice for this diet?

    A. Apples
    B. Rice pudding
    C. Courgette
    D. Bran cereal

Answer: B. Rice pudding is a low-residue food.

7. A patient with cirrhosis would probably have which nutrient restricted to control ascites?

    A. Protein
    B. Calories
    C. Sodium
    D. Calcium

Answer: C. Sodium is restricted to reduce the oedema associated with ascites.

Scoring

★★★   If you answered all seven questions correctly, yippee! When it comes to understanding GI disorders, you're on the right tract.

★★   If you answered four to six questions correctly, keep up the good work! Your understanding of GI disorders is harmonious. It must be the tympany.

★   If you answered fewer than four questions correctly, forge ahead! The malabsorption problems associated with this chapter won't hold you back from future intake.

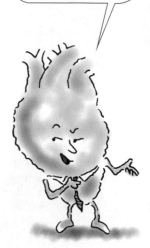

Don't stop now! I'm the star of the next chapter.

⑬ Cardiovascular disorders

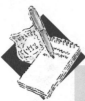

Just the facts

Nutrition can play a major role in the development of cardiovascular disease. In this chapter, you'll learn:

♦ the role of nutrition in cardiovascular disease development

♦ modifiable and nonmodifiable risk factors for cardiovascular disease

♦ nutrition-based preventive and treatment measures for cardiovascular disease.

A look at cardiovascular disease

More than 3.4 million people in Britain have one or more forms of cardiovascular disease (CVD)—the leading cause of death in the UK. CVD kills more people than cancer, chronic obstructive pulmonary disease, pneumonia, influenza, diabetes and acquired immunodeficiency syndrome (AIDS) combined.

Assessment

To plan nutritional therapy for a patient with CVD, first perform a nutrition-focused assessment that includes a health history, a physical examination and diagnostic tests.

Health history

Obtain a history to assess the patient's cardiovascular status and evaluate cardiovascular risk factors. Gather information about the patient's:

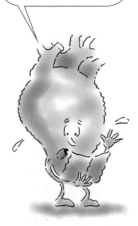

Yikes! Cardiovascular disease is the leading cause of death in the UK.

- dietary intake, especially of foods high in saturated fat and cholesterol
- use of low-fat or low-sodium products
- understanding of the nutrition facts panel on food labels
- knowledge of healthy eating habits
- willingness to change eating habits, if needed
- ability to buy and prepare healthy foods
- frequency of eating out
- physical activity and exercise
- religious and ethnic influences on food choices
- food allergies and intolerances
- use of alcohol, caffeine, tobacco and recreational drugs
- use of nutritional supplements
- current and past medication use
- medical history
- family history of heart disease and diabetes.

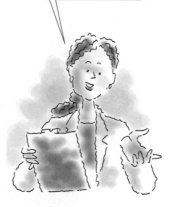

When taking your patient's health history for a nutritional assessment, be sure to gather information on his or her ability to buy and prepare healthy foods.

Assessing cardiovascular risk factors

The Joint British Societies Guidelines (JBS2) for the assessment of risk encompasses the whole atherosclerotic CVD—including acute coronary syndromes (ACSs), stable angina, cerebrovascular disease (non-haemorrhagic atherosclerotic stroke and haemorrhagic stroke, and transient cerebral ischaemia)—and any other arterial atherosclerosis, rather than highlight coronary heart disease (CHD).

The guidelines recommend that CVD prevention should focus equally on people with established CVD, those with diabetes mellitus and those with CVD risk of 20% or greater over 10 years. CVD risk should be calculated as 10-year risk of fatal and nonfatal stroke, including transient ischaemic attack, plus 10-year risk of CHD. CHD risk includes the risks of death from CHD, and nonfatal CHD, including silent myocardial infarction (MI), angina and coronary insufficiency (ACS). National Institute for Clinical Excellence (NICE) recommends that the Framingham 1991 10-year risk equations (as used in the JBS2 risk calculator) should be used to assess CVD risk.

- The JBS2 risk calculator (which is based on the Framingham equations) is not the only risk calculator in use and tends to be less accurate for certain population groups, e.g. women, ethnic minority groups and the socially deprived.
- The JBS2 guidelines recommend that all adults from 40 years onwards who have no history of CVD or diabetes, and who are not already on treatment for blood pressure or lipids, should be considered for an opportunistic comprehensive CVD risk assessment in primary care.
- Adults under 40 years with a family history of premature atherosclerotic disease should also have their cardiovascular risk factors measured.
- The guidelines also recommend recording the pulse rate and rhythm to screen for atrial fibrillation.
- Risk assessment should include ethnicity, smoking habit history, family history of CVD and measurements of weight, waist circumference, blood pressure, nonfasting lipids (total cholesterol and high-density lipoprotein [HDL] cholesterol) and nonfasting glucose.

- The JBS2 cardiovascular risk chart or calculator should be used to estimate total risk of developing CVD over 10 years based on five risk factors: age, gender, smoking habit, systolic blood pressure and the ratio of total cholesterol to HDL cholesterol. (See *Age, gender and cardiovascular risk*.)
- It is becoming recognised that the pulse pressure (PP) is a better independent risk factor in the elderly, and represents an age-related shift in the risk component of blood pressure from diastolic pressure to systolic pressure to PP.
- Total CVD risk should be estimated for the person's current age. A total CVD risk of over 20% over 10 years is defined as high risk.

Other risk factors not included in the CVD risk prediction charts should be taken account of in assessing and managing a person's overall CVD risk:

- In some ethnic groups the risk charts can underestimate, or sometimes overestimate, CVD risk because they have not been derived from these populations. For people originating from the Indian subcontinent, it is reasonable to assume that CVD risk is about 1.4 times higher than predicted from the charts. (See *At greatest risk*.)
- Abdominal obesity (waist circumference: men >102 cm, women >88 cm, and in Asians >90 cm in men and >80 cm in women) increases the risk of type 2 diabetes and CVD.
- Impaired fasting glucose and impaired glucose tolerance are both associated with an increased risk of developing type 2 diabetes and CVD.
- Raised fasting triglyceride (>1.7 mmol/L) increases the risk of CVD.
- A family history of premature CVD (men <55 years and women <65 years) in a first-degree relative increases the risk of developing CVD by about 1.3.
- Women with a premature menopause will also have an increased risk.

Risk indicators

Type 2 diabetes, Framingham risk score and metabolic syndrome are considered risk indicators for CVD.

Lifespan lunchbox

Age, gender and cardio-vascular risk

Typically, cardiovascular disease (CVD) appears in women 10 to 15 years later than it does in men, after age 65. When CVD occurs in younger women, it's generally due to the presence of multiple risk factors and metabolic syndrome. Although CVD is uncommon in both young men (age 20 to 35 years) and women (age 20 to 45 years), high cholesterol levels in this age group may lead to the early onset of CVD in middle age. Early detection of and intervention for high low-density lipoprotein levels can slow or avert the appearance of CVD in the middle and later years.

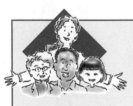

Bridging the gap

At greatest risk

For people originating from the Indian subcontinent, it is reasonable to assume that CVD risk is about 1.4 times higher than predicted from the charts. High blood pressure, left ventricular hypertrophy, type 2 diabetes, cigarette smoking, obesity and lack of physical activity are all more common in this racial group.

CVD–diabetes link

Diabetes mellitus is considered a CVD risk equivalent because a patient with diabetes has the same risk of having a CVD event as someone who already has CVD.

Framing the risk with Framingham

If a person has two or more risk factors (other than high low-density lipoprotein [LDL] cholestrol levels) without CVD or a CVD risk equivalent, Framingham risk scoring is used to estimate the short-term (10-year) risk of heart disease. This scoring system considers the patient's age, total cholesterol level, smoking status, HDL level and systolic blood pressure.

Metabolic mayhem

Metabolic syndrome has emerged as an equal to cigarette smoking in contributing to early heart disease. Also called *syndrome X* or *insulin resistance syndrome*, metabolic syndrome encompasses a cluster of metabolic risk factors that significantly increase the risk of coronary events. The syndrome is diagnosed if the patient has three or more of the following factors:

- increased waist circumference (≥102 cm in men and ≥88 cm in women; ≥90 cm in Asian men and ≥80 cm in Asian women), indicating central obesity
- elevated triglycerides (≥1.7 mmol/L)
- decreased HDL cholesterol (<1.03 mmol/L for men, <1.29 mmol/L for women)
- blood pressure >130/85 mmHg or active treatment for hypertension
- fasting plasma glucose level >5.6 mmol/L or active treatment for hyperglycaemia.

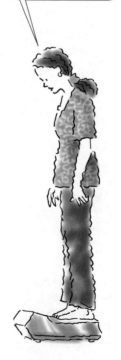

Focus the physical examination on nutrition-related aspects, such as weight and height.

A closer look at the risk factors

Central obesity, or fat contained within the abdominal cavity, is a strong predictor of metabolic syndrome. People with excess weight around their waists (apple-shaped bodies) are at increased risk for the syndrome—even more so than people who are equally overweight but with their weight distributed around the hips (pear-shaped bodies). The reason for this is that intra-abdominal fat tends to be more resistant to insulin than does fat in the periphery of the body. Normally, insulin reduces the amount of free fatty acids in the liver. In people with insulin resistance, the excess free fatty acids that reach the liver cause apolipoprotein B levels to increase, LDL cholestrol levels to increase, HDL levels to decrease and triglyceride levels to increase, producing an abnormal endothelium and atherosclerosis, thereby increasing the risk of CVD.

An elevated fasting blood glucose level greater than 5.6 mmol/L is a hallmark for metabolic syndrome. People with diabetes commonly develop atherosclerotic heart disease at a young age, a condition that affects more

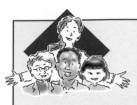

Bridging the gap

Ethnicities and metabolic syndrome

Ethnic groups that are susceptible to metabolic syndrome include South Asians (from the Indian subcontinent), Southeast Asians (for example people of Polynesian and Japanese descent) and Native Americans (such as Pima Indians).

diabetic women than men. Diabetes also increases the risk of macrovascular disease (ischaemic heart disease, stroke and peripheral vascular disease) and is a CHD risk equivalent.

In patients with insulin resistance, cells respond abnormally to insulin. For people who are genetically inclined to insulin resistance, abdominal obesity and sedentary lifestyle promote insulin resistance and metabolic syndrome. Insulin resistance leads to hyperinsulinaemia, hyperglycaemia, abnormal glucose and lipid metabolism, a damaged endothelium and CVD. The combination of insulin resistance, hyperinsulinaemia and abdominal obesity leads to hypertension and its harmful cardiovascular effects. Moreover, insulin resistance promotes salt sensitivity in people with high blood pressure.

Because metabolic syndrome is an independent risk factor in the development of CVD as well as a strong predictor of type 2 diabetes, patients with this syndrome require intensive lifestyle modification. Changes that can prevent or reduce the effects of metabolic syndrome include weight loss, regular exercise and dietary changes. (See *Ethnicities and metabolic syndrome*.)

Physical examination

Be sure to measure the patient's blood pressure and assess for signs and symptoms specific to CVD. However, focus the physical examination on nutrition-related aspects, including:
- patient's height, current weight, usual weight and weight history
- body mass index (BMI)
- waist circumference
- skinfold measurements
- body shape.

Body mass index
The BMI, which describes a person's weight relative to height, gives an acceptable estimate of body fat. (For instructions on calculating the BMI, see Chapter 8.) According to NICE guidelines, a BMI of less than 18.5 kg/m² indicates underweight; 18.5 kg/m² to 24.9 kg/m², normal; 25 to 29.9 kg/m², overweight; and 30 kg/m² and above, obesity.

Waist circumference

Waist circumference reflects body fat distribution. A high distribution of abdominal fat is linked to greater cardiovascular risk than excess lower-body fat. A waist circumference: men >102 cm, women >88 cm (Asians >90 cm in men and >80 cm in women) is considered to be significant. (To determine the patient's waist circumference, see Chapter 8.)

Waist circumference gives a more accurate picture of weight category in patients with large muscle mass, who might be classified as overweight in terms of BMI. For example if a female athlete has a BMI of 27 kg/m2 because of increased muscle mass (which adds to weight); as long as her waist circumference is under 88 cm, she wouldn't be considered overweight despite her high BMI.

Skinfold measurements

Roughly one-half of total body fat is located directly under the skin. For this reason, measuring skinfolds helps assess body fat percentage. Skinfolds are measured with calipers that pinch the skin as it's pulled away from the underlying muscle. Skinfold may be measured at the triceps, biceps, thigh, calf, subscapular or suprailiac areas.

Cardiovascular signs and symptoms

Assess your patient for physical indications of CVD, hypertension and heart failure. Suspect CVD (or high risk of CVD) if the patient has an apple-shaped body or if you note xanthomas—fatty yellow nodules or tumours in the subcutaneous skin layer sometimes seen in patients with high blood cholesterol levels.

Inspect for oedema and measure the patient's blood pressure. Presence of oedema or high blood pressure may indicate hypertension. Oedema, along with ascites and shortness of breath, also may accompany heart failure.

Diagnostic tests

To evaluate a patient for CVD, the doctor may order various laboratory and diagnostic tests, including:
- total cholesterol, LDL cholesterol and HDL cholesterol levels
- serum triglycerides
- C-reactive protein
- blood glucose
- electrocardiogram (ECG)
- stress test
- echocardiography
- cardiac catheterisation.

For a patient with hypertension, the doctor may order tests to check for an underlying cause (such as kidney disease, diabetes or adrenal dysfunction) and studies to detect cardiovascular damage and other complications, such as ECG and chest x-rays.

Diagnostic tests for a patient with suspected heart failure may include:
- ECG
- echocardiogram
- plasma b-type natriuretic peptide assay
- chest x-ray
- pulmonary artery pressure monitoring.

Coronary artery disease

The most common form of CVD, coronary artery disease (CAD) impairs coronary blood flow, leading to a loss of oxygen and nutrients to myocardial tissue. This disease is nearly epidemic in the Western world. It's most prevalent in white, middle-aged men and in elderly patients. CAD is the leading cause of death in the UK in both men and women.

Pathophysiology

Atherosclerosis is the most common cause of CAD. In this condition, fatty fibrous plaques (possibly including calcium deposits) progressively narrow the lumen of the coronary arteries, reducing the flow of blood through them. This can lead to myocardial ischaemia (decreased blood supply to the heart tissue) and infarction (a localised area of necrosis in the heart). (See *Acute coronary syndromes*.)

Atherosclerosis usually results from a high level of cholesterol and other fats in the blood. These fats build up within the arterial walls, causing narrowing of the lumen. The higher the patient's blood cholesterol level, the greater the chance that some cholesterol will be deposited along the arterial walls.

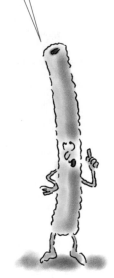

When plaques cause the lumen of the coronary artery to narrow, ischaemia and infarction can occur.

Acute coronary syndromes

Acute coronary syndromes (ACSs) is a general term used to describe a spectrum of disorders, including unstable angina and myocardial infarction (MI), that produce acute myocardial ischaemia and, as a result, chest pain. Patients with ACSs have some degree of coronary artery occlusion. The degree of blockage and the time that the affected vessel remains occluded are major determinants for the type of damage that occurs:

- If a patient has unstable angina, a thrombus partially occludes a coronary vessel. The partially occluded vessel may have distal microthrombi that cause necrosis in some myocytes. This condition may progress to non-ST-segment elevation MI (known as a NSTEMI).
- When a thrombus fully occludes the vessel for a prolonged time, this condition is known as an ST-segment elevation MI (known as a STEMI). In this type of MI, there's a greater concentration of thrombin and fibrin.

Attack of the plaques

In many people, atherosclerosis starts in childhood or adolescence and first appears as fatty streaks in the arteries. With age, these streaks worsen, becoming plaques, or atheromas, that protrude from the inside walls of the arteries and impede blood flow.

Because blood cholesterol is waxy and can't dissolve in water, it mostly travels through the blood in lipoproteins. HDL—the 'good' cholesterol— gathers up excess cholesterol in the blood and carries it to the liver, which reprocesses or excretes it. HDL may also help remove some of the cholesterol deposited along the arterial walls. In contrast, LDL cholesterol—the 'bad' cholesterol—accumulates in body tissues. (See *Classifying cholesterol levels*, page 262.)

Supply-side crisis

As atherosclerosis progresses, arterial narrowing is accompanied by vascular changes that impair the diseased vessel's ability to dilate. This causes a precarious balance between myocardial oxygen supply and demand, threatening the myocardium beyond the lesion. When oxygen demand exceeds what the diseased vessels can supply, localised myocardial ischaemia results.

Transient ischaemia leads to diminishing myocardial function; if left untreated, it can result in tissue injury or necrosis. Left ventricular function then becomes impaired. The strength of contractions in the affected myocardial region decreases as the fibres shorten inadequately with less force and velocity. As wall motion in the ischaemic section becomes abnormal, less blood is ejected from the heart with each contraction.

Pressure and sympathy

Depression of left ventricular function may reduce stroke volume and thus lower cardiac output. Reduction in systolic emptying increases ventricular volumes. As a result, left-sided heart pressure and pulmonary artery wedge pressure rise. Changes in wall compliance induced by ischaemia magnify these pressure increases.

During ischaemia, sympathetic nervous system response causes slight rises in blood pressure and heart rate before the onset of pain. With pain onset, further sympathetic activation occurs.

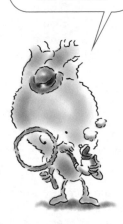

It's elementary, really—just a problem of supply and demand.

What to look for

Angina, the classic sign of ACS, may range from mild and intermittent to pronounced and steady. However, it isn't always present. Some people with ACS, including people with diabetes, are symptom free. The patient may describe chest pain as a burning, squeezing or crushing pain or tightness in the substernal or precordial area that radiates to the left arm, neck, jaw or shoulder blade.

Angina commonly follows physical exertion but may also follow emotional excitement, cold exposure or a large meal. Sometimes, it develops during sleep and awakens the patient.

Stable or unstable?

If the pain is predictable and relieved by rest or nitrates, it's called *stable angina*. If it increases in frequency and duration and is more easily induced, it's called *unstable* or *unpredictable angina*. Left untreated, unstable angina may progress to MI.

Patients typically describe the symptoms of an MI as uncomfortable pressure, squeezing, burning, severe persistent pain or fullness in the centre of the chest lasting several minutes (usually longer than 15 minutes). Pain may radiate to the left arm, shoulders, neck or jaw or may occur in the back between the shoulder blades. The patient may clench his or her fist over his or her chest or rub the left arm when describing it. Pain may be accompanied by nausea, vomiting, fainting, sweating and cool extremities.

Treatment

The primary goal of therapy for a patient with ACS is to lower serum LDL cholesterol levels. Recent clinical trials confirm that lowering LDL cholesterol reduces the short-term risk of heart disease by as much as 40% and brings even greater risk reduction over time.

Lipid modification: Primary and secondary CVD prevention

A target for total cholesterol or LDL cholesterol is not recommended for primary prevention of CVD.

Statin therapy is recommended for adults with clinical evidence of CVD.
- People with ACS should be treated with a higher intensity statin. Any decision to offer a higher intensity statin should take into account the patient's informed preference, comorbidities, multiple drug therapy and the benefits and risks of treatment. Treatment will be managed by your general practitioner or specialist health care professional, according to local protocol and guidance.
- Treatment for the secondary prevention of CVD should be initiated with simvastatin 40 mg. If there are potential drug interactions, or simvastatin 40 mg is contraindicated, a lower dose or alternative preparation such as pravastatin may be chosen.
- In people taking statins for secondary prevention, the dose of simvastatin may be increased or a drug of similar efficacy prescribed if a total cholesterol of less than 4 mmol/L or an LDL cholesterol of less than 2 mmol/L is not attained. Any decision to offer a higher intensity statin should take into account informed preference, comorbidities, multiple drug therapy and the benefit and risks of treatment.
- Medication is supported by new, more powerful lifestyle changes, including increasing physical activity, to improve cholesterol levels.
- People identified with metabolic syndrome are also actively treated earlier.

Matching treatment to risk

The intensity of LDL cholesterol lowering treatment is linked to the patient's cardiovascular risk level. It divides patients with multiple risk factors into

Classifying cholesterol levels

Use the chart below to understand your patient's lipoprotein profile.

Level	Profile
LDL cholesterol	
<2 mmol/L	Optimal
2 to 3.34 mmol/L	Near optimal/above optimal
3.36 to 4.12 mmol/L	Borderline high
4.14 to 4.90 mmol/L	High
≥4.92 mmol/L	Very high
HDL cholesterol	
<1 mmol/L	Low
≥1.55 mmol/L	High (desirable)
Total cholesterol	
<4 mmol/L	Desirable
4 to 6.19 mmol/L	Borderline high
≥6.2 mmol/L	High

Adapted from British Heart Foundation. *Reducing Your Cholesterol*. Available at: *http://www.bhf.org.uk/publications/publications_search_results.aspx?m=simple&q=LDL*

three categories based on their 10-year risk for CVD (see 'Step 4' below). Guidelines focus on a stepped treatment plan, with nine steps progressing according to the patient's cholesterol profile and risk factors.

Step 1

Obtain a complete lipoprotein profile using blood samples drawn after a 9- to 12-hour fast.

Step 2

Identify clinical atherosclerotic disease that confers a high risk of CVD events or a CVD risk equivalent. These include clinical CVD, symptomatic carotid artery disease, abdominal aortic aneurysm and peripheral arterial disease.

Step 3

Count the number of major risk factors a patient has, other than a high LDL cholesterol level. Major risk factors include:
• cigarette smoking
• hypertension (blood pressure of 140/90 mmHg or higher) or use of antihypertensive medication
• HDL level below 1 mmol/L (HDL level greater than 2 mmol/L), which removes a risk factor from the count

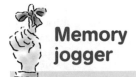

Memory jogger

To remember the major risk factors for CVD, think **ASHHH:**

Age (males 45 or older, females 55 or older)

Smoking

Hypertension

History of CVD in family

HDL level <2 mmol/L.

- family history of premature CVD (CVD in a male first-degree relative under age 55 or in a female first-degree relative under age 65)
- age 45 or older (male) or 55 or older (female).

Step 4

Assess the patient's level of 10-year cardiovascular risk. (Presence of CVD or CVD risk equivalent automatically places the patient in the highest risk category.) Count the number of risk factors the patient has (excluding high LDL cholesterol level and presence of CVD). If he or she has two or more risk factors, the Framingham scoring system is used to determine risk level and intensity of therapy.

The three risk categories are:
- above 20% (CVD and CVD risk equivalent)
- 10% to 20% (two or more risk factors)
- less than 10% (one or zero risk factors).

Step 5

The general practitioner or specialist health care professional will determine the patient's LDL cholesterol goal, need for therapeutic lifestyle changes (TLC) and LDL cholesterol level at which drug therapy should be considered. These include:
- Those with recent MIs or those who have CVD and diabetes, poorly controlled risk factors or metabolic syndrome.
- Those with unusual lipid profile (typically total cholesterol >7.5 mmol/L, LDL cholesterol >4.9 mmol/L) where secondary causes have been ruled out, especially if strong family history of premature CHD is present (family history of MI—aged younger than 50 years in second-degree relative, aged less than 60 in first-degree relative), give dietary advice and seek specialist advice. Confirmation is needed with two measurements of LDL cholesterol. Family screening may be necessary subsequently.
- Absence of clinical signs (for example tendon xanthomata) does not exclude a diagnosis of familial hyperlipidaemia, but their presence makes the diagnosis highly likely.

Step 6

If the patient's LDL cholesterol is above the goal for his or her risk level, initiate TLC, including the TLC diet, weight management and increased physical activity. The TLC diet recommends eating only enough calories to maintain a desirable weight and avoid weight gain. Other highlights include:
- *Cut right down on saturated fats* and replace them with monounsaturated fats and polyunsaturated fats.
- *Reduce the total amount of fat you eat*—especially if you are overweight. (This is because fat is also very high in calories.) For example cut down on foods such as pastries, crisps and biscuits, and replace them with healthier alternatives such as fruits and vegetables. Or, at mealtimes, cut down on the amount of fatty foods you eat by filling up with starchy foods such as bread, pasta or rice instead—particularly the wholegrain versions of these foods.

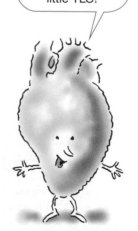

To lower your patient's cholesterol, try a little TLC!

Therapeutic lifestyle change

	Unsaturated fats			Saturated fats	
	Monounsaturated	*Polyunsaturated*	*Omega-3*	*Saturated*	*Trans-fats*
Found in the following foods	Olive oil and rapeseed oil, nuts and seeds (almonds, cashews, hazelnuts and peanuts) and avocado	Corn oil, sunflower oil and soya oil, nuts and seeds (pine nuts, sesame and sunflower seeds)	Fish oil, oily fish such as herring, mackerel and pilchards	Butter, hard cheese, fatty meats, biscuits, cakes, suet, ghee, coconut oil and palm oil	Although less common in the UK than in the US, it can be found in commercially produced cakes and biscuits. Foods containing hydrogenated oils or fat are likely to contain trans-fats

Margarines and spreads may contain differing amounts of monounsaturated, saturated or omega-3 fatty acids

Adapted from British Heart Foundation. *Reducing Cholesterol*. Available at: http://www.bhf.org.uk/publications/publications_search_results.aspx?m5simple&q5cholesterol.

- *Cut down on foods containing trans fats*—this means cutting down on processed foods such as cakes, biscuits and pastries. (See *Therapeutic lifestyle change*.)

Step 7

To maximise cholesterol lowering, TLC should always be maintained when drug therapy is prescribed.

Drug therapy may include:
- statin drugs (such as simvastatin and lovastatin, and pravastatin), which have been shown to be effective in persons with or without CVD (in clinical trials, lowering of LDL cholesterol levels with statins decreased the rate of MI and deaths from CVD by roughly 30%); these drugs may be used in combination with other lipid-lowering drugs
- bile acid sequestrants (such as cholestyramine and colestipol), which also lower LDL cholesterol levels and may be used alone or in combination with statins
- nicotinic acid (niacin), which lowers LDL cholesterol and triglyceride levels and raises HDL levels (however, when taken in doses large enough to lower cholesterol, it can cause adverse effects, so it should be used only under a doctor's supervision)
- fibric acids (such as gemfibrozil and fenofibrate), which are used mainly to treat high triglyceride levels and low HDL levels
- cholesterol absorption inhibitors (ezetimibe), which reduce total cholesterol and LDL cholesterol levels and may slightly increase HDL cholesterol levels
- combination cholesterol absorption inhibitor and statin (ezetimibe/simvastatin), which reduces LDL cholesterol and triglyceride levels and increases HDL cholesterol levels.

Step 8

Assess the patient for the indicators of metabolic syndrome. A patient who meets diagnostic criteria should receive treatment for metabolic syndrome after 3 months of TLC. Therapies centre on addressing obesity, increasing physical activity, lowering blood pressure and serum triglyceride levels, raising HDL levels and using aspirin to reduce prothrombotic states in patients with CVD.

Step 9

A patient with elevated triglyceride levels should take steps to manage weight and increase physical activity, and may be prescribed a lipid-lowering drug.

Dietary management

A heart-healthy diet is essential to controlling and managing CVD. This diet can slow the progression of atherosclerosis. When combined with other heart-healthy strategies, it may even stop or reverse narrowing of arteries. What's more, a heart-healthy diet can help reduce total cholesterol and LDL cholesterol levels, lower blood pressure and blood glucose levels and aid weight management. (See *Sample menu for TLC diet*.)

Menu maven

Sample menu for TLC diet

Breakfast	Lunch	Dinner	Snack
Porridge made with water or skimmed milk	Roast beef sandwich	Tuna	Peaches, canned in water (one portion)
One slice of toast	Wholewheat bun (one medium)	Rice	Water (125 ml)
Soft margarine (2 tsp)	Roast beef, lean Swiss cheese, low fat (1 oz slice)	Sweetcorn	
Jam (1 tbsp)	Lettuce (two leaves)	Mushrooms	
Half grapefruit	Tomato (two medium slices)	Tomatoes	
Orange juice 250 ml	Mustard (2 tsp)	Roll (one small)	
Coffee (250 ml) with fat-free milk (2 tbsp)	Pasta salad	Soft margarine (1 tsp)	
	Pasta noodles	Fresh fruit salad topped with low-fat frozen yoghurt—one pot	
	Mixed vegetables	Fat-free/skimmed milk (250 ml)	
	Olive oil (2 tsp)		
	Apple (one medium)		
	Iced tea, unsweetened (250 ml)		

Based on Food Standards Agency. *Eat Well Be Well Recommendations*. Available at: http://www.eatwell.gov.uk/healthissues/healthyheart.

NutriTips

Tips for eating out

If your patient eats out a lot, pass on these hints to help him or her eat healthier when dining out:

- Choose restaurants that offer low-fat, low-cholesterol menu choices. As a paying customer, don't be afraid to make special requests.
- Don't let the restaurant dictate your portion size, and don't feel compelled to eat everything because you're paying for it. Ask for a small serving, share a dish with a friend or take some home for another meal.
- Limit such extras as gravy, butter, rich sauces and salad dressings. Ask that these items be served on the side, so you can control the amount.
- Avoid fried foods in favour of foods that are baked, grilled or stir-fried.
- Choose extra vegetables and salad whenever possible.
- If you must have dessert, split it so you only eat half the portion.
- At a buffet, choose mostly low-fat foods. If you just can't resist a few higher-fat items, keep portions small.
- At parties, don't fixate on food. Instead, focus on the people and activities.
- Encourage others to help you reduce your fat intake. If you're invited to a friend's home for dinner, ask the friend to include low-fat dishes.
- If you eat too many high-fat foods, don't feel guilty and go on a binge. Just eat lightly the next day to get back on track.

Focus on fat

To help your patient reduce high cholesterol levels, recommend a diet that's low in fat. Advise him or her to restrict total fat intake (saturated, trans-, monounsaturated and polyunsaturated fats) to 25% to 35% of total daily calories and to restrict saturated and trans-fat intake to less than 7%.

Remind the patient that lowering dietary fat intake promotes weight loss. If the patient is overweight, losing excess weight can help lower blood cholesterol as well as high blood pressure—another risk factor for atherosclerosis and heart disease. If the patient eats out a lot, maintaining a heart-healthy diet can pose a challenge. Provide appropriate suggestions. (See *Tips for eating out*.)

Top tips to prevent heart disease

- Eat five portions of fruits and vegetables each day, avoiding fruits and vegetables that are very sweet such as parsnips and strawberries.
- Reduce the amount of fat you eat by changing to low-fat dairy products, removing skin from meat before cooking, trimming off all visible fat from

cuts of meat, using a spoon to measure oil when cooking and cutting down on snacks like crisps and chocolate.
• Eat oily fish. It's rich in omega-3, a polyunsaturated fatty acid which is good for the heart. Aim for at least two portions of oily fish. Fish can be fresh, frozen or canned (canned fish may be high in salt!)
• Skip the salt by trying to remove salt from the table and cooking. Choose foods labelled 'no added salt', and limit intake of salty snacks such as crisps, Bombay mix, pickles and readymade processed foods.

Cut the cholesterol

Point out to the patient that cholesterol comes in two different types—blood (serum) cholesterol and dietary cholesterol. Dietary cholesterol is found in foods of animal origin, including egg yolks, organ meats and full-fat dairy products. Blood cholesterol is a waxy substance that occurs naturally in the body.

Many patients think that just avoiding foods high in cholesterol will lower their serum cholesterol level. However, the body continues to make cholesterol no matter what kind of diet a person eats. Controlling *total* fat intake—and saturated fat in particular—has a more direct impact on blood cholesterol levels.

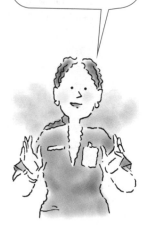

If it sounds too good to be true, it probably is. Make sure your patient understands that fat free usually doesn't mean calorie free.

Dish out the dietary do's, not the don'ts

To help the patient succeed with a heart-healthy diet, focus on what he or she *can* eat rather than what he or she can't. Stress that a well-balanced diet—one that relies on fruits, vegetables, wholegrains, legumes, lean meat, low-fat dairy products and a minimum amount of added fat—is the key. Emphasise that the goal is to *lower* fat intake—not eliminate fats entirely. Fats play an important role in the body, providing storage of calories for energy, insulation and a means for transporting fat-soluble vitamins.

Fat-free fallacies

Tell the patient that limiting calories is important, too—especially if he or she must lose excess weight. Point out that fat-free foods aren't calorie free. Many fat-free and low-fat foods and beverages have added sugars to make them taste better. These sugars increase calories—that's why a fat-free or low-fat food may still be high in calories. In fact, some fat-free foods contain nearly the same number of calories as their high-fat counterparts.

Serving savvy

When teaching your patient about a heart-healthy diet, recommend the following measures:
• Eat at least two servings of fruits or vegetables at each meal. Choose fruits as between-meal snacks. They're the healthiest 'fast food'. (In cultures where people consume a lot of fruits, vegetables and grains and relatively little meat,

CAD rates are far lower than in cultures that consume a lot of meat and high-fat, high-sugar foods.)

- Eat more wholegrains, such as wholegrain breads, brown rice, barley, oatmeal and soluble fibre.
- Pay attention to total fat intake. Choose low-fat dairy products and lean meats. Watch out for high-fat desserts and snacks.
- Reduce intake of saturated fat and fats that act like saturated fat, such as hydrogenated fat and trans-fat. (See *Fat facts: The good, the bad and the ugly*.)
- Use more monounsaturated fats (canola oil and olive oil).
- Taste food before adding salt. A yen for salt is a learned taste—it can be unlearned, too. Getting used to less salty foods takes about 6 weeks.
- Mind portion size. Just about any food can be consumed in moderation.
- Make balanced meals. The meat portion should take up no more than one-third of the plate.

Two servings of vegetables and one serving of starch should accompany the main course. Adding a green, leafy salad with additional raw vegetables tossed in, topped with a light or fat-free salad dressing, earns an 'A'.

Fat facts: The good, the bad and the ugly

Fats (fatty acids) come in many varieties—some good, some bad and some really bad. To help your patient plan a heart-healthy diet, make sure you understand the various types.

Good	Bad	Ugly
Monounsaturated fats	*Saturated fats*	*Trans-fatty acids*
Monounsaturated fats are found mainly in canola oil, olive oil, peanut oil and avocados. These fats are liquid at room temperature.	Saturated fats are found chiefly in animal sources, such as meat, poultry, whole or reduced-fat milk and butter. Some vegetable oils, such as coconut oil, palm kernel oil and palm oil, are saturated. Saturated fats are usually solid at room temperature.	Trans-fatty acids (trans-fats for short) form when vegetable oils are processed into margarine or shortening. Sources of trans-fats in the diet include snack foods and baked goods made with partially hydrogenated vegetable oil or vegetable shortening. Trans-fatty acids also occur naturally in some animal products, such as dairy products.
Polyunsaturated fats	*Dietary cholesterol*	
Polyunsaturated fats are found in soybean, sesame, sunflower and safflower seeds and their oils. They're also the main fats found in seafood. These fats are liquid or soft at room temperature. Specific polyunsaturated fatty acids, such as linoleic acid and alpha-linoleic acid, are called essential fatty acids because they're necessary for cell structure and making hormones. Essential fatty acids must be obtained from foods.	Dietary cholesterol is found in foods of animal origin, such as meat, pork, poultry, fish, eggs and full-fat dairy products.	

Vitamins for healthy vessels

Numerous studies from around the world suggest that getting enough folic acid and vitamins B_6 and B_{12} can help maintain a healthy heart and blood vessels. Folic acid and vitamins B_6 and B_{12} work in combination to reduce the blood level of homocysteine, a natural product of protein breakdown in the blood. Scientific evidence shows that lower blood homocysteine levels are associated with reduced risk of heart disease.

The leading sources of folic acid are ready-to-eat cereals, enriched breads, fruits, vegetables, citrus juice and dry beans. In 2009 the Food Standards Agency endorsed the scientific advisory committee on nutrition recommendation for the compulsory fortification of bread and flour in the UK. This is currently being reviewed by the Minister for Health.

Vitamin B_6 is widely distributed in foods. Significant sources include meats, wholewheat products, vegetables and nuts. Vitamin B_{12} is found in animal products only—particularly meat, milk, eggs, fish and cheese.

Fibre-ific facts

Only plant foods, such as fruits, vegetables and grains, contain fibre. The part of the plant fibre that's consumed, called *dietary fibre*, is an important part of a heart-healthy diet.

Dietary fibre comes in two main types—insoluble and soluble. Soluble fibre forms a gel when mixed with liquid, whereas insoluble fibre passes through the GI tract largely intact. Both types of fibre are important in the diet and help maintain regular bowel movements.

Soluble fibre has additional cardiovascular health benefits. It has been proven to reduce blood cholesterol levels, which may help reduce the risk of heart disease.

Set your sights on psyllium

Soluble fibre is found in oats, peas, beans, certain fruits and a grain called *psyllium*, found in some cereal products, dietary supplements and bulk fibre laxatives. Instruct the patient to read food, dietary supplement and drug labels carefully to check for psyllium. (See *How much fibre?*)

Judging a food by its label

Food labels have two important parts: the Nutrition Facts panel and the ingredients list. Instruct the patient to read the Nutrition Facts panel to check the amount of saturated fat, trans-fat, total fat, cholesterol and calories in one serving of the product and then compare similar products to find the one with the lowest amounts. If he or she has high blood pressure, he or she should do the same for sodium.

Tell the patient that the ingredients are listed in descending order by weight. For instance if sugar is listed first on a cereal product, the cereal has more sugar than any other ingredient. To choose foods low in saturated fat

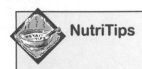

NutriTips

How much fibre?

Health experts recommend that people eat 25 to 38 g of fibre each day, including soluble and insoluble fibre. The average British person eats only 12 to 17 g/day; about one-fourth is soluble fibre. This means the average person eats only 3 to 4 g/day of soluble fibre—less than half of the recommended 5 to 10 g/day. Daily intake of 3 g of soluble fibre from oats or 7 g from psyllium has been shown to lower blood cholesterol levels.

or total fat, advise the patient to limit food products that list any fat or oil first—or that list many fat and oil ingredients. If the patient is watching their sodium intake, tell them to do the same for sodium or salt.

Hypertension

Blood pressure is defined as the amount of pressure exerted on the walls of the arteries as the blood moves through them. It is measured in millimetres of mercury (mmHg).

There are two measurements used to assess blood pressure:
- *Systolic pressure* is the blood pressure that is exerted when the heart beats and forces blood around the body. This is the top reading.
- *Diastolic pressure* is the measure of blood pressure when the heart is resting between beats. This is the bottom reading.

Hypertension (high blood pressure) is a consistent blood pressure of 140/90 mmHg or higher. Suggest to individuals that they contact their general practitioner for advice if their blood pressure is greater than 120/80 mmHg. The major types of hypertension are essential (also called *primary* or *idiopathic*) and secondary.

The cause of essential hypertension, the most common type, involves several interacting homoeostatic mechanisms. Hypertension is classified as secondary if it's related to a systemic disease that raises peripheral vascular resistance or cardiac output. Malignant hypertension is a severe fulminant form of the disorder that may arise from either primary or secondary hypertension.

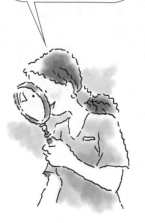

Tell your patient to read the fine print! If sugar is listed first, there's more sugar than any other ingredient!

No news isn't good news

Hypertension is often called a *silent killer* because it causes few, if any, symptoms. A person may have it for years without knowing it. Hypertension can lead to vascular disease including CHD, stroke, diabetes and kidney disease. This currently affects the lives of over 4 million people in England. It causes 36% of deaths (170,000 a year in England) and is responsible for a fifth of all hospital admissions. It is the largest single cause of long-term ill-health and disability, impairing the quality of life for many people. The burden of these conditions falls disproportionately on people living in deprived circumstances and on particular ethnic groups, such as South Asians.

The British Hypertensive Society supports the creation of a new category, called prehypertension, which includes blood pressure readings of 120/80 to 139/89 mmHg, levels previously considered normal or high normal. Normal blood pressure is defined as less than 120/80 mmHg. Research indicates that people with prehypertension are twice as likely to develop CVD as people with blood pressure values less than 120/80 mmHg. For each increase of 20/10 mmHg, the risk of developing CVD doubles.

Classifying blood pressure readings

The revised categories are based on the average of two or more readings taken on separate visits after an initial screening. They apply to adults aged 18 and older. (If the systolic and diastolic pressures fall into different categories, use the higher of the two pressures to classify the reading. For example a reading of 160/92 mmHg should be classified as grade 2.)

Normal blood pressure with respect to cardiovascular risk is characterised by a systolic reading below 120 mmHg and a diastolic reading below 80 mmHg. Patients with prehypertension are at increased risk for developing hypertension and should follow health-promoting lifestyle modifications to prevent cardiovascular disease.

In addition to classifying stages of hypertension based on average blood pressure readings, clinicians should also take note of target organ disease and additional risk factors, such as diabetes, left ventricular hypertrophy and chronic renal disease. These additional factors are important in assessing the patient's true cardiovascular health.

Classification of blood pressure levels of the British Hypertension Society:

Category	Systolic (mmHg)		Diastolic (mmHg)
Optimal	<120	AND	<80
Normal	<130	AND	<85
High normal	130 to 139	OR	85 to 89
Hypertension Grade 1	140 to 159	OR	90 to 99
Grade 2	160 to 179	OR	100 to 109
Grade 3	≤180		≤110

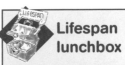

Lifespan lunchbox

Isolated systolic hypertension in elderly patients

In elderly people, systolic blood pressure may be elevated, even when diastolic blood pressure is not. This condition, known as isolated systolic hypertension (ISH), was once believed to be a normal part of ageing and commonly went untreated. However, atherosclerosis causes a loss of elasticity in large arteries, which can cause ISH. Results of the Systolic Hypertension in the Elderly Program found that treating ISH with antihypertensive drugs lowered the incidence of stroke, coronary artery disease and left-sided heart failure.

The risk of death from heart disease and stroke rises with increasing blood pressure readings, starting as low as 115/75 mmHg. (See *Classifying blood pressure readings*.)

Pathophysiology

Hypertension may result from increases in cardiac output or total peripheral resistance or both. Cardiac output rises from conditions that increase the heart rate or stroke volume. Peripheral resistance rises from factors that increase blood viscosity or reduce vessel lumen size. (See *Isolated systolic hypertension in elderly patients*.)

Essentially preventable

Essential hypertension usually starts insidiously as a benign disease and progresses slowly to a malignant state. If untreated, even mild cases can cause major complications and death. Carefully managed treatment, which may include lifestyle changes and drug therapy, improves prognosis.

In theory...

Various theories help explain the development of hypertension. For example it's thought to arise from:
- changes in the arteriolar bed that cause increased resistance
- abnormally increased tone in the sensory nervous system that arises in the vasomotor centres, increasing peripheral vascular resistance
- greater blood volume resulting from renal or hormonal dysfunction
- increase in arteriolar thickening caused by genetic factors, leading to increased peripheral vascular resistance
- abnormal renin release, resulting in the formation of angiotensin II, which constricts the arterioles and increases blood volume.

Not-so-secondary considerations

Secondary hypertension may result from pre-existing diseases or use of certain drugs:
- renal vascular or parenchymal disease
- pheochromocytoma
- primary hyperaldosteronism
- Cushing's syndrome
- diabetes mellitus
- dysfunction of the thyroid, pituitary or parathyroid gland
- aortic coarctation
- pre-eclampsia—a significant blood pressure rise during the last 3 months of pregnancy
- neurologic disorders
- use of certain cold remedies, decongestants, over-the-counter pain relievers and prescription drugs (including hormonal contraceptives)
- cocaine and amphetamine use.

The pathophysiology of secondary hypertension varies with the underlying disorder. For example in chronic renal disease, insult to the kidney from renal artery stenosis or chronic glomerulonephritis interferes with sodium excretion, the renin–angiotensin–aldosterone system or renal perfusion. As a result, blood pressure rises.

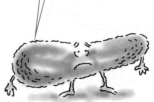

Oh my! Diabetes mellitus is a risk factor for CAD and secondary hypertension.

Out of my hands

Four major risk factors for hypertension can't be controlled. They include:

 increasing age

race (hypertension is more common in ethnic minorities, particularly in South Asian rather than in Caucasian populations)

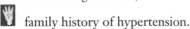 gender (in young adulthood and early middle age, more men have high blood pressure; rates are equal from ages 55 to 64; at age 65 and older, women have higher rates)

family history of hypertension.

In the driver's seat

Hypertension risk factors that a person can control or manage include:
* obesity
* inactivity
* tobacco use (chemicals in tobacco damage the lining of the arterial wall, causing the arteries to accumulate plaques; nicotine constricts blood vessels and forces the heart to work harder)
* sodium sensitivity (increased sensitivity to sodium causes increased sodium retention, leading to fluid retention and higher blood pressure)
* low potassium levels (potassium helps balance the amount of sodium in cells)
* excessive alcohol intake
* stress (high stress levels can lead to a temporary but steep blood pressure rise).

Chronic illnesses—including hypercholesterolaemia, diabetes mellitus, sleep apnoea and heart failure—can also increase the risk of hypertension.

What to look for

Patients with hypertension may complain of a dull ache in the back of the head when they awaken in the morning. Some patients also experience dizziness and nosebleeds. However, these symptoms typically don't occur until hypertension is severe. In fact, most people with hypertension—even those with the highest blood pressure readings—have no signs or symptoms until vascular changes in the heart, brain or kidneys occur. As severely elevated blood pressure damages the inner lining of small blood vessels, fibrin accumulates in the vessels and local oedema occurs. Some patients also experience intravascular clotting. Signs and symptoms depend on the location of the damaged vessels:
* brain—stroke, transient ischaemic attacks
* retina—blindness
* heart—MI
* kidneys—proteinuria, oedema and, eventually, renal failure.

Because hypertension increases the heart's workload, the patient may also experience left ventricular hypertrophy and, later, left-sided heart failure, pulmonary oedema and right-sided heart failure.

Treatment

Treatment of secondary hypertension focuses on correcting the underlying cause and controlling hypertensive effects. For essential hypertension, the NICE recommends the following approach:

• Help the patient make necessary lifestyle changes, such as weight loss, sodium restriction, moderation of alcohol intake, regular physical exercise, smoking cessation and adoption of a healthy diet.

• Many people will be prescribed medication to help control their blood pressure. Thiazide-type diuretics, alone or in combination with other classes of antihypertensive drugs, are recommended for most patients with uncomplicated hypertension. Individulas should be advised to still drink plenty of fluids when on diuretics as they can become dehydrated if they restrict their fluid intake as well. If a patient has compelling indications, other antihypertensive drugs may be used first, such as angiotensin-converting enzyme (ACE) inhibitors, beta-adrenergic blockers, calcium channel blockers and angiotensin receptor blockers. A combination of two or more drugs may be necessary to achieve blood pressure control. Other drugs that can be used include angiotensin II antagonists, alpha$_1$-receptor blockers, alpha–beta blockers and vasodilators.

• If the patient fails to achieve the desired blood pressure or make significant progress, the doctor may increase the drug dosage, substitute a drug in the same class or add a drug from a different class.

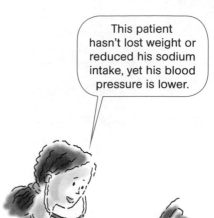

This patient hasn't lost weight or reduced his sodium intake, yet his blood pressure is lower.

Dietary management

Nutrition therapy for hypertension focuses on reducing sodium intake, losing any excess weight, moderating alcohol intake and increasing physical activity. (See *Tips to reduce sodium intake*.)

Heart failure

Heart failure refers to the inability of the myocardium to pump effectively enough to meet the body's metabolic needs. Typically, loss in pumping action reflects an underlying heart problem such as CVD. Pump failure usually occurs in a damaged left ventricle but may also affect the right ventricle. Usually, left-sided heart failure develops first.

Heart failure is classified in the following ways:
• acute or chronic
• left-sided or right-sided
• diastolic or systolic.

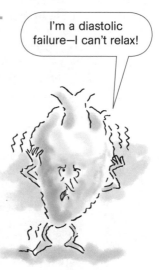

I'm a diastolic failure—I can't relax!

Systolic or diastolic?

Systolic failure occurs when the heart's ability to contract decreases. The heart can't pump with enough force to pump a sufficient amount of blood int circulation. Diastolic failure occurs when the heart has a problem relaxing. The heart can't properly fill with blood because the muscle has become stiff.

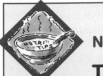

NutriTips

Tips to reduce sodium intake

Only a small amount of sodium occurs naturally in foods. Most sodium is added to foods during processing in the form of sodium chloride. To help your patient cut down their sodium intake, provide the following suggestions.

Read those labels

- Read food labels for sodium content.
- Use food products with reduced sodium or no added salt.
- Be aware that soy sauce, broth and foods that are pickled or cured have high sodium contents.

Now you're cookin'

- Instead of cooking with salt, use herbs, spices, cooking wines, lemon, lime or vinegar to enhance food flavours.
- Cook pasta and rice without salt.
- Rinse canned foods, such as tuna, to remove some sodium.
- Avoid adding salt to foods, especially at the table.
- Avoid condiments such as soy and teriyaki sauces and monosodium glutamate (MSG)—or use lower-sodium versions.

You are what you eat

- Eat fresh poultry, fish and lean meat rather than canned, smoked or processed versions (which typically contain a lot of sodium).
- Whenever possible, eat fresh foods rather than canned or convenience foods.
- Limit intake of cured foods (such as bacon and ham), foods packed in brine (pickles, olives and sauerkraut) and condiments (mustard, ketchup, horseradish and Worcestershire sauce).
- When dining out, ask how food is prepared. Ask that your food be prepared without added salt or MSG.

Pathophysiology

Heart failure may result from a primary abnormality of the heart muscle, such as MI, that impairs ventricular function and prevents the heart from pumping enough blood. It can also result from problems unrelated to MI, including:

- mechanical disturbances in ventricular filling during diastole, which occur because blood volume is too low for the ventricle to pump
- systolic hemodynamic disturbances (such as excessive cardiac workload caused by volume or pressure overload) that limit the heart's pumping ability.

Get smart about salt terms

Food manufacturers use various terms to indicate that a product has a low sodium content. The chart below lists interpretations of these terms. Reduced-sodium alternatives contain less sodium than standard salt and taste similar. But they are not sodium free—sodium is the part of salt that can lead to high blood pressure if you have too much. Salt substitutes are not suitable for some people, so always check the label. Also, because these alternatives taste salty, they don't help people to get used to less salty flavours. It's better to gradually reduce the amount of salt in cooking and eating until finally the individual uses hardly any—or none at all.

What the label says

Next time you go shopping, compare the labels on different foods to help you choose those that are lower in salt. Look at the figure for salt per 100 g.

High is more than 1.5 g salt per 100 g (or 0.6 g sodium).

Low is 0.3 g salt or less per 100 g (or 0.1 g sodium).

If the amount of salt per 100 g is in between these figures, then that is a medium level of salt.

Remember that the amount you eat of a particular food affects how much salt you will get from it. Foods such as bacon, cheese, anchovies, pickles and smoked fish tend to be quite salty, so it's better not to eat too much as this will increase your salt intake.

Adapted from FSA, available online at http://www.eatwell.gov.uk/healthydiet/fss/salt/checkinglabelforsalt/

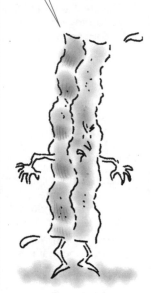

I don't want to sound bitter but your patients should keep the salt off me!

Failure factors

Certain conditions can predispose a patient to heart failure, especially if he or she has underlying heart disease. These conditions include:
• arrhythmias that reduce ventricular filling time, disrupt filling synchrony or reduce cardiac output
• pregnancy and thyrotoxicosis, which increase cardiac output
• pulmonary embolism, which raises pulmonary arterial pressures, causing right ventricular failure
• infections, which increase metabolic demands and further burden the heart
• anaemia, which leads to increased cardiac output to meet tissue oxygen needs
• heart valve problems
• heart infections
• genetic abnormalities
• increased salt or water intake, emotional stress or failure to comply with a prescribed treatment regimen for underlying heart disease.

Core complications

Eventually, fluid may enter the lungs, causing pulmonary oedema, a life-threatening condition. Decreased perfusion to the brain, kidneys and other major organs may cause them to fail. MI also may result because the oxygen demands of the overworked heart can't be met.

Worth the risk?

Heart failure is closely associated with major risk factors for CVD: smoking, high cholesterol levels, hypertension, diabetes mellitus and obesity. A single risk factor may be sufficient to cause heart failure, but a combination of factors dramatically increases the risk. Advanced age adds to the potential impact of any heart failure risk.

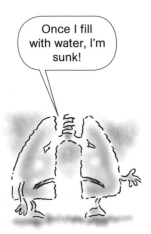

Once I fill with water, I'm sunk!

What to look for

Early signs and symptoms of heart failure include:
- fatigue
- exertional, paroxysmal and nocturnal dyspnoea
- neck vein engorgement
- hepatomegaly.

Later signs and symptoms include:
- tachypnoea
- palpitations
- dependent oedema
- unexplained, steady weight gain
- nausea
- chest tightness
- slowed mental response
- anorexia
- hypotension
- diaphoresis
- narrow PP
- pallor
- oliguria
- gallop rhythm and inspiratory crackles on auscultation
- dullness over the lung bases
- haemoptysis
- cyanosis
- marked hepatomegaly
- pitting ankle oedema
- sacral oedema in bedridden patients.

Treatment

Heart failure will be managed by the general practitioner, heart failure nurse specialist and other specialists according to local protocol. Management includes a range of prescription drugs:
- ACE inhibitor (first-line treatment which prolongs life, delays progression and improves symptoms)

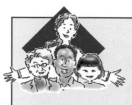

Bridging the gap

Ethnicity and drug response

A patient's ethnicity may affect how his or her body responds to the drugs used to treat heart failure. For example almost half of all Asian patients develop a cough while taking an angiotensin-converting enzyme (ACE) inhibitor. In America it has been recognised that although the majority of hypertensive drugs work well in Black American patients, some of these drugs are more dependable and produce effects with lower doses in this population.

African-Caribbean hypertensives tend to have low renin levels and are particularly salt sensitive. They respond better to thiazide/thiazide-like diuretics or calcium channel blockers than to beta blockers, ACE inhibitors or angiotensin receptor blockers.

- diuretics (can provide rapid symptomatic relief; in severe heart failure, spironolactone added to other treatments in a low dose (e.g. 25 mg daily) can reduce mortality and morbidity; careful monitoring for hyperkalaemia and hypovolaemia is required especially for people taking other diuretics and/or ACE inhibitors)
- a beta-blocker (in people with controlled heart failure, beta-blockers started in low doses can reduce mortality when used with other treatments, e.g. ACE inhibitors, diuretics and digoxin; should usually be initiated by a consultant)
- nitrates and hydralazine (for people in whom ACE inhibitors are not tolerated)
- digoxin (does not reduce mortality but may reduce symptoms and hospital admission for worsening heart failure)
- avoiding aggravating factors (e.g. advise low-salt diet and reduced/no alcohol, review other medication, e.g. NSAIDs and short-acting calcium channel blockers).

Lifestyle changes and drug therapy can improve the patient's quality of life and survival. Some ethnic groups will respond differently to drug regimens. (See *Ethnicity and drug response*.) For instance the patient can minimise the effects of heart failure by controlling cardiovascular risk factors, stopping smoking and losing weight if necessary, abstaining from alcohol and reducing dietary sodium and fat intake.

Dietary management

The dietary management for a patient with heart failure centres around encouraging a healthy balanced diet and reducing salt intakes, easing oedema (fluid retention) and minimising the cardiac workload. Reducing salt intakes is difficult as people may be very unaware of how much salt they are consuming. To visualise this, keep in mind 1 tsp of table salt contains about 2,400 mg of sodium. Salt is also known as sodium chloride. (See *Get smart about salt terms*, page 276.)

Most people in the UK are probably eating more salt than the maximum of 6 g/day recommended for adults. But there are lots of ways to reduce the amount of salt that is consumed. It's not just a case of adding less at the table, although this will help, because about three-quarters of the salt we eat is already in the food we buy. (See *Sample menu for reducing salt intake: Reducing sodium*, page 280.)

For example some types of bread, breakfast cereals, savoury biscuits, sauces, tinned vegetables and soups can be high in salt, as well as ready meals.

When shopping, advise the individual to try comparing the labels on similar foods—sometimes there can be a big difference in the amount of salt they contain.

Here are some other ways to cut down on salt:

• Be sparing with sauces, especially cooking sauces, soy sauce, brown sauce and tomato ketchup, because these can be high in salt.
• Cut down on salty snacks, such as crisps and salted nuts.
• Go for low-salt snacks, such as dried fruit, sticks of vegetables and unsalted nuts.
• Try to eat less of heavily salted foods, such as bacon, cheese, pickles and smoked fish.
• Choose canned vegetables and pulses that are marked 'no added salt'.
• Make your own stock or choose lower-salt stock cubes, because stock cubes tend to be high in salt.
• Add less salt to food when cooking.
• Use herbs and spices to add flavour to cooking, instead of salt.
• Get out of the habit of adding salt at the table—try to remember to taste food first.

Some people will also have to restrict their fluid intakes, but this should happen only after advice from a doctor. Speaking with registered dietitian can help a person to make informed food choices.

Pour on the potassium

If your patient is taking a thiazide (potassium-wasting) diuretic or a cardiac glycoside, make sure the diet provides adequate potassium to replace losses. Foods high in potassium include:

• bananas
• citrus fruits and their juices
• melons
• raisins
• apricots
• avocados
• potatoes
• tomatoes and tomato products
• dried peas and beans
• green leafy vegetables
• spinach
• carrots
• corn

Menu maven

Sample menu for reducing salt intake: Reducing sodium

If your patient must restrict his or her sodium intake, a registered dietitian can provide a sample menu such as the one below. Be sure to emphasise that he or she shouldn't add any salt to these items.

Breakfast

- orange juice
- rice cereal with banana
- wholewheat toast with margarine and jelly
- coffee with no more than 2 tsp sugar and skimmed milk

Lunch

- apple or cranberry juice (one glass)
- roast turkey sandwich with lettuce and tomato
- carrot and raisin salad (no salt added)
- low-fat frozen yoghurt (vanilla)

Dinner

- pork tenderloin
- baked sweet potato
- fresh steamed mixed vegetables
- dinner roll with margarine
- fresh fruit salad and jelly dessert
- decaffeinated coffee with no more than 2 tsp sugar and skimmed milk

Snack

- unsalted pretzels
- apple juice

- wholegrains
- fresh meat
- milk
- yoghurt
- ice cream.

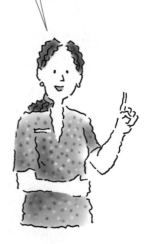

Drug therapy can be used in conjunction with other treatments to control heart failure quickly. For longer-term effects, though, tell your patient to consider quitting smoking and cutting down on salt intake.

Spice, not salt

Advise the patient to use no-salt spices and seasonings instead of table salt. Tell him or her to avoid food products whose labels state 'convenient', 'instant' or 'prepared'. The high sodium content of most of these products makes them nearly impossible to work into a low-sodium diet.

Caution the patient that various nonfood products also contain sodium—including certain medications, toothpastes, mouthwash and drinking water. (See *Sodium content of nonprescription drugs*.)

Other ways to ease the workload

If your patient is overweight, recommend the patient to lose weight to help reduce cardiac workload. Provide five to six small meals per day, with no more

Sodium content of nonprescription drugs

The chart below lists the sodium content of some commonly used nonprescription (over-the-counter) drugs.

Medication	Dosage	Sodium content (mg)
Alka-Seltzer	Two tablets	1,040
Milk of magnesia	2 tbsp	3
Tums	Two tablets	6
Vicks cough syrup	5 ml	54
Vicks Formula 44 D	5 ml	68

than 3 L/day of fluid (or as specified by the doctor) to increase intake without overstressing the heart. Recommend nonirritating and non-gas-forming foods to minimise gastric distension and pressure on the heart.

Advise the patient to restrict caffeine intake to avoid stimulating the heart. Tell him or her to avoid alcohol.

Stop those fluids

If a patient has oedema that is not resolving, a doctor may advise the patient to reduce their fluid intake. This should be done only on medical advice. An obese patient requires a calorie-controlled diet.

If a patient has been asked to reduce their fluid intake, advise the patient to plan fluid consumption throughout the day. Recommend that he or she fill a clear jug each morning with the amount of fluid he or she's permitted to have daily. Each time he or she consumes fluid, he or she should pour the same amount of water out of the jug to keep track of the remaining fluid allowance.

No roughage in the house

To lessen heartburn, abdominal distension and flatulence, encourage the patient to eat slowly and avoid gulping food. To reduce the amount of chewing required, encourage the patient to eat a soft diet—one consisting of plain, soft foods that are low in roughage.

Less is more

Patients with heart failure commonly complain of feeling congested and, as a result, find it difficult to muster an appetite. If your patient has a poor appetite, instruct them to try smaller, more frequent meals—but tell them they should never force themself to eat. A registered dietitian can advise on a diet that may be required if the appetite is very poor. Remember, though, that a patient who can eat solid foods shouldn't use oral supplements.

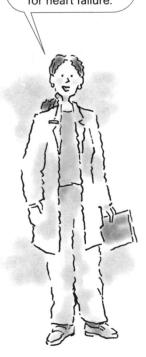

Fluid restriction is a key component to nutrition therapy for heart failure.

Perplexing cachexia

If the patient has poor nutritional intake and has been using long-term medication, he or she may develop cardiac cachexia—a type of malnutrition that causes anorexia and fat and muscle wasting with oedema. Patients with cardiac cachexia need a diet higher in calories, protein and nutrients but may still need to restrict salt intakes. A calorie- and nutrient-dense diet maximises intake.

Quick quiz

1. Janet, age 60, is a white female with no family history of heart disease. Her LDL cholesterol level is 6.2 mmol/L, HDL cholesterol level 0.9 mmol/L and blood pressure 148/96 mmHg. How many risk factors for CVD does Janet have?

    A. 1
    B. 2
    C. 3
    D. 4

Answer: D. Risk factors for CVD include a high LDL cholesterol level (4.4 mmol/L or higher), a low HDL cholesterol level (under 1 mmol/L), hypertension and postmenopausal status.

2. The TLC diet recommends that calories from saturated fat should be what percentage of total intake?

    A. Less than 7%
    B. Less than 10%
    C. 12%
    D. 20%

Answer: A. The TLC diet recommends that less than 7% of calories come from saturated fat.

Scoring

✩✩✩ If you answered both questions correctly, hopping hearts! You perform well under pressure.

✩✩ If you answered one question correctly, keep it up! Run to the fridge and grab a snack; then move on to the next chapter.

✩ If you answered none of the two questions correctly, don't get disheartened. Take a break and then review the chapter!

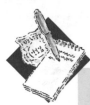

14 Renal disorders

Just the facts

The renal system is responsible for the excretion of body wastes. In this chapter, you'll learn:

♦ the structure and functions of the renal system

♦ pathophysiology, signs, symptoms and treatments for common renal disorders

♦ nutrition therapy for common renal disorders and kidney transplants.

A look at the renal system

The renal system, teamed with the urinary system, serves as the body's water treatment plant. These systems work together to collect the body's waste products and expel them as urine.

Filtration system

The kidneys, located on each side of the abdomen near the lower back, contain an amazingly efficient filtration system that filters about 180 L of fluid per day. (See *Kidney function declines with age*, page 284.) The by-product of this filtration process is urine, which contains water and waste products. After it's produced by the kidneys, urine passes through the urinary system and is expelled from the body.

Other structures of the system, extending downwards from the kidneys, include:
• ureters—muscular tubes that contract rhythmically (peristalsis) to transport urine from each kidney to the bladder
• urinary bladder—a sac with muscular walls that collects and holds urine that's expelled from the ureters every few seconds
• urethra—a narrow passageway, surrounded by the prostate gland in men, from the bladder to the outside of the body through which urine is excreted.

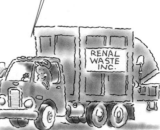

We kidneys are good at taking out the trash!

Kidney role

The kidneys perform vital functions, including:
- maintaining fluid and acid–base balance
- regulating electrolyte concentration
- detoxifying the blood and eliminating wastes
- regulating blood pressure
- aiding red blood cell (RBC) production (erythropoiesis)
- regulating vitamin D and calcium formation.

Assessment

To plan the diet for a patient with kidney disease, first perform a nutrition-focused assessment. This assessment should include a health history, a physical examination and diagnostic tests.

Health history

Obtain a history to assess the patient's kidney status. Focus the health history on the patient's eating habits, weight, blood pressure, past illnesses and pre-existing conditions. Gather information about the patient's:
- dietary intake, especially of high-sodium foods
- use of low-protein or low-sodium products
- understanding of the Nutrition Facts panel on food labels
- knowledge of healthy eating habits
- willingness to change eating habits, if needed
- ability to buy and prepare healthy foods
- frequency of eating out
- physical activity and exercise
- religious and ethnic influences on food choices
- food allergies and intolerances
- use of alcohol, caffeine, tobacco and recreational drugs
- use of nutritional supplements
- use of herbal supplements
- current and past medication use
- medical history
- family history of kidney disease and hypertension.

Physical examination

Focus the physical examination on nutrition-related aspects, such as the patient's weight and height, vital signs, skin condition and mental status.

Weighing in on kidney health

Weighing the patient can provide information about fluid status and is important for patients with kidney disorders or kidney failure, especially those receiving dialysis. Ask the patient about recent weight changes.

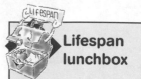

Lifespan lunchbox

Kidney function declines with age

After age 40, kidney function may diminish. If a person lives up to age 90, kidney function may have decreased by as much as 50%. This change is reflected by a decline in the glomerular filtration rate caused by age-related changes in renal vasculature that disturb glomerular haemodynamics. Renal blood flow decreases by 53% from reduced cardiac output and age-related atherosclerotic changes. Tubular reabsorption and renal concentrating ability also decline because the size and number of functioning nephrons decrease.

Additionally, as a person ages, the bladder muscles weaken, which can result in incomplete bladder emptying and chronic urine retention, predisposing the bladder to infection.

They ain't called *vital* for nothin'

Evaluate your patient's vital signs, which can provide clues about kidney dysfunction. For example a patient's vital signs might reveal hypertension, which can cause kidney dysfunction if it's uncontrolled. Be sure to check blood pressure in each arm.

Get the skinny on the skin

Examine your patient's skin. Inspect for oedema especially. Presence of oedema could indicate fluid retention and kidney dysfunction.

Stable status?

Observing the patient's behaviour can give you clues about his or her mental status. Does he or she have trouble concentrating, have memory loss or seem disoriented? Kidney dysfunction can cause these symptoms. Progressive chronic kidney failure can cause lethargy, confusion, disorientation, stupor, convulsions and coma.

Diagnostic tests

To evaluate a patient for kidney disease, the doctor may order various laboratory and diagnostic tests, including:
- blood urea nitrogen (BUN) level
- creatinine level
- albumin level
- electrolyte levels
- haemoglobin level
- haematocrit level
- parathyroid hormone level
- phosphorus and calcium levels
- renal scan
- urinalysis.

Renal calculi

Renal calculi, or kidney stones, may form anywhere in the urinary tract but usually develop in the renal pelvis or calices. Calculi form when substances that normally dissolve in the urine precipitate. They vary in size, shape and number.

The incidence of renal calculi is increasing in the UK. This is almost certainly due to increased dietary protein intake, which increases urinary excretion of phosphates and magnesium and reduces urinary citrate concentration. Symptomatic stones occur in 27 to 34 per 100 population per annum in adults, occurring three times more commonly in the south than in the north of the country. In the adult population, males are affected four times more often than females. The incidence is lower in children (1 to 2 per million per year), and in this age group, boys are more frequently affected than girls.

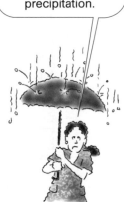

Hail stones and kidney stones are both forms of precipitation.

Pathophysiology

Renal calculi are more common in the south of the UK. Although their exact cause is unknown, there are several predisposing factors:

- *Dehydration*—Decreased water and urine excretion concentrate calculus-forming substances.
- *Infection*—Infected, scarred tissue, such as that formed from a urinary tract infection, provides a site for calculus development. Calculi may become infected if bacteria are the nucleus in calculi formation. Calculi that result from *Proteus* infections may lead to the destruction of kidney tissue.
- *Changes in urine pH*—Consistently acidic or alkaline urine provides a favourable medium for calculus formation.
- *Obstruction*—Urinary stasis allows calculus constituents to collect and adhere, forming calculi. Obstruction also encourages infection, which compounds the obstruction.
- *Immobilisation*—Immobility from spinal cord injury or other disorders allows calcium to be released into the circulation and, eventually, to be filtered by the kidneys.
- *Diet*—Increased intake of animal protein or oxalate-rich foods encourages calculi formation.
- *Metabolic factors*—Hyperparathyroidism, renal tubular acidosis, elevated uric acid (usually with gout), defective oxalate metabolism, a genetic defect in cystine metabolism and excessive intake of vitamin D or dietary calcium may predispose a person to renal calculi.

Disturbing a delicate balance

Renal calculi usually arise because the delicate excretory balance breaks down. Here's how it happens:

Urine becomes concentrated with insoluble materials.

Crystals form from these materials and then consolidate, forming calculi. These calculi contain an organic mucoprotein framework and crystalloids, such as calcium, oxalate, phosphate, urate, uric acid, struvite, cystine and xanthine.

Mucoprotein is reabsorbed by the tubules, establishing a site for calculi formation.

Calculi remain in the renal pelvis and damage or destroy kidney tissue, or they enter the ureter.

Large calculi in the kidneys may cause tissue damage (pressure necrosis).

In certain locations, calculi obstruct urine, which collects in the renal pelvis (hydronephrosis). These calculi also tend to recur. Intractable pain and serious bleeding can result.

Memory jogger

To remember how renal calculi formation happens, think **U**nusual **C**hanges **M**ean **T**hat **L**iquid **U**nder **P**ressure **G**athers:

Urine concentrates

Crystals form

Mucoprotein is reabsorbed

Tissue is damaged

Large calculi may form

Urine collects

Pressure builds

GFR falls.

Initially, hydrostatic pressure increases in the collection system near the obstruction, forcing nearby renal structures to dilate as well. The farther the obstruction from the kidney, the less serious the dilation because the pressure is diffused over a larger surface area.

With a complete obstruction, pressure in the renal pelvis and tubules increases, the glomerular filtration rate (GFR) falls and a disruption occurs in the junctional complexes between tubular cells. If left untreated, tubular atrophy and destruction of the medulla leave connective tissue in place of glomeruli, causing irreversible damage.

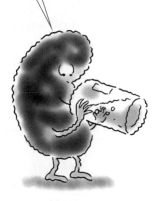

Ninety percent of renal calculi may pass naturally with vigorous hydration. So bottoms up!

What to look for

The key symptom of renal calculi is severe pain, which usually occurs when large calculi obstruct the opening of the ureter and increase the frequency and force of peristaltic contractions. Pain may travel from the lower back to the sides, and then to the pubic region and external genitalia. Pain intensity fluctuates and may be excruciating at its peak.

The patient with calculi in the renal pelvis and calices may complain of more constant, dull pain. He or she also may report back pain from an obstruction within a kidney and severe abdominal pain from calculi travelling down a ureter. Severe pain is typically accompanied by nausea, vomiting and, possibly, fever and chills.

It isn't just painful

Other signs and symptoms include:
- haematuria (when stones abrade a ureter)
- abdominal distension
- oliguria (from an obstruction in urine flow).

Treatment

Ninety percent of renal calculi are smaller than 5 mm in diameter and may pass naturally with vigorous hydration (3 L/day). Other treatments may include drug therapy for infection or other effects of illness and measures to prevent recurrence of calculi. If calculi are too large for natural passage, they may be removed by surgery or other means.

Drug duty

Drug therapy may include:
- antimicrobial agents for infection (varying with the cultured organism)
- analgesics, such as morphine, for pain
- diuretics to prevent urinary stasis and further calculi formation
- thiazides to decrease calcium excretion in the urine
- methenamine mandelate to suppress calculi formation when infection is present.

Canning the calculi

Calculi lodged in the ureter may be removed by inserting a cystoscope through the urethra and then manipulating the calculi with catheters or retrieval instruments. A flank or lower abdominal approach may be needed to extract calculi from other areas, such as the kidney calyx or renal pelvis. Percutaneous ultrasonic lithotripsy and extracorporeal shock wave lithotripsy shatter the calculi into fragments for removal by suction or natural passage.

Prevention techniques

Measures to prevent recurrence of renal calculi include:
- oxalate-binding cholestyramine for absorptive hypercalciuria
- parathyroidectomy for hyperparathyroidism
- allopurinol for uric acid calculi.

Nutrition management

Increasing fluid intake, thereby diluting urine, is the most effective nutritional support for treating and preventing renal calculi. High urine output helps flush calculi from the urinary system and also decreases the risk of recurrence. Fluid intake should be increased to 2.5 to 3 L/day. At least 250 ml of water should be consumed before bedtime because urine becomes more concentrated at night. (See *Cranberry juice controversy*.)

Hold the oxalate

Patients with calculi typically need to restrict their intake of oxalate. Foods high in oxalate include:
- beetroot
- asparagus
- rhubarb
- chocolate
- berries
- leeks
- parsley
- spinach
- celery
- almonds, peanuts and cashew nuts
- soy products
- grains, such as oatmeal, wheat germ and wholewheat.

In addition, vitamin B_6 supplements have been shown to reduce oxalate production by 50%. Therefore, supplementation may be helpful.

Other limits

To prevent developing a uric acid stone, reduce the amount of meat, poultry and fish in the diet and limit sodium intake to 2 g/day.

Cranberry juice controversy

Cranberry juice may be effective in preventing urinary tract infections, which can lead to calculi formation. An ingredient in the juice prevents bacteria such as *Escherichia coli* from adhering to the lining of the urinary tract, promoting their excretion. Unfortunately, not all bacteria are sensitive to the juice. Also, the juice's protective feature lasts only as long as the juice is consumed regularly.

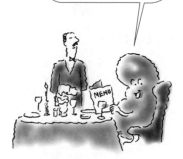

Garçon, give me the special but hold the beets, nuts and spinach, and put the soy on the side. While you're at it, can you throw in a little extra B_6?

Acute kidney failure

Acute kidney failure is the sudden interruption of kidney function. It can be caused by obstruction, poor circulation or kidney disease. It's potentially reversible; however, if left untreated, permanent damage can lead to chronic kidney disease (CKD).

Pathophysiology

Acute kidney failure may be classified as prerenal, intrarenal or postrenal. Each type has its own causes:
• *Prerenal failure* results from conditions that diminish blood flow to the kidneys. Examples include hypovolaemia, hypotension, vasoconstriction or inadequate cardiac output. One condition, prerenal azotaemia (excess nitrogenous waste products in the blood), accounts for 40% to 80% of all cases of acute renal failure. Azotaemia occurs as a response to renal hypoperfusion. Usually, it can be rapidly reversed by restoring renal blood flow and glomerular filtration.
• *Intrarenal failure*, also called *intrinsic* or *parenchymal renal failure*, results from damage to the filtering structures of the kidneys, usually from acute tubular necrosis (a disorder that causes cell death) or from nephrotoxic substances such as certain antibiotics.
• *Postrenal failure* results from bilateral obstruction of urine outflow, as in prostatic hyperplasia or bladder outlet obstruction.

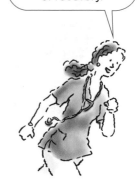

In acute kidney failure, early intervention improves the chance of recovery.

Phasing out

With treatment, each type of acute renal failure passes through three distinct phases:

 oliguric (decreased urine output)

 diuretic (increased urine output)

recovery.

Going down

The oliguric phase is marked by decreased urine output (less than 400 ml/ 24 hours). Prerenal oliguria results from decreased blood flow to the kidneys. Before damage occurs, the kidneys respond to decreased blood flow by conserving sodium and water. Once damage occurs, the kidneys' ability to conserve sodium is impaired. Untreated prerenal oliguria may lead to acute tubular necrosis.

During this phase, BUN and creatinine levels rise and the ratio of BUN to creatinine falls from 20:1 (normal) to 10:1. Hypervolaemia also occurs, causing oedema, weight gain and elevated blood pressure.

Going up

The diuretic phase is marked by urine output that can range from normal levels to as high as 5 L/day. High urine volume has two causes:

 inability of the kidney to conserve sodium and water

 osmotic diuresis produced by high BUN levels.

During this phase, BUN and creatinine levels slowly rise, and hypovolaemia and weight loss result. This phase lasts from several days to 1 week. These conditions can lead to deficits of potassium, sodium and water that can be deadly if left untreated. If the cause of the diuresis is corrected, azotaemia gradually disappears and the patient improves greatly—leading to the recovery phase.

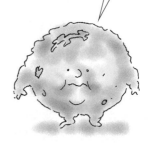

During the oliguric phase of acute renal failure, hypervolaemia occurs. Boy am I full!

Riding the road to recovery

The recovery phase is reached when BUN and creatinine have returned to normal and urine output is between 1 and 2 L/day.

Getting complicated

Primary damage to the renal tubules or blood vessels results in kidney failure (intrarenal failure). The causes of intrarenal failure are classified as nephrotoxic, inflammatory or ischaemic.

When the damage is caused by nephrotoxicity or inflammation, the delicate layer under the epithelium (basement membrane) becomes irreparably damaged, commonly proceeding to CKD. Severe or prolonged lack of blood flow (ischaemia) may lead to renal damage (ischaemic parenchymal injury) and excess nitrogen in the blood (intrinsic renal azotaemia).

What to look for

The signs and symptoms of prerenal failure depend on the cause. If the underlying problem is a change in blood pressure and volume, the patient may have:
- oliguria
- tachycardia
- hypotension
- dry mucous membranes
- flat neck veins
- lethargy progressing to coma
- decreased cardiac output and cool, clammy skin in a patient with heart failure.

As renal failure progresses, the patient may show signs and symptoms of uraemia, including:
- confusion
- GI complaints

- fluid in the lungs
- infection.

About 5% of all hospitalised patients develop acute renal failure. The condition is usually reversible with treatment, but if it isn't treated, it may progress to end-stage renal disease, excess urea in the blood (prerenal azotaemia or uraemia) and death.

Treatment

Supportive measures for acute kidney failure include:
- establishment and maintenance of fluid and electrolyte balance
- diuretic therapy during the oliguric phase
- renal-dose dopamine to increase renal perfusion
- monitoring for signs of uraemia
- antibiotics to prevent or treat infection.

If the above measures fail to control uraemia, the patient may require haemodialysis, continuous renal replacement therapy or peritoneal dialysis.

Halting hyperkalaemia

Meticulous electrolyte monitoring is needed to detect excess potassium in the blood (hyperkalaemia). Symptoms include malaise, anorexia, numbness and tingling, muscle weakness and electrocardiogram changes. If these symptoms occur, I.V. hypertonic glucose, insulin and calcium polystyrene sulphonate (Calcium Resonium) are given by mouth or rectum.

Dietary management

Adequate calories are required in patients with acute renal failure to prevent weight loss and body protein catabolism. Caloric needs for most adults with acute renal failure are 30 to 50 kcal/kg/day.

Patients with acute renal failure may require enteral or parenteral feedings if they're unable to consume enough calories orally. Special enteral feeds are available for patients with renal failure. These feeds are low in potassium and phosphorus and high in calories.

Patients who have acute renal failure accompanied by diabetes mellitus frequently must have their insulin or antidiabetic drug dosages adjusted to meet the nutritional demands of renal failure.

Protein controversy

Some health care providers believe that protein should be restricted in acute kidney failure because restricting protein may help preserve kidney function. Others believe that high-protein intake is important to correct the negative nitrogen balance. Those who aren't receiving dialysis are typically restricted to 0.8 g/kg/day. As the patient's kidney function returns to normal or dialysis begins, the protein allowance is increased to 1.4 to 1.6 g/kg/day.

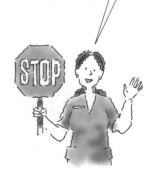

Stop uraemia in its tracks to avoid haemodialysis, renal replacement therapy and peritoneal dialysis.

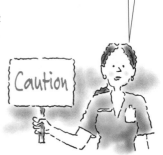

Be sure to adjust insulin or antidiabetic drug dosages for diabetic patients who also have acute renal failure!

Fluid in phases

Fluid intake for patients in the oliguric and diuretic phases of acute kidney failure should be 400 to 500 ml greater than their 24-hour urine output. For example if the patient's urine output is 2,500 ml, then the patient should consume at least 2,900 ml of fluid.

Hold the potassium

Hyperkalaemia may occur during the oliguric phase of acute kidney failure. This electrolyte imbalance results when potassium is retained and tissue catabolism occurs, causing potassium to leave the cells and enter the serum. During this phase, intake of potassium will be dictated by the serum level of the individual, but generally the patient should restrict the intake of potassium to 2 g or less per day. During the diuretic phase, potassium is excreted and supplementation may be necessary.

The salt story

During the oliguric phase of acute kidney failure, sodium may be restricted to 500 to 1,000 mg/day. Sodium intake is adjusted according to the patient's urine output, serum sodium level and need for dialysis. Sodium is excreted during the diuretic phase and supplementation may be required.

Chronic kidney disease (CKD)

The overall aim is to prevent malnutrition, hyperkalaemia, hyperphosphataemia and obesity and to aid the treatment of hypertension and (as CKD advances) alleviate uraemic symptoms. All of this must occur in the context of any other dietary restriction a person might be following, such as a diabetic diet, to ensure a balanced healthy diet to meet individual nutritional requirements. CKD, a usually progressive and irreversible condition, is the end result of gradual tissue destruction and loss of kidney function. Occasionally, CKD results from rapidly progressing disease of sudden onset that destroys the nephrons and causes irreversible kidney damage.

Pathophysiology

CKD typically progresses through four stages:

- Reduced renal reserve—GFR is 35% to 50% of the normal rate.

- Renal insufficiency—GFR is 20% to 35% of the normal rate.

- Renal failure—GFR is 20% to 25% of the normal rate.

- End-stage renal disease—GFR is less than 20% of the normal rate.

It may result from:
- chronic glomerular disease, such as glomerulonephritis, which affects the capillaries in the glomeruli
- chronic infections, such as chronic pyelonephritis and tuberculosis
- congenital anomalies such as polycystic kidney disease
- vascular diseases, such as hypertension and nephrosclerosis, which cause hardening of the kidneys
- obstructions such as renal calculi
- collagen diseases such as lupus erythematosus
- nephrotoxic agents such as long-term aminoglycoside therapy
- endocrine diseases such as diabetic neuropathy.

Nephrons lose the battle

Nephron damage is progressive. Once damaged, nephrons can no longer function. Healthy nephrons compensate for destroyed nephrons by enlarging and increasing their clearance capacity. The kidneys maintain relatively normal function until about 75% of the nephrons are nonfunctional.

Eventually, the healthy glomeruli are so overburdened that they become sclerotic and stiff, leading to their destruction. If this condition continues unchecked, toxins accumulate and produce potentially fatal changes in all major organ systems.

Everlasting effects

Even if the patient can tolerate life-sustaining maintenance dialysis or a kidney transplant, he or she may still have anaemia, nervous system effects (peripheral neuropathy), cardiopulmonary and GI complications, sexual dysfunction and skeletal defects.

What to look for

Few symptoms develop until more than 75% of glomerular filtration is lost. Then the remaining normal tissue deteriorates progressively. Symptoms worsen as kidney function decreases. Profound changes affect all body systems. Major findings include:
- hypervolaemia (abnormal increase in plasma volume)
- hyperkalaemia
- hypocalcaemia
- hyperphosphataemia
- azotaemia
- metabolic acidosis
- anaemia
- peripheral neuropathy.

The progression of CKD can sometimes be slowed, but it's ultimately irreversible, culminating in end-stage kidney disease. Although it's fatal without treatment, dialysis or kidney transplant can sustain life.

Treatment

Treatment for CKD consists of haemodialysis, peritoneal dialysis, or renal transplantation and drug therapy. Drugs used to treat CKD include:
- loop diuretics such as furosemide (if some renal function remains) to maintain fluid balance
- cardiac glycosides to increase the heart's contractility and mobilise fluids that cause oedema
- antihypertensives to control blood pressure and oedema
- antiemetics to relieve nausea and vomiting
- histamine-2 receptor antagonists such as famotidine to reduce gastric irritation
- stool softeners such as docusate to prevent constipation
- iron and folate supplements or RBC transfusions to treat anaemia
- synthetic erythropoietins to stimulate bone marrow to produce RBCs
- antipruritics such as trimeprazine to relieve itching
- phosphate binders to lower serum phosphorus levels
- calcimimetic drugs to treat secondary hyperparathyroidism in patients on dialysis.

Emergency measures

Potassium levels in the blood must be monitored closely to detect hyperkalaemia. Emergency treatment includes dialysis therapy, oral or rectal administration of cation exchange resins such as calcium polystyrene sulphonate (Calcium Resonium) and I.V. administration of calcium gluconate, sodium bicarbonate, 50% hypertonic glucose and regular insulin.

Dietary management

NICE has published clinical practice guidelines for nutrition in chronic renal disease in primary and secondary care. Referral to a renal dietitian for dietary advice is important.

Protein

In the past, a low-protein diet was often recommended to slow down the steady deterioration of kidney function that occurs in some patients. It is now recommended that a moderate protein diet is one that contains 0.8 to 1 g protein per kg of ideal body weight. The richest sources of protein are *animal protein*—meat, fish, cheese, eggs and milk—and *vegetable protein*—nuts, pulses (beans, lentils, etc.), tofu and quorn.

Why not low protein?

- Modern treatments, especially improved blood pressure treatments, have made any extra benefit from low-protein diets much smaller.
- Low-protein diets don't taste good, and this may reduce calories too.
- There is a significant risk of long-term malnutrition in those on low-protein diets.

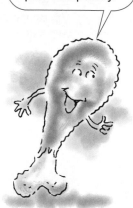

Half of the protein consumed by the patient with CKD should be high biological value protein, which can be found in such foods as beef, egg whites, fish, milk, pork and poultry.

Why not high protein?

- High-protein intake in CKD makes the body more acidic, and this can lead to increased muscle breakdown.
- High-protein intake means high-phosphate intake too (see below).
- In animals and probably humans, large amounts of protein may damage kidneys.

Supplements and high-protein diets may be harmful if your patient has CKD

- Don't follow the Atkins diet or other high-protein diets for weight loss if you have CKD.
- Don't take protein supplements unless a renal dietitian agrees you need them.
- Don't take creatine or similar supplements for muscle development.

Sometimes low-protein diets are useful

In patients who do not want dialysis, or cannot have it for some reason, low-protein diets may cut down symptoms, but should be monitored by a renal dietitian.

Counting on calories

Adequate calorie intake is necessary to prevent weight loss and protein catabolism. Failure to consume adequate calories can cause BUN levels to rise because body protein is broken down for energy. Those who don't require dialysis should consume 35 kcal/kg/day. Patients receiving peritoneal dialysis should decrease their calorie intake by 680 kcal/day to compensate for the calories absorbed from the dialysate.

Sweet tooths, celebrate!

In many cases, patients with CKD must consume simple carbohydrates in order to provide enough calories without adding extra protein to the diet. Sources of protein-free calories include fruit drinks and punches, chewy fruit snacks, sorbet, lemonade, honey, corn syrup and butter or margarine. (See *Slowed growth*.)

How much water and salt?

Sodium and fluid restrictions are determined by the patient's blood pressure, electrolyte levels, urine output and weight. Most patients can successfully consume 2 to 4 g of salt daily. (See *Spicing up foods*, page 296.)

In patients who have normal blood pressure, no oedema and normal serum sodium levels, fluid intake should be 500 ml greater than the patient's 24-hour urine output. For example if the patient's urine output is 600 ml over the past 24 hours, then the patient can safely consume 1,100 ml of fluid. If the patient is receiving dialysis, the goal is to limit weight gain to 0.9 kg between treatments. (See *Dining out*, page 297.)

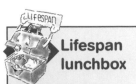

Lifespan lunchbox

Slowed growth

Children with CKD typically experience growth retardation. This failure to grow may be permanent if not corrected before puberty. Aggressive calcium and vitamin D supplementation may be used to boost calcium uptake by the bones and subsequent bone growth. Phosphate binders and human growth hormone may also be prescribed.

NutriTips

Spicing up foods

Because patients with renal failure must limit salt (sodium) intake, food commonly tastes bland. Inform the patient that the following seasonings can be used to spice up foods in place of salt:

- allspice
- anise
- basil
- bay leaf
- caraway seed
- chives
- cilantro
- cinnamon
- cloves
- cumin
- curry
- ginger
- horseradish root
- nutmeg
- onion powder
- oregano
- paprika
- pepper
- poppy seed
- rosemary
- saffron
- sage
- sesame seeds
- tarragon
- thyme
- turmeric
- vinegar.

Potassium parity

Typically, patients with renal insufficiency and those receiving peritoneal dialysis don't need to restrict their potassium intake. Patients who have hyperkalaemia and undergo haemodialysis should restrict their potassium intake to 2 to 3 g/day. (See *Avoiding potassium-rich foods*, page 298.)

Bone protection

Vitamin D deficiency is common in patients with CKD because the kidneys are unable to convert vitamin D to its active form. Calcium, magnesium and phosphorus metabolism are altered, leading to hyperphosphataemia, bone demineralisation, bone pain and possible soft tissue calcification. These complications may be prevented by limiting the intake of phosphorus and providing vitamin D supplements and phosphorus binders. (See *Avoiding phosphorus-rich foods* and *Commonly prescribed phosphorus binders*, page 299.)

Vital vitamins

Patients with CKD usually have deficiencies of the water-soluble vitamins. Inadequate intake caused by anorexia and dietary restrictions, altered metabolism caused by uraemia and medications, or increased losses of vitamins caused by dialysis are responsible.

Whew! patients with renal insufficiency don't usually need to restrict their potassium intake.

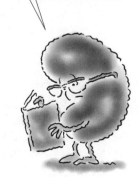

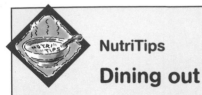

NutriTips

Dining out

Patients with CKD can still enjoy dining out. However, they need to plan ahead and make wise menu choices. Here are a few tips to help make dining out easier.

Menu choices

- Instruct the patient to choose meats without sauces or gravies.
- Explain that baked or grilled fish, broiled steaks, chicken, hamburgers, roast beef and turkey are all good choices.
- Cold cuts, such as salami and hot dogs, should be avoided.
- Tell the patient that a small house salad is acceptable; however, it shouldn't contain tomatoes and should be served with oil and vinegar dressing. A serving of cooked vegetables without sauce is an acceptable alternative.
- When choosing bread products, the patient should choose French, Italian, white, rye or sourdough bread. English muffins and bagels are also acceptable.
- The choice of starches is somewhat limited. Instruct the patient to choose plain rice, plain noodles or mashed potatoes.

Restaurant choices

- Eating at a Mexican restaurant is acceptable; however, avocados, beans, sour cream and fresh tomatoes should be avoided. Fajitas, tacos, beef or chicken enchiladas, and meat-filled burritos are wise choices.
- Eating at an Italian restaurant is somewhat difficult. Tomato sauces and cream sauces should be avoided. Plain pasta can be ordered with butter or olive oil and meat.
- Chinese food is acceptable; however, it should be made without monosodium glutamate. Extra soy sauce should be avoided. The patient should be instructed to avoid courses containing nuts.

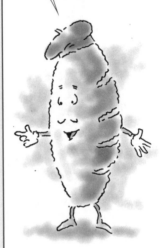

C'est magnifique! A patient with CKD can safely eat several kinds of bread—including me!

Boy, could I go for a tall glass of B_6 right about now?

Both dialysed patients and those who don't require dialysis should receive supplementation according to Reference Nutrient Intake (RNI). Specialist renal dietitians can advise on this according to protocol. Patients may need vitamin B_6 and folic acid in amounts greater than the RNI to promote RBC production. Vitamin C intake should be limited to 100 mg to prevent the occurrence of kidney stones.

They may be trace, but they're important

Deficiencies in trace minerals such as zinc may occur in patients undergoing dialysis. Supplementation is suggested if a zinc deficiency is identified. Iron supplements may be necessary to treat anaemia. However, they shouldn't be taken with calcium supplements.

NutriTips

Avoiding potassium-rich foods

When preparing the patient with CKD for discharge, make sure he or she understands the importance of avoiding foods rich in potassium. The list below contains some examples of potassium-rich foods.

Fruits

- avocados
- bananas
- cantaloupe
- grapefruit juice
- honeydew melon
- oranges
- orange juice
- fresh peaches
- dried fruit

Beans

- baked beans
- black beans
- black-eyed peas
- butter beans
- chickpeas
- crowder peas
- Great Northern beans
- kidney beans
- lentils
- lima beans
- navy beans

- pinto beans
- split peas

Vegetables

- broccoli
- lettuce greens
- spinach
- tomatoes
- tomato soup
- tomato juice

Potatoes

- baked white potato
- baked sweet potato
- potato chips
- French fries
- instant potato mixes
- home fries
- yams

Miscellaneous foods

- molasses
- nuts
- salt substitutes

Nutrition therapy for transplant recipients

Transplant recipients are typically malnourished. In the immediate post-operative period, the patient should be encouraged to consume a healthy diet with adequate protein and calories for recovery. The goal of long-term nutrition management is to help reduce adverse effects and complications related to immunosuppressant therapy.

If temporary or permanent rejection occurs, resulting in uraemia, the patient must resume dietary restrictions for CKD.

Consumed with calories

Calories should be consumed in amounts necessary to maintain moderate body weight. Certain drugs cause anorexia, nausea, vomiting and diarrhoea,

NutriTips

Avoiding phosphorus-rich foods

Advise patients with CKD to avoid foods high in phosphorus. Examples of high-phosphorus foods are listed here.

Bread group

- bran

Vegetable group

- artichoke (boiled)

Milk group

- milk (1%, 2%, skimmed and whole)
- yoghurt
- cheese
- ice cream

Meat and beans group

- kidney beans
- split peas
- lentils
- beef
- salmon
- chicken
- pork
- nuts
- peanut butter

Miscellaneous

- cocoa, beer and cola beverages

which cause weight loss. Corticosteroids, on the other hand, contribute to obesity. Fat intake should be limited to 30% of the total calories.

How much protein?

Patients typically require 1 to 1.2 g/kg of protein daily. Protein intake should be adjusted as needed. Higher amounts may be necessary to surpass the catabolic effects of corticosteroid therapy. Lower amounts may be necessary if symptoms of uraemia return. A renal dietitian will advise on protein restrictions.

Old salt

Sodium intake should be limited and individuals advised not to add table salt to their food to help prevent fluid retention and hypertension.

Commonly prescribed phosphorus binders

Phosphorus binders, alone or in combination, may be prescribed to reduce high-phosphorus levels in a patient with CKD. Some common phosphorus binders include:

- calcium carbonate
- calcium acetate
- sevelamer hydrochloride
- lanthanum carbonate.

Patients should avoid salt substitutes because many replace sodium with potassium.

Adjusting potassium

Potassium intake should be adjusted according to serum potassium levels and diuretic therapy.

Got milk?

Patients should be encouraged to consume 800 to 1,500 mg of calcium per day to prevent bone demineralisation. The patient with hyperphosphataemia may need to limit intake of milk and other dairy products and as such need to include other sources of calcium in their diet.

Quick quiz

1. Which of the following foods is high in oxalate and should be avoided in patients with renal calculi?
   A. Green beans
   B. Beetroots
   C. Peaches
   D. Apples

Answer: B. Beetroots should be avoided in patients with renal calculi because they contain high levels of oxalate.

2. A patient develops kidney failure that's complicated by hyperkalaemia. Which high-potassium food should the patient avoid?
   A. Rhubarb
   B. Strawberries
   C. Honeydew melon
   D. Grapes

Answer: C. Honeydew melon is very high in potassium and should be avoided in patients with hyperkalaemia.

3. Teaching about salt restriction has been effective for the kidney transplant patient when they state that they should restrict their salt intake to what amount?
   A. 2 to 3 g/day
   B. Not adding salt
   C. 4 to 5 g/day
   D. 5 to 6 g/day

Answer: B. Renal transplant recipients should restrict salt intake by not adding salt to control hypertension and weight gain.

Scoring

☆☆☆ If you answered all three questions correctly, what a whiz! You really know your renal.

☆☆ If you answered two questions correctly, great! You're skilled at transplanting knowledge.

☆ If you answered fewer than two questions correctly, don't worry! Unlike CKD, these results are reversible. Review the chapter and try again.

15 Neurologic disorders

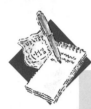

Just the facts

Because the neurologic system coordinates the functions of all other body systems, nutrition can be a major component of neurologic care. In this chapter, you'll learn:

♦ the structure and function of the neurologic system

♦ pathophysiology, signs, symptoms and treatments for common neurologic disorders

♦ nutrition therapy for common neurologic disorders.

A look at the neurologic system

The neurologic, or nervous, system is the body's communication network. It coordinates and organises the functions of all other body systems. This intricate network has two main divisions:

The central nervous system (CNS), made up of the brain and spinal cord, is the body's control centre.

The peripheral nervous system, containing cranial and spinal nerves, provides communication between the CNS and remote body parts.

Neuron your own

The neuron, or nerve cell, is the nervous system's fundamental unit. This highly specialised conductor cell receives and transmits electrochemical nerve impulses. Delicate, threadlike nerve fibres called *axons* and *dendrites* extend from the central cell body and transmit signals. Axons carry impulses away from the cell body; dendrites carry impulses to the cell body. Most neurons have multiple dendrites but only one axon.

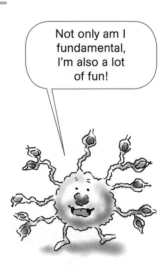

Not only am I fundamental, I'm also a lot of fun!

Living computer network

This intricate network of interlocking receptors and transmitters, along with the brain and spinal cord, forms a living computer that controls and regulates every mental and physical function. From birth to death, the nervous system efficiently organises the body's affairs, controlling the smallest actions, thoughts and feelings.

Central intelligence

The CNS consists of the brain and spinal cord. The fragile brain and spinal cord are protected by the bony skull and vertebrae, cerebrospinal fluid (CSF) and three membranes—the dura mater, the arachnoid mater and the pia mater.

Leading role

The *cerebrum*, the largest part of the brain, houses the nerve centre that controls sensory and motor activities and intelligence. The outer layer of the cerebrum, the cerebral cortex, consists of neuron cell bodies (grey matter). The inner layer consists of axons (white matter) plus basal ganglia, which control motor coordination and steadiness.

Supporting roles

Other main parts of the brain are the cerebellum and the brain stem:
• The *cerebellum* lies beneath the cerebrum, at the base of the brain. It coordinates muscle movements, controls posture and maintains equilibrium.
• The *brain stem* includes the midbrain, pons and medulla oblongata. It houses cell bodies for most of the cranial nerves. Along with the thalamus and hypothalamus, it makes up a nerve network called the *reticular formation*, which acts as an arousal mechanism.

Two-way conduction system

The spinal cord extends downwards from the brain to the second lumbar vertebrae. The spinal cord functions as a two-way conduction pathway between the brain stem and the peripheral nervous system.

Assessment

To plan nutritional support for a patient with neurologic disease, first perform a nutrition-focused assessment that includes a health history, a physical examination and diagnostic test findings.

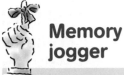

Memory jogger

To remember the basic areas of the brain, think **N**erves **C**an **C**ontrol **B**ody **R**eactions:

Neurons

Cerebrum

Cerebellum

Brain stem

Reticular formation.

Health history

Obtain a history to assess the patient's neurologic status. Focus the health history on the patient's eating habits, weight, and past illnesses and pre-existing conditions. Gather information about the patient's:

- dietary intake
- knowledge of healthy eating habits
- willingness to change eating habits, if needed
- ability to buy and prepare healthy foods
- frequency of eating out
- physical activity and exercise
- religious and ethnic influences on food choices
- food allergies and intolerances
- use of alcohol, caffeine, tobacco and recreational drugs
- use of nutritional supplements
- current and past medication use
- medical history
- family history of neurologic disease.

Physical examination

Focus the physical examination on nutrition-related aspects, such as the patient's weight and height and his or her ability to feed themself and swallow. Evaluate your patient's vital signs and mental status. These observations will provide clues about neurologic dysfunction.

Observing the patient's behaviour can give you clues about his or her mental status. Does the patient have trouble concentrating, memory loss or seem disoriented?

Diagnostic tests

To evaluate a patient for neurologic disease, the doctor may order various laboratory and diagnostic tools, including:

- calcium levels
- glucose levels
- EEG
- computed tomography scan
- magnetic resonance imaging.

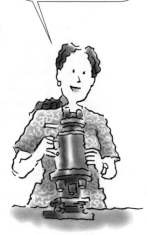

Calcium and glucose are two important lab tests for neurologic disease.

Alzheimer's disease

Alzheimer's disease, also referred to as *primary degenerative dementia*, is a progressive degenerative disorder of the cerebral cortex. Cortical degeneration is most marked in the frontal lobes, but atrophy occurs in all areas of the cortex. It accounts for more than half of all cases of dementia. An estimated 5% of people over age 65 have a severe form of the disease, and 12% suffer from mild to moderate dementia.

Because this is a primary progressive dementia, the prognosis is poor. The average duration of illness before death is 8 years.

Pathophysiology

The cause of Alzheimer's disease is unknown, but several factors are thought to be implicated in the disease, including:
- neurochemical factors, such as deficiencies in the neurotransmitters acetylcholine, somatostatin, substance P and norepinephrine (noradrenalin)
- environmental factors
- genetic factors.

Genetic studies show that an autosomal dominant form of Alzheimer's disease is associated with early onset and death. A family history of Alzheimer's disease and the presence of Down's syndrome are two known risk factors.

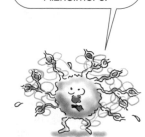

Neurofibrillary tangles cause a mess of symptoms in a patient with Alzheimer's.

The brain tissue issue

The brain tissue of patients with Alzheimer's disease has three distinguishing features:
- neurofibrillary tangles, formed out of proteins, in neurons
- neuritic plaques
- granulovascular degeneration of neurons.

Degeneration of the neurophil

The disease causes degeneration of neurophils (dense complexes of interwoven cytoplasmic processes between nerve cells and neuroglial cells), especially in the frontal, parietal and occipital lobes. It also causes enlargement of the ventricles (cavities within the brain filled with CSF).

Early cerebral changes include formation of microscopic plaques, consisting of a core surrounded by fibrous tissues. Later on, atrophy of the cerebral cortex becomes strikingly evident.

Plaque attack

If a patient has a large number of neuritic plaques, the dementia will be more severe. The plaques contain amyloid, which may exert neurotoxic effects. Evidence suggests that plaques play an important part in bringing about the death of neurons.

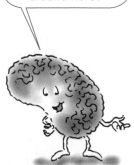

What's a brain got to do to get a little acetylcholine around here?

Acetylcholine shortage

Problems with neurotransmitters and the enzymes associated with their metabolism may play a role in the disease. The severity of dementia is directly related to reduction in the amount of the neurotransmitter acetylcholine.

On autopsy, the brains of Alzheimer's patients may contain as little as 10% of the normal amount of acetylcholine and are typically atrophic, weighing less than 1,000 g. The weight of a normal brain is commonly about 1,380 g.

What to look for

Alzheimer's disease has an insidious onset. Initially, the patient undergoes almost imperceptible changes. These changes may include forgetfulness, recent memory loss, difficulty learning and retaining new information, inability to concentrate, and deterioration in personal hygiene and appearance. As the disease progresses, signs and symptoms indicate a degenerative disorder of the frontal lobe. They may include:
• difficulty with abstract thinking and activities that require judgement
• progressive difficulty with communicating
• severe deterioration of memory, language and motor function progressing to coordination loss and an inability to speak and write
• irritability, mood swings, hostility and combativeness.

Neurologic examination commonly reveals an impaired sense of smell (usually an early symptom), an inability to recognise and understand the form and nature of objects by touching them, gait disorders and tremors.

In the final stages, urinary or faecal incontinence, twitching and seizures commonly occur.

Treatment

Therapy consists of the anticholinesterase drugs galantamine, donepezil and rivastigmine to help improve symptoms. Memantine, an *N*-methyl-D-aspartate antagonist, can be prescribed to treat symptoms of moderate-to-severe Alzheimer's disease, but routine prescription is not recommended by the NICE guidelines. Vitamin E may help protect brain cells from damage. Other drugs can be used, as needed, to control behavioural symptoms, such as anxiety, agitation, sleep disturbances and depression.

Dietary management

Although there's no evidence that Alzheimer's disease changes nutritional requirements, it does have significant effects on the patient's nutritional status. Initially, the patient may have difficulty purchasing and cooking food. The patient may forget to eat or may forget he or she has eaten and eat again. Mood swings may cause fluctuations in appetite. Food preferences change with alterations in the patient's sense of smell. Agitation may increase calorie requirements by as much as 1,600 kcal/day.

All choked up

The patient with Alzheimer's disease may hoard food or may forget to chew food thoroughly, which places him or her at risk of choking. Therefore, mealtimes should be closely supervised. Food temperatures should be monitored to prevent burns.

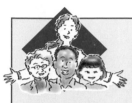

Bridging the gap

Sticking to the patient's personal routine

Sticking to a routine is important when caring for a patient with Alzheimer's disease. However, make sure it's as close to the patient's personal routine as possible. Be aware that certain beliefs may play a part in that routine.

Religion tends to have a great impact on eating habits, even greater than nationality and culture. Orthodox Jews, for example, eat Kosher foods, and use separate dishes and utensils for meat and dairy. Question the family about the patient's religious practices surrounding food. Remember, religious practices can vary significantly, even among denominations of the same faith.

Follow a routine

Meals should be served at the same time each day in familiar surroundings. Distractions should be kept to a minimum. It may be necessary to offer one food at a time because a whole plate or tray of food can be overwhelming. (See *Sticking to the patient's personal routine*.)

Consistency counts

It may be necessary to modify food consistency to prevent choking. Food should be cut into small pieces and the patient reminded to chew, as necessary. Easy-to-consume snacks, such as finger foods, should be offered between meals. When the patient can no longer take in food orally, tube feeding may be initiated. However, this choice needs to be discussed with the family.

Epilepsy

Also known as *seizure disorder*, epilepsy is a brain condition that's characterised by recurrent seizures. Seizures are paroxysmal events associated with abnormal electrical discharges of neurons in the brain. The discharge may trigger a convulsive movement, an interruption of sensation, an alteration in level of consciousness or a combination of these symptoms. In most cases, epilepsy doesn't affect intelligence.

Under control

Over 440,000 people have epilepsy in the UK. It is the most serious neurologic condition and is a major long-term disability, with similar numbers of people affected as Type 1 diabetes. The condition appears most commonly in early childhood, early adolescence and advanced age. About 80% of patients have good seizure control with strict adherence to prescribed treatment.

Pathophysiology

In about half the cases of epilepsy, the cause is unknown and the patient has no other neurologic abnormality. In other cases, however, possible causes of epilepsy include:
- birth trauma (inadequate blood supply to the brain)
- anoxia (after respiratory or cardiac arrest)
- infectious diseases (meningitis, encephalitis or brain abscess)
- ingestion of toxins (mercury, lead or carbon monoxide)
- brain tumour
- fever
- head trauma or injury.

Hyperactivity

This is what happens during a seizure:

The electronic balance of the neuronal level is altered, causing the neuronal membrane to become susceptible to activation.

Increased permeability of the cytoplasmic membranes helps hypersensitive neurons fire abnormally. Abnormal firing may be activated by hyperthermia, hypoglycaemia, hyponatraemia, hypoxia or repeated sensory stimulation.

Once the intensity of a seizure discharge has progressed sufficiently, it spreads to adjacent brain areas. The midbrain, thalamus and cerebral cortex are most likely to become epileptogenic.

Excitement feeds back from the primary focus and to other parts of the brain.

The discharges become less frequent until they stop.

Getting complicated

Depending on the type of seizure, injury may result from a fall at the onset of a seizure or afterwards, when the patient is confused. Injury may also result from the rapid, jerking movements that occur during or after a seizure. Anoxia can occur due to airway occlusion by the tongue, aspiration of vomit or traumatic injury. A continuous seizure state known as *status epilepticus* can cause respiratory distress and even death.

What to look for

Signs and symptoms of epilepsy vary depending on the type and cause of the seizure.

Complex partial seizure

Signs and symptoms of a complex partial seizure are variable but usually include purposeless behaviour, a glassy stare, aimless wandering and lip-smacking. An aura may occur first, and seizures may last a few seconds to 20 minutes. Afterwards, mental confusion may last for several minutes.

Absence seizure

Absence seizure occurs most often in children. It usually begins with a brief change in the level of consciousness, signalled by blinking or rolling of the eyes, a blank stare and slight mouth movements. The patient retains his or her posture and continues preseizure activity without difficulty. Seizures last from 1 to 10 seconds, and impairment is so brief that the patient may be unaware of it. However, if not properly treated, these seizures can recur up to 100 times per day and progress to a generalised tonic–clonic seizure.

Generalised tonic–clonic seizure

Typically, a generalised tonic–clonic seizure begins when the patient's body stiffens (tonic phase). It then alternates between episodes of muscle spasm and relaxation (clonic phase). The patient may fall to the ground and lose consciousness. Tongue biting, incontinence, laboured breathing, apnoea and cyanosis may also occur.

The seizure stops in 2 to 5 minutes, when abnormal electrical conduction of the neurons is completed. Afterwards, the patient regains consciousness but is somewhat confused. The patient may have difficulty talking and may have drowsiness, fatigue, headache, muscle soreness and arm or leg weakness. He or she may fall into a deep sleep afterwards.

Treatment

Common first-line antiepileptic medications include carbamazepine, ethosuximide, oxcarbazepine, phenytoin and valproic acid. Medications that can be added to or replace first-line medications include felbamate, gabapentin, lamotrigine, levetiracetam, tiagabine, topiramate and zonisamide. Other medications used to treat epilepsy include benzodiazepines, phenobarbital and primidone.

Distress call

Some drugs used to treat epilepsy cause GI distress. Encourage the patient to take the drug with food to minimise distress, if appropriate.

Other treatments for epilepsy may include surgery to remove a focal lesion or correct the underlying problem or insertion of a vagal nerve stimulator.

Medication meddler

If the patient taking phenytoin requires enteral feedings, separate dosing and feeding times as much as possible and by no less than an hour. Enteral feeding may interfere with the absorption of oral suspension.

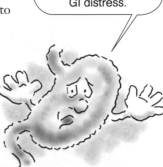

Some drugs used to treat epilepsy cause GI distress.

Dietary management

Most patients with epilepsy don't require dietary changes. However, those patients who don't attain seizure control through the use of antiseizure medications are sometimes prescribed ketogenic diets in conjunction with their medications. The diet is most effective when used for children.

Children selected for ketogenic therapy typically experience at least two seizures per week despite receiving two antiseizure medications. Research has shown that elevated blood ketone levels in these children reduce the incidence of seizure activity, sometimes to the point that antiseizure medications are no longer needed.

Change in the popularity poll

Initially studied in the 1920s, the ketogenic diet was used to treat intractable seizures. As different seizure medications were developed, fewer people were encouraged to follow this diet. Recently, however, there has been a resurgence of its use.

What? High fat, low carb and low protein?

This high-fat, low-carbohydrate, low-protein diet causes ketosis as the body is forced to use fatty acids instead of glucose for energy. This reaction causes mild starvation and dehydration. In addition, the diet places the patient at risk for hypoglycaemia.

A dietitian uses the patient's age and weight to calculate the caloric needs. The patient's calorie allotment for the diet is restricted and based on the patient's age and activity level. When the patient begins the diet, he or she's usually started at a ratio of 4 parts fat to 1 part carbohydrate and protein. Children under age 15 months or obese children may be started on a 3:1 ratio.

The brink of drink

Fluid intake is restricted to 75% of the patient's typical intake. As a rule, the patient should consume no more millilitres of fluid per day than the number of calories prescribed in the diet. For example if the patient is prescribed a 1,500 cal diet, he or she should consume no more than 1,500 ml of fluid per day. Fluid intake should be spread over the course of the day, and no more than 120 ml should be consumed in a 2-hour period. Urine specific gravity is maintained between 1.020 and 1.025. Beverages containing aspartame or caffeine must be avoided because they inhibit ketosis.

Don't get caught short

A dietitian calculates the patient's protein allowance, making sure that the patient consumes the reference nutrient intake. The diet is supplemented daily with calcium; a sugar-free, lactose-free multivitamin; and fluoride, if indicated. (See *On the way to ketosis*.)

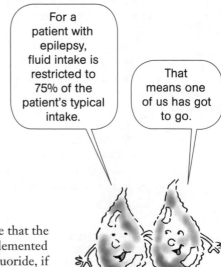

For a patient with epilepsy, fluid intake is restricted to 75% of the patient's typical intake.

That means one of us has got to go.

On the way to ketosis

When a patient requires a ketogenic diet to control seizures, a dietitian uses age and weight to determine caloric needs. Then the dietitian uses formulas to determine fat, protein and carbohydrate needs. When the individual diet plan is formulated, the patient prepares for admission to the hospital to initiate treatment. The day before hospitalisation, the patient consumes a low-carbohydrate diet and, after dinner, fasts with the exception of water. The typical postadmission treatment plan is outlined here.

Day 1

- Patient continues to fast with the exception of fluids.
- Oral intake is increased to three to four times the maintenance level; patient consumes water or diet, caffeine-free fizzy drinks.
- Family meets with the dietitian.
- Baseline laboratory tests such as serum antiseizure medication level, lipoprotein level and electrolyte levels are obtained.
- Baseline EEG is obtained.
- Antiseizure medication doses are decreased because levels may rise during the fasting period.
- I.V. therapy is initiated.
- Parent or other family member is instructed to keep a seizure diary and an accurate record of the patient's intake.

Your responsibilities

- Maintain strict intake and output.
- Monitor urine for ketones after every void.
- Monitor blood glucose levels every 4 to 6 hours as ordered.
- Weigh the patient after the first void in the morning.
- Monitor vital signs every 4 hours.
- Measure the child's head circumference, if age appropriate.
- Instruct the family about checking urine for ketones and monitoring blood glucose levels.
- Explain to the patient and family that the patient can't use toothpaste or mouthwash with sugar or carbohydrate in them.

Day 2

- Dietitian develops meal plans.
- Patient receives I.V. normal saline solution, if needed.
- Family begins learning how to plan and prepare meals.
- Urine ketone levels become elevated (4+ is target value).
- Laboratory tests such as serum electrolytes and antiseizure medication levels are obtained.

Your responsibilities

- Monitor blood glucose and urine ketone levels.
- Monitor weight after first morning void.
- Monitor vital signs.

Day 3

- Patient is in ketosis.
- Food is reintroduced to meet one-third of the child's requirements.
- Family continues learning dietary planning and food preparation.
- Serum antiseizure medication levels and electrolyte levels are obtained.

Your responsibilities

- Monitor blood glucose and urine ketone levels.
- Monitor weight after first morning void.
- Monitor vital signs.
- Have parents perform a return demonstration of blood glucose and ketone testing.

Day 4

- Meals are progressed to two-third requirements.
- Family education regarding meal planning and preparation continues.
- Serum antiseizure medication levels and electrolyte levels are obtained.

Your responsibilities

- Monitor weight, vital signs, and blood and ketone levels.
- Reinforce family education.

Day 5

- Patient begins full diet.
- Serum antiseizure medication levels and electrolyte levels are obtained.
- If the patient's condition is stable and the family understands dietary teaching, the patient can be discharged.

Your responsibilities

- Monitor weight and vital signs.
- Review discharge teaching.

Menu maven

Serving up a ketogenic diet

Meal preparation for the patient receiving a ketogenic diet can be difficult. The patient's family must be educated about the type and amount of food allowed at each meal because any deviation can easily prevent ketosis. The menu below shows the types of food consumed on the diet. The amount of food consumed is highly individualised.

Breakfast

- scrambled eggs with butter
- diluted cream
- orange juice

Lunch

- spaghetti squash with butter and Parmesan cheese
- lettuce leaf with mayonnaise
- orange diet sparkling drink mixed with whipped cream

Dinner

- sausage slices with sugar-free ketchup
- asparagus with butter
- chopped lettuce with mayonnaise

Snack

- sugar-free vanilla ice cream

Family education is the key to success. The patient's family is taught meal planning and preparation and blood glucose and ketone monitoring during the patient's hospitalisation. (See *Serving up a ketogenic diet*.)

Parkinson's disease

Parkinson's disease produces progressive muscle rigidity, loss of muscle movement (akinesia) and involuntary tremors. The patient's condition may deteriorate for about 10 years until death finally ensues.

Parkinson's disease is one of the most common crippling diseases in the UK. It affects men and women equally and usually occurs in middle age or later, striking 1 in every 100 people over age 60. (See *Young-onset Parkinson's disease*.)

Pathophysiology

In most cases, the cause of Parkinson's disease is unknown. However, some cases result from exposure to toxins, such as manganese dust and carbon monoxide, that destroy cells in the substantia nigra of the brain.

Dopamine pathway defect...

Parkinson's disease affects the extrapyramidal system of the brain, which influences the initiation, modulation and completion of movement. The

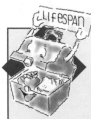

Lifespan lunchbox

Young-onset Parkinson's disease

Young-onset Parkinson's disease is the appearance of Parkinsonian symptoms before age 40. Although young patients experience all the typical symptoms, dystonic spasms are more common and may appear before the onset of other characteristic symptoms of Parkinson's disease. Younger patients are also less likely to experience tremors than people who develop Parkinson's disease after age 60. Levodopa is effective in treating symptoms in younger patients; however, younger patients are more likely to develop dyskinesia while taking this drug.

extrapyramidal system includes the corpus striatum, subthalamic nucleus, substantia nigra and red nucleus.

In Parkinson's disease, a dopamine deficiency occurs in the basal ganglia, the dopamine-releasing pathway that connects the substantia nigra to the corpus striatum.

...causes neurotransmitter imbalance

Reduction in dopamine in the corpus striatum upsets the normal balance between the inhibitory dopamine and excitatory acetylcholine neurotransmitters. This prevents affected brain cells from performing their normal inhibitory function within the CNS and causes most Parkinsonian symptoms.

What to look for

Important signs of Parkinson's disease include:
- muscle rigidity
- akinesia
- unilateral pill-rolling tremor.

Muscle rigidity results in resistance to passive muscle stretching, which may be uniform (lead-pipe rigidity) or jerky (cogwheel rigidity).

Akinesia causes a masklike facial expression and gait and movement disturbances. The patient walks with his or her body bent forward, takes a long time initiating movement when performing a purposeful action, pivots with difficulty and easily loses balance.

Pill-rolling tremor is insidious. It begins in the fingers, increases during stress or anxiety and decreases with purposeful movement and sleep.

Supplemental symptoms

Other signs and symptoms of Parkinson's disease include:
- high-pitched, monotone voice
- drooling

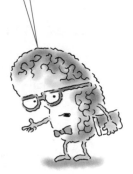

Dopamine reduction prevents my cells from doing their job and causes most Parkinsonian symptoms.

- dysarthria (impaired speech due to disturbance in muscle control)
- dysphagia (difficulty swallowing)
- fatigue.

Compiling the complications

Common complications of Parkinson's disease include injury from falls, food aspiration due to impaired voluntary movements, urinary tract infections and skin breakdown due to increased immobility.

Treatment

Because Parkinson's disease has no cure, treatment aims to relieve symptoms and keep the patient functional as long as possible. Treatment consists of drugs, physical therapy and, in severe cases that are unresponsive to drugs, stereotactic surgery or foetal cell transplantation (controversial).

A look at levodopa

Drug therapy usually includes levodopa, a dopamine replacement that's most effective during the early stages of treatment. It's given in increasing doses until symptoms are relieved or adverse effects develop. Because adverse effects can be serious, levodopa is frequently given along with carbidopa to halt peripheral dopamine synthesis. Unfortunately, levodopa doesn't prevent the progressive brain changes found in Parkinson's disease.

Other drugs that can be used include anticholinergics, antihistamines, amantadine, entacapone, selegiline and catechol-*O*-methyl transferase inhibitors.

Is neurosurgery next?

When drug therapy fails, stereotactic neurosurgery is sometimes effective. In this procedure, electrical coagulation, freezing, radioactivity or ultrasound destroys the ventrolateral nucleus of the thalamus to prevent involuntary movement. Such neurosurgery is most effective in comparatively young, otherwise healthy people with unilateral tremor or muscle rigidity. Like drug therapy, neurosurgery is a palliative measure that can only relieve symptoms.

Other treatments include brain stimulator implantation, foetal cell transplantation (controversial) and neurotransplantation.

Exercise expectations

The patient with Parkinson's disease should be encouraged to exercise at least three times per week while he or she's able. The exercise regimen should include aerobic, strengthening and stretching exercises.

Easy PT

Physiotherapy helps maintain the patient's normal muscle tone and function. It includes active and passive range-of-motion exercises, routine daily activities, walking, and baths and massage to help relax muscles.

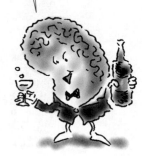

Here's to levodopa and carbidopa. They make a beautiful pair!

Dietary management

Constipation, a common complication of Parkinson's disease, can interfere with the uptake of drugs such as levodopa. Patients should be encouraged to consume a high-fibre diet. High-fibre foods should be gradually substituted for refined, low-fibre foods to avoid symptoms of intolerance (gas, diarrhoea and cramping).

Coffee, tea or...lemon water?

The patient should also increase their fluid intake to at least 8 to 10 glasses daily. Encourage the patient to drink hot coffee, tea or lemon water to stimulate peristalsis. Encourage the intake of prunes or prune juice, which have laxative effects.

Vivacious vitamin D

The gait disturbance associated with Parkinson's disease places the patient at risk for falls. This, combined with inadequate intake of vitamin D and calcium, places the patient at increased risk for fractures. Consuming adequate amounts of vitamin D helps promote calcium absorption and prevent bone density loss.

Be smart about B₆

Excessive intake of pyridoxine (vitamin B_6) can reduce the effectiveness of levodopa. If the patient takes over-the-counter supplements, discuss the interaction. Encourage the patient to limit the intake of foods fortified with vitamin B_6.

Levodopa, an amino acid, competes for absorption with other amino acids found in dietary protein. Absorption of levodopa may be reduced, lessening the drug's effectiveness. Excess protein intake should be avoided, and the majority of the daily allowance of protein should be consumed during the evening meal. (See *Ineffective mix*.)

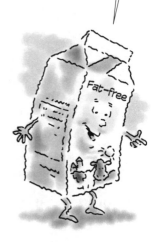

Consuming adequate amounts of vitamin D helps to promote calcium absorption and prevent bone density loss.

Ineffective mix

Carbidopa–levodopa (Sinemet) is absorbed in the small bowel. Any condition that delays stomach emptying can reduce the absorption of carbidopa–levodopa. Many people will feel nauseous on the drugs used to treat Parkinson's disease due to the action of the drug in the central nervous system. Some foods that are high in protein compete with the drug for entry into the brain. When less carbidopa–levodopa enters the brain, the exacerbation of Parkinsonian symptoms occurs.

To help maintain adequate protein intake and drug absorption, the patient should take these precautions:

- Restrict protein intake if typical intake is higher than the recommended daily allowance.
- Eat small amounts of protein divided evenly throughout the day, or restrict protein intake to the evening meal to get the full effects of medication during the day.

Difficult going down

Eating, and especially swallowing, may be difficult for the patient with Parkinson's disease. An speech and language therapist can suggest the appropriate consistency for a patient, and the dietitian can suggest appropriate foods to meet nutritional requirements at that consistency. This might include pudding, custard, scrambled eggs, hot cereals and yoghurt.

Slowing down

Patients with Parkinson's disease may eat very slowly. Using insulated dishes or a warming tray helps keep food warm. Distractions can cause the elderly patient with Parkinson's disease to lose focus while eating. If interrupted during eating, patients may have trouble starting again. It's best to plan uninterrupted mealtimes. Because hand coordination becomes poor, plate guards and special eating utensils may be helpful. Soft-textured foods may be necessary for those who have difficulty chewing.

Parkinson's disease also slows gastric motility, prolonging digestion. Food takes less time to digest when consumed in small amounts. Encourage the patient to consume small, frequent meals instead of consuming three larger meals per day.

Weighing in on weight loss

Weight loss can be a problem for patients with Parkinson's disease. Patients sometimes become so diligent about limiting protein and fat intake that they deprive themselves of necessary calories. Encouraging an appropriate diet and nutrition supplements, as necessary, can combat calorie deprivation.

Quick quiz

1. Which characteristic increases the likelihood of a patient with Alzheimer's disease experiencing weight loss?
    A. A slow shuffling gait
    B. Loss of fine motor coordination
    C. Agitation
    D. Lethargy

Answer: C. Agitation increases caloric needs, leading to weight loss.

2. How does the ketogenic diet control seizures?
    A. By forcing ketone production
    B. By limiting the number of circulating ketones
    C. By increasing the amount of dopamine available to the brain
    D. By increasing acetylcholine levels

Answer: A. The ketogenic diet induces mild starvation and dehydration, forcing the body to produce ketones, which have naturally occurring seizure-suppressing properties.

3. The patient prescribed a ketogenic diet should avoid which of the following foods?
A. Butter
B. Oatmeal biscuits
C. Eggs
D. Mayonnaise

Answer: B. The ketogenic diet is high in fat and protein and low in carbohydrates. Foods that contain sugar, such as oatmeal biscuits, should be avoided. A small deviation in the diet can prevent ketosis.

4. Why might a doctor suggest that a patient with Parkinson's disease limit protein intake to one meal per day?
A. Protein competes with levodopa for entry into the brain.
B. Protein potentiates the effect of levodopa.
C. Protein delays gastric emptying.
D. Protein induces ketosis when consumed with levodopa.

Answer: A. Protein and levodopa compete for entry into the brain. The less levodopa that gets to the brain, the less symptom control the patient receives. Consuming protein during the last meal of the day allows adequate protein intake while maintaining adequate drug levels.

Scoring

☆☆☆ If you answered all four questions correctly, congratulations! You've got a head for this kind of information.

☆☆ If you answered three questions correctly, good job! Your neuro-logic is right on track.

☆ If you answered fewer than three questions correctly, that's okay! Reading about neurologic disorders can be a real brain drain. Review the chapter and try again.

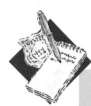

16 Diabetes mellitus

Just the facts

Nutrition is an important factor in the development and treatment of diabetes mellitus. In this chapter, you'll learn:

♦ the relationship between glucose metabolism and dietary intake

♦ the role of medications, exercise and diet in blood glucose control

♦ nutrition therapy guidelines for patients with diabetes.

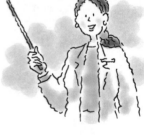

Your biggest impact on a patient with diabetes may be teaching self-care skills.

A look at diabetes mellitus

Diabetes mellitus is a chronic disease of insulin deficiency or resistance in which disturbances in carbohydrate, protein and fat metabolism lead to hyperglycaemia (increased blood glucose level). It affects 3.86% of the UK population, or roughly 2.5 million people. Half of those affected are undiagnosed.

Squeezing the pound

Diabetes cost the NHS £1 million per hour, this does not include the costs to the lives of the people affected. Good diabetes management can reduce the risk of complications, but when not well-managed it is associated with complications including heart disease, blindness, kidney disease, nerve damage and amputations leading to disability and premature mortality.

• By the time they are diagnosed, half the people with type 2 diabetes show signs of complications.

• Complications may begin 5–6 years before diagnosis of diabetes.

However, some experts estimate that nearly 99% of diabetes outcomes depend on patient self-care. So teaching your patients good self-care skills gives them an excellent chance of avoiding diabetes complications.

Type writers

In 2000, the Diabetes UK recommended health care professionals to adopt the WHO revised diabetes classification system. Currently, there are five main types of diabetes:
- type 1
- type 2
- impaired glucose tolerance (IGT)
- impaired fasting glycaemia (IFG)
- gestational (diabetes during pregnancy).

Diagnosing diabetes

The patient has diabetes symptoms (i.e. polyuria, polydipsia and unexplained weight loss) plus
- a random venous plasma glucose concentration of 11.1 mmol/L

or
- a fasting plasma glucose concentration of 7.0 mmol/L (whole blood 6.1 mmol/L)

or
- plasma glucose concentration of 11.1 mmol/L 2 hours after 75 g anhydrous glucose has been administered in an oral glucose tolerance test (OGTT).

With no symptoms, diagnosis should not be based on a single glucose determination but requires confirmatory plasma venous determination. At least one additional glucose test result on another day with a value in the diabetic range is essential, either fasting, from a random sample or from the 2-hour postglucose load. If the fasting or random values are not diagnostic, the 2-hour value should be used.

Three's company

To aid evaluation and check for complications, three other tests may also be done:
- Glycosylated haemoglobin (HbA_{1c}) tests monitor long-term effectiveness of therapy in a patient previously diagnosed with diabetes. These tests show variants in haemoglobin levels that reflect average blood glucose levels over the previous 2 to 3 months.
- Ophthalmologic examination may show diabetic retinopathy.
- Urinalysis determines presence of acetone in the urine.

Caught in the middle

Some people have *prediabetes*, an intermediate state between normal glucose metabolism and diabetes. Prediabetes increases the risk of developing diabetes, heart attack and stroke. About 1 million people in the UK have *prediabetes*.

There are two forms of prediabetes:
- IGT is a stage of impaired glucose regulation (fasting plasma glucose 7.0 mmol/L and OGTT 2-hour value 7.8 to 11.1 mmol/L).

Diabetes screening guidelines

Use these guidelines to screen at risk groups for prediabetes and diabetes in asymptomatic patients:

- people who have previously been found to have impaired glucose regulation (impaired glucose tolerance and/or impaired fasting glycaemia)
- women who have had gestational diabetes and have tested normal following delivery
- white people aged over 40 years and people from Black, Asian and minority ethnic groups aged over 25 years who:
  - have a first-degree relative with diabetes and/or
  - are overweight (BMI > 25 kg/m^2) and have a sedentary lifestyle and/or
  - have ischaemic heart disease, cerebrovascular disease, peripheral vascular disease or hypertension
- women with polycystic ovary syndrome who are obese.

- IFG has been introduced to classify individuals who have fasting glucose values above the normal range but below those diagnostic of diabetes (fasting plasma glucose 6.1 to 7.0 mmol/L).

Sugar, get yourself screened

Guidelines are available to screen for diabetes in patients who are asymptomatic. (See *Diabetes screening guidelines*.)

Type 1 and type 2 diabetes

Type 1 and type 2 diabetes are the most common forms of diabetes mellitus. Type 1, which accounts for approximately 5% to 10% of diabetes cases, can occur at any age. Usually, though, it's detected before age 30 in people with normal or below-normal weight. The cause isn't known, although experts suspect that multiple factors, including genetic susceptibility, are involved.

Type 2 diabetes is the most common diabetes form in adults, accounting for more than 90% of diabetes cases in the UK. It's associated with multiple factors, including a family history of the disease, advancing age, obesity and lack of exercise. Type 2 diabetes is more common in Asian and African people. (See *Diabetes in South Asians*.)

Breaking the mould

Type 2 diabetes doesn't always fit into set patterns. For example some patients have an ideal weight and no family history of the disease. Type 2 diabetes can also occur in children. In fact, childhood type 2 diabetes is an emerging epidemic linked to obesity, poor eating habits and a sedentary lifestyle.

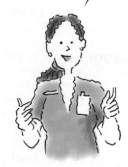

Diabetes is hard to typecast. Types 1 and 2 can both occur at any age.

Pathophysiology

Normally, insulin allows glucose to travel into cells where it's used for energy and stored as glycogen. Insulin also stimulates protein synthesis and free fatty acid storage in adipose tissue. When insulin is deficient, tissues can't access essential nutrients for fuel and storage.

Diabetes mellitus results from insulin deficiency, although the pathophysiology differs with the type of diabetes.

What goes wrong in type 1?

In type 1 diabetes, suppression or destruction of the pancreatic beta cells (which produce insulin) impairs insulin production, preventing normal food metabolism. As a result, the blood glucose level rises and cells can't use glucose for energy. Eventually, glucose spills into the urine.

Total lack of insulin leads to build-up of ketone bodies (ketosis). Unless treated, ketosis reduces blood pH, resulting in diabetic ketoacidosis (DKA), a life-threatening form of metabolic acidosis.

Attack on beta cells

Type 1 diabetes is subdivided into *idiopathic diabetes* (which has an unknown cause) and *immune-mediated diabetes*. In immune-mediated diabetes, the body's immune system destroys the beta cells. This causes an inflammatory response in the pancreas, called *insulitis*.

By the time type 1 diabetes becomes apparent, 80% of beta cells are gone. Some experts believe beta cells aren't destroyed by the antibodies but are disabled—and might be reactivated later. Islet cell antibodies may be present long before symptoms appear. These immune markers also precede evidence of beta cell deficiency. Autoantibodies against insulin have also been noted.

What goes wrong in type 2?

Experts have identified three aetiologies for type 2 diabetes:

resistance to insulin action in target tissues

abnormal insulin secretion

inappropriate hepatic gluconeogenesis (carbohydrate formation from non-carbohydrate molecules).

Insulin resistance and abnormal insulin secretion eventually lead to IGT. The pancreas simply can't produce enough insulin to drive blood glucose and other nutrients into body tissues and shut off the liver's glucose production.

Complications

Research shows that glucose readings don't have to be as high as previously thought for complications to develop. Two acute diabetes complications—DKA

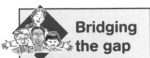

Bridging the gap

Diabetes in South Asians

South Asian people who live in the UK are up to six times more likely to have type 2 diabetes than the white European population, and with diabetes prevalence in England predicted to increase by 47% by 2025, the condition will continue to have a considerable impact on South Asian communities across the UK.

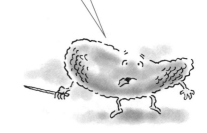

Even though the patho differs from type to type, diabetes mellitus essentially results from insulin deficiency.

and hyperosmolar hyperglycaemic nonketotic syndrome (HHNS)—can lead to shock, coma and even death. Hypoglycaemia (low blood sugar) can also occur.

DKA

DKA occurs most often with type 1 diabetes—and sometimes is the first sign of the disease. The condition is triggered by extremely high blood glucose levels. Ketone build-up causes metabolic acidosis, and severe hyperglycaemia leads to dehydration. Although life threatening, DKA is reversible.

Hyperosmolar hyperglycaemic nonketotic syndrome (HHNS)

HHNS is most common in patients with type 2 diabetes, although it can occur in anyone whose insulin tolerance is stressed and in patients who have undergone certain therapeutic procedures (such as peritoneal dialysis, haemodialysis, tube feedings or total parenteral nutrition).

As with DKA, HHNS is triggered by insulin deficiency. However, HHNS doesn't involve ketosis. Nonetheless, coma can occur if extremely high blood glucose levels (often over 40 mmol/L) cause dehydration of brain tissues.

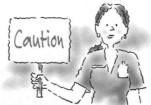

Diabetes complications can lead to shock, coma and even death.

Hypoglycaemia

Acute hypoglycaemia may occur if a diabetic patient:
- eats too little
- exercises too much
- drinks alcohol without eating enough carbohydrates
- takes too much antidiabetic medication
- doesn't prepare or inject insulin properly.

Signs and symptoms include weakness, confusion, syncope, diaphoresis (profuse sweating) and heart palpitations. Untreated, hypoglycaemia can cause seizures, brain damage, coma and death.

Long-term complications

Patients with diabetes mellitus are at higher risk for chronic complications affecting virtually all body systems. The most common complications are cardiovascular disease such as atherosclerosis, peripheral vascular disease, retinopathy, nephropathy (kidney disease), diabetic dermopathy (skin disease) and peripheral and autonomic neuropathy.

In addition, because hyperglycaemia impairs resistance to infection, diabetes may cause skin and urinary tract infections as well as vaginitis. Glucose content of the skin and urine encourages bacterial growth.

The paths of neuropathies

Peripheral neuropathy usually affects the hands and feet and may cause numbness or pain. Autonomic neuropathy may manifest in several ways, including gastroparesis (leading to delayed gastric emptying and nausea and fullness after meals), nocturnal diarrhoea, impotence and postural hypotension.

What to look for

The body eliminates excess glucose in urine. As it does so, it excretes a large volume of water, causing the patient with hyperglycaemia to become dehydrated and extremely thirsty. Although he or she may be consuming adequate calories, glucose isn't being absorbed or used properly, so the patient becomes very hungry and may lose weight.

Patients with type 1 diabetes usually report rapid symptom onset, including muscle wasting and subcutaneous fat loss. With type 2 diabetes, symptoms usually are vague, long-standing and of gradual onset. Typically, the patient reports a family history of diabetes, gestational diabetes, delivery of a baby weighing more than 4 kg, severe viral infection or use of drugs that increase blood glucose levels. Obesity, especially in the abdominal area, is also a common finding.

Trying triad

With either type 1 or type 2 diabetes, as the body tries to eliminate excess glucose and ketones, the patient may experience the classic symptom triad of:

 polyuria—excessive urination

 polydipsia—excessive thirst

 polyphagia—excessive eating. (See *Diabetes symptoms in elderly patients*.)

Beyond the triad

Other signs and symptoms of diabetes may include:
- weakness and fatigue
- irritability
- vision changes

Lifespan lunchbox

Diabetes symptoms in elderly patients

In older adults, two of the classic symptoms of diabetes—polydipsia and polyuria—may be absent. Nonspecific complaints may be the only clues to the disease. Older adults and their caregivers may report appetite loss, weight loss, unexplained fatigue, slow wound healing, mental status changes, incontinence and decreased vision. Constipation or abdominal bloating may result from gastric hypotonicity. Recurrent bacterial or fungal infections of the skin, urinary tract infections and pruritus vulvae (in women) may also occur.

Memory jogger

The three **P**s of the classic symptom triad may help you identify a patient with type 1 or type 2 diabetes mellitus:

Polydipsia

Polyphagia

Polyuria.

- muscle wasting
- weight loss
- dry, itchy or cool skin
- dry mucous membranes
- slow peripheral pulses
- decreased reflexes
- poor wound healing
- vaginal discomfort.

In addition, patients with DKA may have a fruity breath odour from increased acetone production.

Treatment

Diabetes treatment should include the patient, family and an interdisciplinary health care team. Treatment varies with the diabetes type and any coexisting medical problems. For type 1 and type 2 diabetes, the goal is to normalise blood glucose levels and decrease complications. Treatment emphasises lifestyle changes involving diet and exercise. Some patients also require medication.

In type 1 diabetes, lack of insulin production by the pancreas may make the blood glucose level particularly hard to control, so food intake and exercise patterns must be consistently matched to insulin administration.

Medication

All patients with type 1 diabetes receive drug therapy. With type 2 diabetes, the need for medication depends on individual factors.

Drug therapy for type 1

The patient with type 1 diabetes must receive insulin by subcutaneous or intravenous injection to survive. Treatment requires a strict regimen that includes daily insulin injections along with a carefully calculated diet, planned physical activity and home blood glucose testing several times per day.

Types for type 1

Current forms of insulin replacement include single-dose, mixed-dose, split-mixed-dose and multiple-dose regimens. Patients on multiple-dose regimens may use an insulin pump, which can administer variable rates throughout the day.

Choice of insulin and insulin regimen

NICE guidance recommends that the prescribed type of insulin allows an individual to achieve optimal well-being using multiple insulin injection regimens in adults who prefer an integrated package with education, food, skills training and appropriate self-monitoring.

For people who are prone to hypoglycaemia at night, a twice-daily insulin regimen, often biphasic rapid-acting insulin analogue pre-mixes, is beneficial. This is useful for people who find adherence to lunchtime insulin

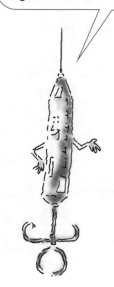

Patients with type 1 diabetes require insulin injections for glucose control.

injections difficult or who have a learning impairment. Insulin preparations can be of three types:

- those of *short* duration, which have a relatively rapid onset of action, namely soluble insulin and the rapid-acting insulin analogues, insulin aspart, insulin glulisine and insulin lispro
- those with an *intermediate* action, e.g. isophane insulin
- those whose action is slower in onset and lasts for *long* periods, e.g. protamine zinc insulin, insulin detemir and insulin glargine.

The insulin regimen recommended by NICE includes:

- *Mealtime insulin*: use unmodified (soluble) insulin or rapid-acting insulin analogues. However use rapid-acting insulin analogues rather than unmodified insulin:
    - where nocturnal or late, between meals (interprandial) or, hypoglycaemia is a problem
    - to avoid need for snacks, while maintaining equivalent blood glucose control.
- *Basal/nocturnal insulin supply*: use isophane (NPH) insulin or long-acting insulin analogues (insulin glargine) for basal/nocturnal insulin supply (isophane [NPH] insulin given at bedtime, or given twice daily with mealtime insulin analogues). Use long-acting insulin analogues (insulin glargine) when:
    - nocturnal hypoglycaemia is a problem on isophane (NPH) insulin
    - morning hyperglycaemia on isophane (NPH) insulin results in difficult daytime blood glucose control
    - rapid-acting insulin analogues are used for mealtime blood glucose control.
- If the individual has a dietary intake and activity pattern that vary considerably from day to day, advise them to consult diabetic nurse specialists. Their blood glucose monitoring or insulin regimen may need to be reviewed and modified accordingly.

In addition to insulin

The insulin dosage must be balanced with food intake and daily activities. Blood glucose levels must be monitored closely. Most people in the UK do not use an insulin pump and must inject insulin at least twice per day to achieve adequate glucose control overnight without causing daytime drowsiness.

Drug therapy for type 2

For many patients with type 2 diabetes, dietary regulation and adequate exercise may sufficiently control the blood glucose level. Otherwise, the patient may require insulin or, more commonly, oral antidiabetic agents. The most commonly used drugs include:

- Sulphonylureas, which are considered for patients who have some pancreatic beta cell activity, who are not overweight or in whom metformin is contraindicated or not tolerated. Several sulphonylureas are available, and the choice is determined by side effects and the duration of action as well as the patient's age and renal function. The long-acting sulphonylureas chlorpropamide and

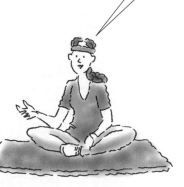

For patients with type 2 diabetes, diet and exercise may be all the therapy that's necessary.

glibenclamide are associated with a greater risk of hypoglycaemia; for this reason they should be avoided in the elderly, and shorter-acting alternatives, such as gliclazide or tolbutamide, should be used instead.
• metformin (Glucophage), a biguanide that decreases glucose production by the liver and improves glucose uptake.

In addition some people may be prescribed other medication including the following:
• alpha-glucosidase inhibitors (starch blockers), such as acarbose (Glucobay), which slow digestion and absorption of starches and sugars, thus countering the rapid blood glucose rise that follows eating
• thiazolidinedione, insulin sensitisers, such as rosiglitazone (Avandia) and pioglitazone (Actos), which increase glucose uptake in tissues and lower serum glucose levels in patients with insulin resistance
• meglitinides, repaglinide (Prandin) and nateglinide (Starlix), which are taken before meals to stimulate the release of insulin, act very quickly and may cause hypoglycaemia.

Some patients receive combinations of these drugs—for instance metformin with sulphonylureas.

Dietary approaches

Treatment of diabetes requires a diet planned to meet a patient's nutritional needs, control his or her blood glucose level and help him or her reach and maintain an appropriate weight. Obesity increases the body's need for insulin to compensate for the extra glucose consumed with a higher food intake. So even a moderate weight loss (for example 4.5 to 9 kg) can lower blood glucose levels and counter insulin resistance. For more details on dietary approaches, see 'Nutrition support for Diabetes,' page 331.

Exercise

In type 1 diabetes, exercise doesn't improve glycaemic control. However, it yields cardiovascular and other important benefits.

In patients with type 2 diabetes, exercise helps control blood glucose levels. The muscles use more glucose during vigorous physical activity. Exercise improves glucose tolerance and makes body cells more sensitive to insulin, allowing them to use available insulin stores more efficiently. Also, exercise helps the patient reach and maintain a healthy weight and can delay or even help prevent cardiovascular disease—the leading cause of death among diabetic patients.

Advise the patient to warm up before exercise and cool down afterwards. Instruct him or her to exercise 5 days/week for optimal glycaemic control. Stress that even a short period of physical activity—30 minutes at a time—provides benefits.

Exercise-induced hypoglycaemia

If your patient takes insulin or oral antidiabetics, caution him or her about the possibility of exercise-induced hypoglycaemia. During exercise, blood insulin levels can rise from increased insulin sensitivity and glucose levels reduce due to increased utilisation.

Exercise tips for patients with diabetes

Exercise frequency and intensity should be tailored to the patient's needs. The lists below are exercise tips for type 1 and type 2 diabetes.

Type 1 tips

- Exercise decreases blood glucose levels, which can lead to hypoglycaemia. Eat a light carbohydrate snack about 30 minutes before exercising and carry fast-acting carbohydrates or glucose tablets to take in case hypoglycaemia occurs.
- Consume an additional 10 to 15 g of carbohydrates for each hour of moderate exercise and an extra 20 to 30 g for each hour of vigorous exercise.
- Time exercise sessions so they don't coincide with peak insulin effects.
- Exercise within 2 hours of eating to help prevent hypoglycaemia.
- Check the blood glucose level before and after exercise. With poorly controlled type 1 diabetes, exercise may actually worsen hyperglycaemia. Avoid exercise if the fasting glucose level exceeds 16.65 mmol/L (or 13.88 mmol/L when ketosis is present).

Type 2 tips

- Exercise for 20 to 45 minutes at least three times per week.
- If taking an oral antidiabetic or insulin, exercise within 2 hours of eating.
- Stop exercising if hypoglycaemia signs or symptoms occur.

For planned exercise, the patient may need to decrease the insulin dosage. Moderate exercise increases the muscles' glucose uptake by 2 to 3 mg/kg of body weight per minute above resting levels. Higher-intensity activity can raise glucose uptake by as much as 6 mg/kg of body weight per minute. (See *Exercise tips for patients with diabetes*.)

Exercise agonies

If your patient has diabetic retinopathy, tell him or her that strenuous exercise may lead to retinal haemorrhage or detachment. If the patient has neuropathy, advise him or her that exercise may cause foot injury.

Self-monitoring

Because blood glucose changes may cause misleading signs and symptoms—or none at all—a patient with diabetes must monitor their blood glucose levels closely to determine if they needs to adjust their medication, diet or exercise. Self-monitoring allows the patient to determine metabolic status quickly. It's especially useful for those on a tight-control regimen.

Custom-made monitoring

Test method, timing and frequency are tailored to a patient's needs. Generally, blood should be tested before meals and at bedtime. More frequent monitoring may be necessary:

- during stress, illness or surgery
- during pregnancy
- after a change in the medication dosage, meal plan or activity level
- when a patient starts a new medication.

Advise a patient to record blood glucose values in a log, noting any changes in diet, medication or activity level as well as stress, illness or insulin reactions. Emphasise that a blood glucose level should be less than 9 mmol/L. If a patient's level is higher, instruct them to check their urine for ketones and to call the diabetic clinic or general practitioner for further instructions.

Monitoring long-term glucose control

The consultant or general practitioner may request an HbA_{1c} test every 12 weeks to determine long-term blood glucose control. Test results reveal average blood glucose levels over a 3-month period. After a patient has achieved treatment goals, testing may be done twice per year.

Ur-ine for something

Although urine glucose testing is used less commonly than in the past, it can detect ketone bodies—particularly important for the ketosis-prone patient.

Also, diabetic patients should have their urine tested for albumin every year to screen for kidney disease. If albumin is detected, the dietary protein allowance may need to be decreased. Although research isn't conclusive on how much protein is optimal for these patients, some experts recommend 0.6 to 0.8 g/kg of body weight.

Treatment of acute complications

Meticulous control of blood glucose levels is crucial in preventing both acute and chronic diabetes complications. Make sure your patient knows what to do in case an acute complication occurs.

Treating hypoglycaemia

If the blood glucose level drops below 1.11 mmol/L, brain damage can occur if glucose isn't administered within minutes. If the blood glucose level is less than 4.44 mmol/L, scheduled insulin shouldn't be given until the level rises from carbohydrate consumption.

If the patient is unconscious, a glucagon injection raises the blood glucose level rapidly. Once conscious, and levels have improved, give oral carbohydrate when safe and continue to closely observe for relapse.

If the patient is conscious, advise them to take any available glucose/sucrose substance that can be swallowed.

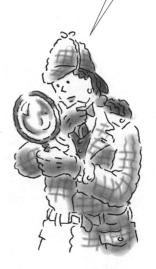

Diabetic patients must stay focused on blood glucose levels in case medication, diet or exercise adjustments are needed.

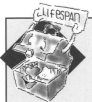

Lifespan lunchbox

Hypoglycaemia in young children

Many children under age 7 experience hypoglycaemic unawareness due to immature counter-regulatory mechanisms (hormonal and neural responses). These young children don't have the cognitive ability to identify the symptoms of hypoglycaemia or take action to treat symptoms. As a result, they're at great risk for hypoglycaemia and its complications.

When choosing target blood glucose goals in this age group, the risk of hypoglycaemia must be taken into account. NICE (2004) recommend that for the children with type 1 diabetes the blood glucose should be:

- before meals: 4 to 8 mmol/L
- 2 hours after meals: less than 10 mmol/L.

Alternatives include:
- placing honey on the tongue
- squeezing cake-decorating icing between the gum and the cheek
- drinking 150 ml regular Coca-Cola
- giving 6 jelly beans, or 10 gumdrops. (See *Hypoglycaemia in young children*.)

Rule of 15, really?

Many clinicians recommend that diabetic patients use the Rule of 15 to treat hypoglycaemia. (See *Rule of 15*, page 330.)

Instruct a diabetic patient to carry fast-acting carbohydrates (such as glucose sweets or fruit pastilles) at all times. Make sure others in the patient's household know how to treat hypoglycaemia because a patient who becomes unconscious or confused needs help administering treatment.

Treating DKA and HHNS

Emergency treatment for DKA or HHNS may include insulin and I.V. fluid administration, along with correction of electrolyte imbalances.

Preventing long-term complications

Preventing long-term diabetic complications requires stringent glycaemic monitoring and control, along with measures to prevent specific complications. If the patient smokes, urge him or her to stop.

Don't get disheartened

Because diabetes mellitus increases the risk of heart disease, the patient should eat a heart-healthy diet (see Chapter 13), control

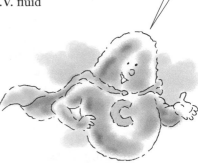

Advise your patient with diabetes to carry me around in a chocolate bar. I act fast and taste sweet!

Rule of 15

To treat hypoglycaemia, teach your patient the Rule of 15:

- If the blood glucose level is below 3.89 mmol/L, eat 15 g of an easily absorbable carbohydrate. If the level is below 2.78 mmol/L, ingest 30 g of carbohydrate instead of 15 g.
- Wait 15 minutes and then recheck the blood glucose level.
- If the level hasn't risen, repeat the process of eating 15 g (or 30 g) of carbohydrate and rechecking the level after 15 minutes, until the blood glucose level registers above 4.4 mmol/L.
- Then eat a meal containing carbohydrate, protein and fat.

Sugar therapy

Examples of 15 g of easily absorbable carbohydrates include:

- three glucose tablets
- six or seven hard sweets
- 1 tbsp sugar
- 2 tbsp raisins
- 177 ml of a nondiet soft drink
- 118 ml of fruit juice.

Low-fat and no-fat carbohydrate foods work faster because they're broken down more easily.

blood pressure and cholesterol levels, maintain a normal weight and exercise regularly.

Visualise yearly eye exams

To safeguard vision, advise the patient to get annual eye examinations to detect retinopathy-related damage before symptoms appear. Taking measures to control blood glucose and blood pressure levels can decrease the risk and progression of diabetic retinopathy.

Dental do's

To minimise dental complications, such as gum disease and abscesses, instruct the patient to have regular dental check-ups and follow good home care. Tell them to brush their teeth after every meal, floss daily and report bleeding, pain or soreness in the gums and teeth immediately.

Keeping a clean bill of health for the kidneys

To help prevent kidney disease, advise the patient to keep blood pressure and blood glucose levels under control and get prompt treatment for urinary tract infections.

Saving skin

Because skin breaks increase the infection risk, tell the patient to check his or her skin daily for cuts and irritated areas. Tell him or her to bathe daily with warm water and a mild soap and to apply a lanolin-based lotion afterwards to prevent dryness. Advise the patient to pat the skin dry thoroughly, especially between the toes and in skinfolds. Instruct him or her to wear cotton underwear to let moisture evaporate and help prevent skin breakdown.

Solid footing

Proper foot care can improve blood circulation to the feet, helping to prevent gangrene and infection. Tell the patient to avoid foot injury and temperature extremes. Instruct them to wash their feet daily with warm water and mild soap and to dry them thoroughly. Advise them to trim toenails to match the shape of the toes—but not too short. Instruct the patient to wear only soft, clean and absorbent socks of a natural fabric or stockings and avoid tight-fitting shoes.

Emphasise the need to examine their feet daily for cuts, scrapes, cracks, bruises, corns, calluses, swelling and redness—and to call the practitioner if these appear.

Other treatments

The consultant may recommend pancreas transplantation for certain patients with type 1 diabetes. This procedure may eliminate the need for exogenous insulin, frequent daily blood glucose level measurement and certain dietary restrictions. It also may prevent episodes of acute hypoglycaemia and hyperglycaemia. However, pancreas transplantation is only partially successful in reversing long-term neurologic and renal complications.

Experimental explorations

Experimental approaches to treating or curing diabetes include:
- islet cell transplantation
- artificial pancreas implantation
- genetic manipulation (transplanting a fat or muscle cell with a human insulin gene into a patient with type 1 diabetes).

Nutrition support for diabetes

The cornerstone of diabetes treatment, a proper diet is essential for effective control of the blood glucose level. A patient must carefully regulate consumption of carbohydrates, fats and proteins through a personal meal plan based on food preferences, health concerns and drug therapy. If he or she's overweight, weight reduction is a primary goal. To assess the effectiveness of nutrition support, blood glucose levels, lipid levels and weight must be monitored regularly.

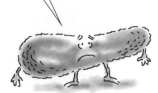

Pancreas transplantation is only partially successful in reversing long-term neurologic and renal complications.

Dear diary

Whether your patient has type 1 or type 2 diabetes, encourage him or her to keep a food diary (including specific foods and portions eaten) to determine whether and where he or she needs to make dietary changes. Keeping a food record can yield a wealth of information about the patient's intake.

Nutrition in type 1 diabetes

People with diabetes should try to maintain a healthy weight and eat a diet that is:
- low in fat (particularly saturated fat)
- low in sugar
- low in salt
- high in fruit and vegetables (at least five portions a day)
- high in starchy carbohydrate foods, such as bread, chapatti, rice, pasta and yams (these should form the base of meals)—choose wholegrain varieties when possible.

There are no foods that people with diabetes should never eat. And there is no need to cut out all sugar. But, like everyone, people with diabetes should try to eat only small amounts of foods that are high in sugar or fat or both. If you have diabetes you can eat cakes and biscuits sparingly, as part of a balanced diet.

Fruit juice is high in fructose (fruit sugar), so it can cause blood sugar levels to rise quickly. Because of this, it's best for people with diabetes to drink juice with a meal and avoid having more than one small glass a day.

If you are prone to low blood sugar (hypoglycaemia), you might sometimes need to increase your blood sugar level quickly. If you suffer from a hypoglycaemic episode, you should have some fast-acting carbohydrate, such as a sugary drink or some glucose tablets, and follow this up with a starchy snack, such as a sandwich.

Guidelines galore

Also provide the following nutritional guidelines:
- Limit total fat to reduce the risk of heart disease.
- Don't be afraid of sugar—but use it cautiously. It is no longer taboo for diabetic patients. Sugar can be substituted by other carbohydrates as long as the overall diet is healthy.
- Restrict salt intake to 2 to 4 g/day to help control blood pressure and maintain cardiovascular health.
- Eat a variety of lean protein foods, such as lean meat, fish, poultry, tofu, egg whites and low-fat dairy products. (See *Dealing out protein*).
- Limit starches—especially quickly absorbable starches, such as those in potatoes and white and processed flours. Get most starches from beans and whole unprocessed grains. Replace some starch with low-fat protein and monounsaturated fats.

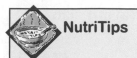

NutriTips

Dealing out protein

To help your patient track the amount of protein they're getting, inform them that one meat serving (85 g) is about the size of a deck of playing cards. Likewise, they can track cheese intake by thinking of one cheese serving as one individually wrapped slice or one cube about the size of a dice.

Recommend a variety of lean protein foods, such as lean meat, poultry, tofu, egg whites and, well, (gulp!) me.

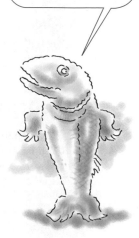

- Eat 20 to 35 g of fibre daily to help prevent constipation and reduce cholesterol levels.
- Consume plenty of fresh vegetables and fruits—but not fruit juices, which are high in sugar.
- Restrict alcohol to two drinks per day, and only if the blood glucose level is well controlled. To avoid hypoglycaemia, always ingest food along with alcohol. Also, don't reduce food intake to compensate for alcohol calories. (A patient who is pregnant or has a history of alcohol abuse should abstain from alcohol completely.)
- Coordinate meal timing with the insulin schedule and insulin type.

For example if the patient is taking a fast-acting insulin (such as Lispro) to provide coverage before meals, he or she should eat within 15 minutes of the injection to avoid hypoglycaemia.

Nutrition in type 2 diabetes

For a patient with type 2 diabetes, the goal of nutrition support is to maintain a balanced diet while achieving or maintaining a reasonable weight and normal levels of blood glucose and cholesterol.

If the patient is overweight, the diet should promote weight loss. Research shows that even a minimal weight loss—4.5 or 7 kg—can improve glycaemic control. Typically, the practitioner recommends therapeutic lifestyle changes, including:

- moderate calorie restriction (for example 600 fewer average daily intake)
- reduction in total fat intake, especially saturated fat
- increased physical activity.

Rules to eat by

Provide the following nutritional guidelines for a patient with type 2 diabetes:
- Get about 50% of total daily calories from complex carbohydrates, including grains, wholegrain bread, beans and other legumes, and vegetables and fruits (but not fruit juices).
- Allow roughly 12% to 20% of daily calories to come from protein (less if kidney disease is present).
- Eat a variety of lean protein foods, such as lean meat, fish, poultry, tofu, egg whites and low-fat dairy products.
- Limit total fat intake to less than 30% of daily calories, with less than 10% of calories coming from saturated fats.
- Cut back on concentrated simple sugars, such as sucrose, honey, fruit juices or corn syrup. (See *Softening the blow of soft drinks*.)
- Be stingy with starches. Get most starch from beans and whole unprocessed grains (rather than potatoes or white or processed flours). Replace some starch with low-fat protein and monounsaturated fats.
- Substitute any alcohol intake for fat calories, with one alcoholic beverage replacing two fat exchanges. (However, alcohol should be avoided if the patient is trying to lose weight, has a high triglyceride level, is pregnant or has a history of alcohol abuse.)

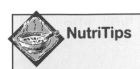 **NutriTips**

Softening the blow of soft drinks

A good way for a diabetic patient to cut back on calories is to cut down on nondiet soft drinks. On average, a 355-ml can of nondiet soft drink provides about 150 cal. So drinking just a few cans per day adds hundreds of extra calories.

Encourage your patient to turn to low-calorie or no-calorie alternatives, such as diet soft drinks, sugar-free squash and water.

Think small and think often

Proper meal timing can help prevent extreme blood glucose levels. Many type 2 diabetics achieve good glycaemic control by eating smaller food portions more often—five to six small meals daily instead of three larger ones—or small meals combined with high-protein or complex carbohydrate snacks throughout the day. This practice offers several advantages:
- The body processes smaller amounts of glucose more easily than larger amounts.
- Eating before hunger sets in usually leads to better food choices than eating in a ravenous rush.

Type 2 diabetic patients who take insulin should coordinate meals with the type and timing of insulin administration. Patients on oral antidiabetics should avoid skipping meals but don't need the tight schedule required by those on insulin. For better results, though, these patients should adhere to a consistent pattern, eating meals of approximately the same composition at about the same time each day.

Meal planning

Options for helping a patient plan better meals include exchange lists, carbohydrate counting and the menu approach. (See *Sample menu for a diabetic patient*.) The patient should work with a dietitian and a health care provider to determine which type of meal planning best fits his or her condition and preferences.

Glycaemic index

The glycaemic index (GI) is a ranking of foods based on their overall effect on blood glucose levels. Slowly absorbed foods have a low GI rating, whilst foods that are more quickly absorbed will have a higher rating. This is important because choosing slowly absorbed carbohydrates can help even out blood glucose levels when you have diabetes.

What's your GI number...

Foods are given a GI number according to their effect on blood glucose levels. Glucose or white bread is used as the standard reference (GI 100), and other foods are measured against this. The effect on blood glucose levels of a portion of the test food containing 50 g of carbohydrate is compared with the effect of the reference food (white bread or glucose) over a 3-hour period.

Because meals including low-GI foods allow the body to absorb carbohydrate more slowly, they help to maintain even blood glucose levels between meals and can therefore help avoid 'hypos'. The effect of a low-GI meal can run into the following meal, which helps keep blood glucose more even during the whole day.

Menu maven

Sample menu for a diabetic patient

Combining foods with different GIs alters the overall GI of a meal. Your patient can maximise the benefit of GI by including a low-GI food with each meal or snack, to lower the overall effect on the blood glucose levels. There are, of course, multiple combinations of foods that the patient could pick, but a few suggestions are given below.

Breakfast

- Use an oat-based breakfast cereal and eat some fruit
- Try Muesli, All-Bran, Sultana Bran and Special K.

Snacks

Get into the habit of eating

- fruit as a snack (as well as part of a main meal)
- yoghurt (choose low-fat varieties)
- popcorn
- smaller portions of lower GI foods like chocolate and nuts, which have a high fat content, especially if you are trying to lose weight.
- a slice of Rye bread or fruit loaf (again, watch the amounts, especially if you are trying to lose weight)

Lunch

- Add baked beans to your jacket potato.
- Try a lentil-based soup.
- Add variety with different breads, e.g. pitta bread, pumpernickel and bread made with a substantial amount of mixed grains.
- Try grilled chicken, salad, rice and peas.

Evening meal

- Try basmati rice, sweet potato, buckwheat, bulgar wheat, pearl barley and noodles with your meal.
- Include more vegetables with your meal.
- Eat more pasta-based meals.
- Include more beans and pulses (dal).

Slow-acting carbohydrates will also reduce the peaks in blood glucose that often follow a meal, and this may have a role in helping to prevent or reduce the risk of getting type 2 diabetes in those at risk. There are also benefits for weight loss. Low-GI foods can help you control your appetite by making you feel fuller for longer, with the result that you eat less. Research has shown that people who have an overall low-GI diet have a lower incidence of heart disease.

Lower GI diets have also been associated with improved levels of 'good' cholesterol. One or two small changes can make all the difference. (See *Understanding the GI of some common foods*, page 336.)

Carbohydrate counting

Carbohydrate counting emphasizes eating a consistent amount of carbohydrates rather than restricting the *type* of carbohydrate. It lets the patient swap an occasional high-sugar food for other carbohydrate-containing foods. The system is based on two concepts:
- The amount of carbohydrate consumed determines the blood glucose level after a meal or snack. (Carbohydrate is the main nutrient affecting blood

Carbohydrate counting emphasises the amount of carb intake rather than the type of carbs.

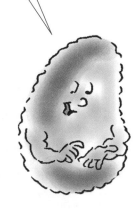

Understanding the GI of some common foods

Low GI	Medium GI	High GI
Apples, oranges, pears and peaches	Honey	Glucose
Beans and lentils	Jam	White and wholemeal bread
Pasta (all types made from durum wheat)	Shredded wheat	
	Weetabix	Brown rice, cooked
Sweet potato, peeled and boiled	Ice cream	White rice, cooked
Sweetcorn	New potatoes, peeled and boiled	Cornflakes
Porridge		Baked potato
Custard	White basmati rice, cooked	Mashed potato
Noodles	Pitta bread	
All-Bran, Special K and Sultana Bran	Couscous	

sugar. Within an hour or two of consumption, most carbohydrate changes to blood glucose.)
• Eating equal amounts of sugar or starch raises the blood glucose level by roughly the same amount.

It's all in the label

Carbohydrate information on food labels has simplified carbohydrate counting. The system is easier to learn than the exchange lists system, gives the patient more flexible food choices and provides a better estimate of how much the blood glucose level will rise after a meal or snack. Also, if the patient takes insulin, carbohydrate counting can be helpful in determining insulin dosages. (See *Carb counting for kids*.)

If your patient counts carbohydrates, emphasise the importance of keeping accurate food logs and recording blood glucose levels before and after eating.

Menu approach

In the menu approach, the patient and dietitian collaborate to develop menus tailored to the patient's needs and preferences. As the patient desires, menus may be relatively flexible or more rigid, dictating specific foods and the amounts that the patient must eat at specific times.

The menu approach is best for patients who have fairly regimented eating habits or who want to be told exactly what and how much to eat. It isn't ideal for those who want or need flexibility.

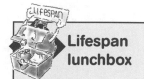

Lifespan lunchbox

Carb counting for kids

Carbohydrate counting can be particularly effective in helping children stick to their recommended diet while meeting caloric needs. In addition to allowing more flexibility in food choices, this meal-planning approach provides extra calories in the form of fat and protein—which most active, growing children need.

Adjusting diet to exercise, illness and stress

Patients with diabetes may need to adjust their diet for exercise, illness and stress.

Exercise adjustments

Instruct the patient to check blood glucose levels before, during and after exercise. If the pre-exercise level exceeds 4.4 mmol/L, he or she should base dietary adjustments on the anticipated duration and intensity of exercise:
- For short-duration, low-intensity exercise, no extra carbohydrate is needed.
- For longer-lasting, higher-intensity exercise, he or she should consume an additional 15 to 30 g of carbohydrate for every 30 to 60 minutes of exercise.

Illness adjustments

Illnesses as minor as a cold may cause hyperglycaemia. During illness, glucagon and adrenalin secretion increases, contributing to higher blood glucose levels. As a result, intracellular glucose, fluid and electrolytes may be lost, leading to dehydration, electrolyte imbalance and nutrient loss. To prevent these problems, the patient needs to adjust food intake.

Review these sick-day guidelines with the patient:
- Maintain adequate food intake. Don't skip meals.
- As a general rule, consume 15 g of carbohydrate every 1 to 2 hours. If you can't tolerate solid food, drink liquids containing carbohydrates (such as nondiet cola, milk, fruit juice or tomato juice). (See *Serving up an adequate diet to an ill diabetic patient*, page 338.)
- Keep taking insulin, if prescribed, but adjust the dosage as needed.
- Increase fluid intake if vomiting, diarrhoea or fever occurs.
- During periods of illness, even if you are not eating, insulin is still needed, and it is important never to stop taking your insulin. You should do more frequent blood glucose testing. Diabetes UK recommends that you test at least four times a day during periods of illness. Ask your care team for help if you are worried.
- Call the practitioner if the illness lasts more than 2 days.

Stress adjustments

As with illness, the hormonal changes that occur in response to pronounced stress can affect glycaemic control. Recommend that the patient learn effective stress-management techniques, especially if he or she takes insulin.

Adjusting to eating out

If the patient eats out often, make sure they understand their meal-planning system. Advise them to choose restaurants with an appropriate food selection. Instruct them to plan ahead so that they can adjust their food intake before and after a meal out according to their overall dietary allowances.

Also provide the following guidelines:
- Eat only small portions, even if the restaurant serves large ones.

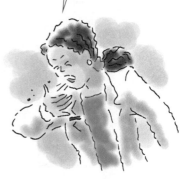

Achoo! Illnesses as minor as a cold may cause hyperglycaemia in patients with diabetes.

Order roasted, baked or grilled meat, fish or poultry instead of fried, sautéed or breaded entrées.

NutriTips

Serving up an adequate diet to an ill diabetic patient

When illness strikes, the appetite may go AWOL. For a diabetic patient, though, skipping meals can be especially dangerous. To help your diabetic patient consume adequate carbohydrates during illness, urge them to substitute liquids for solid foods if their appetite is poor. Advise them to choose among the high-carbohydrate foods listed below.

Food	Serving (ml)	Carbohydrate (g)
Milk	250	12
Apple juice	125	15
Grape juice	125	15
Orange juice	125	15
Pineapple juice	125	15
Prune juice	80	15
Tomato juice	125	5
Nondiet cola	125	13
Nondiet ginger ale	194	16

• Use oil and vinegar (or fresh lemon juice) instead of regular salad dressing, or ask for dressing on the side.
• Order roasted, baked or grilled meat, fish or poultry instead of fried, sautéed or breaded entrées.
• Avoid sweetened juices, fried vegetables, creamed or thick soups, stews and casseroles.
• Order potatoes, rice and noodles plain, steamed, baked or boiled—not fried.
• Choose fresh fruit rather than pastry for dessert.

Making travel adjustments

Advise the patient to talk to the dietitian when planning a trip. Instruct them to find out which foods will be available at their destination and on the way there. If they plan to fly, they can order a diabetic diet from the airline.

Here are some other travel guidelines to relay:
• Always carry appropriate snacks and quick-acting carbohydrates.
• Plan for any time-zone changes.
• Wear medical identification jewellery.

- If you take medication, have the general practitioner write a letter covering the prescription and insulin syringes.
- Make sure travel companions know signs, symptoms and treatment for hypoglycaemia and other acute diabetes complications.

Other forms of diabetes

Besides type 1 and type 2 diabetes, the two other major categories of diabetes mellitus are:
- gestational diabetes (diabetes during pregnancy)
- other specific types of diabetes—a group of disorders marked by altered glucose metabolism.

Gestational diabetes

Approximately 650,000 women give birth in England and Wales each year, and 2% to 5% of pregnancies involve women with diabetes. Approximately 87.5% of pregnancies complicated by diabetes are estimated to be due to gestational diabetes (which may or may not resolve after pregnancy), with 7.5% being due to type 1 diabetes and the remaining 5% being due to type 2 diabetes.

Gestational diabetes may lead to congenital malformations, increased birth weight and a higher risk of prenatal mortality. Strict metabolic control may reduce these risks.

Gestational diabetes is more common in women of African, Black Caribbean, South Asian, Middle Eastern and Chinese family origin. Obesity also increases the risk.

Managing gestational diabetes

Women- and baby-centred care for a patient with gestational diabetes promotes a healthy pregnancy and delivery for mother and child. Initially, the disorder is managed by diet and then, if necessary, by insulin therapy. About 6 weeks after delivery, the patient should be re-evaluated for diabetes.

Other specific types of diabetes

Other specific types of diabetes account for 1% to 5% of diagnosed diabetes cases. They include eight specific causes of altered glucose metabolism:
- genetic defects of beta cells
- genetic defects in insulin action
- certain pancreatic diseases (such as pancreatitis and cystic fibrosis) or pancreas injury or removal
- certain endocrine diseases, such as Cushing's syndrome, hyperthyroidism and polycystic ovary syndrome
- infections, such as measles in a foetus or newborn (congenital rubella) and cytomegalovirus

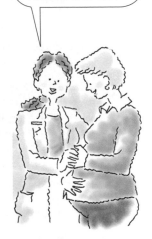

Medical care for gestational diabetes promotes a healthy pregnancy and delivery for mother and child.

- certain rare immune disorders
- other genetic syndromes, such as Down's syndrome, Klinefelter's syndrome and Huntington's disease
- drug- or chemical-induced injury to the pancreas (drugs that can cause diabetes include glucocorticoids, thyroid hormone, diazoxide, beta-adrenergic agonists, thiazides and phenytoin).

Managing other specific types of diabetes

Depending on the body's ability to produce insulin and the degree to which insulin resistance plays a role in altered metabolism, some patients may require exogenous insulin.

Quick quiz

1. What's a long-term complication of diabetes?
   A. Retinal detachment
   B. Skeletal deformities
   C. Heart disease
   D. Deafness

Answer: C. Heart disease is a long-term complication of diabetes.

2. Diabetes meal planning should include:
   A. a minimal amount of carbohydrates
   B. no meat
   C. salty snacks for fluid volume management
   D. a balance of carbohydrates, proteins and fats

Answer: D. The patient with diabetes must carefully regulate consumption of carbohydrates, fats and proteins.

3. A good way for a patient with type 2 diabetes to reduce calories is to:
   A. cut out all carbohydrates
   B. eliminate high-carbohydrate beverages, such as regular soft drinks and juices
   C. eat only vegetarian meals
   D. eat only one meal per day

Answer: B. Because 355 ml of regular soft drink or juice provides approximately 150 cal, eliminating these beverages from the diet is a good way to reduce caloric intake.

Scoring

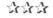 If you answered all three questions correctly, awesome! You're hyperintelligent when it comes to hyperglycaemia.

If you answered two questions correctly, keep up the good work! There's no doubting your diabetic knowledge.

If you answered fewer than two questions correctly, it seems your information level is low! Grab a biscuit and a glass of orange juice, and dig in for a chapter review.

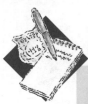

17 Human immunodeficiency virus

Just the facts

Human immunodeficiency virus (HIV) disease significantly alters the patient's nutritional status. In this chapter, you'll learn:

♦ the pathophysiology and signs and symptoms of HIV disease

♦ treatments and nutritional therapy for HIV disease

♦ alternative treatment options.

Understanding HIV disease

HIV can affect anybody, but in the UK most people with HIV come from several groups:
*   men who have sex with men
*   people of sub-Saharan African origin.

There are 73,000 people who are estimated to be living with HIV in the UK, including one-third who are unaware of their diagnosis. An estimated 43% of those living with HIV are men who have sex with men, and 35% are people born in sub-Saharan Africa. Although gay men are the group most affected by HIV in the UK, since 2003 more of the people newly diagnosed with HIV in the UK became infected through heterosexual sex than through gay sex.

Immune impairer

HIV disease, characterised by progressive immune system impairment, destroys T cells and, therefore, the cell-mediated immune response. This immunodeficiency makes the patient more susceptible to infections and unusual cancers. (See *Facts about AIDS*, page 342.)

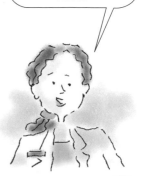

Most experts believe that everyone infected with HIV will develop AIDS.

The CDC has established criteria for making a diagnosis of HIV disease. The course of HIV disease can vary, but it usually results in death from opportunistic infections. Most experts believe that virtually everyone infected with HIV eventually develops AIDS. (See *Classifying HIV infection*.)

Pathophysiology

HIV is a ribonucleic acid–based retrovirus that requires a human host to replicate. The average time between HIV infection and development of AIDS is 8 to 10 years.

Classifying HIV infection

In the UK, classification of HIV is based primarily on presenting symptoms (WHO, 2007) and to a lesser extent on the Centres for Disease Control and Prevention (CDC)'s (America) revised 1993 guidelines for human immunodeficiency virus (HIV)-infected adolescents and adults.

WHO clinical staging

Clinical stage 1
- asymptomatic
- persistent generalised lymphadenopathy

Clinical stage 2
- moderate unexplained weight loss (<10% of presumed or measured body weight)
- recurrent respiratory tract infections such as sinusitis, tonsillitis, otitis media and pharyngitis)
- herpes zoster
- angular cheilitis
- recurrent oral ulceration
- papular pruritic eruptions
- seborrhoeic dermatitis
- fungal nail infections

Clinical stage 3
- unexplained severe weight loss (>10% of presumed or measured body weight)
- unexplained chronic diarrhoea for longer than 1 month
- unexplained persistent fever (above 37.6°C intermittent or constant, for longer than 1 month)
- persistent oral candidiasis
- oral hairy leukoplakia
- pulmonary tuberculosis (current)
- severe bacterial infections (such as pneumonia, empyema, pyomyositis, bone or joint infection, meningitis or bacteraemia)
- acute necrotising ulcerative stomatitis, gingivitis or periodontitis
- unexplained anaemia (<8 g/dl), neutropaenia (<0.5 × 109 per L) or chronic thrombocytopaenia (<50 × 109 per L)

Facts about AIDS

HIV is the fastest growing serious health condition in the UK. These are some of the statistics:

- Around 97,400 cases of HIV have been reported since the early 1980s.
- Over 18,000 people with HIV have died since the early 1980s.
- There were 7,734 new diagnoses in 2007.
- In 2007, it was estimated that 28% of people living with HIV did not know about their infection.
- Thirty-one per cent of people diagnosed with HIV in 2007 were diagnosed late.

Classifying HIV infection (continued)

Clinical stage 4

- HIV wasting syndrome
- pneumocystis pneumonia
- recurrent severe bacterial pneumonia
- chronic herpes simplex infection (orolabial, genital or anorectal of more than 1 month's duration or visceral at any site)
- oesophageal candidiasis (or candidiasis of trachea, bronchi or lungs)
- extrapulmonary tuberculosis
- Kaposi's sarcoma
- cytomegalovirus infection (retinitis or infection of other organs)
- central nervous system toxoplasmosis
- HIV encephalopathy
- extrapulmonary cryptococcosis including meningitis
- disseminated non-tuberculous mycobacterial infection
- progressive multifocal leucoencephalopathy
- chronic cryptosporidiosis (with diarrhoea)
- chronic isosporiasis
- disseminated mycosis (coccidioidomycosis or histoplasmosis)
- recurrent non-typhoidal *Salmonella bacteraemia*
- lymphoma (cerebral or B-cell non-Hodgkin) or other solid HIV-associated tumours
- invasive cervical carcinoma
- atypical disseminated leishmaniasis
- symptomatic HIV-associated nephropathy or symptomatic HIV-associated cardiomyopathy
- The CDC classification system identifies where the patient lies in the progression of the disease and helps guide treatment.

Ranges of CD4$^+$ T-lymphocytes

- category 1: CD4$^+$ cell count greater than or equal to 500 cells/mm^3
- category 2: CD4$^+$ cell count of 200 to 499 cells/mm^3
- category 3: CD4$^+$ cell count less than 200 cells/mm^3.

World Health Organization. *WHO Case Definitions of HIV for Surveillance and Revised Clinical Staging and Immunological Classification of HIV-Related Disease in Adults and Children.* 2007. Available at: www.who.int/hiv/pub/guidelines/HIVstaging150307.pdf. Accessed 28 May 2010.

Centers for Disease Control and Prevention. 1993 Revised classification system for HIV infection and expanded surveillance case definition for AIDS among adolescents and adults. *MMWR Recommendations and Reports.* 1992, December 18;41 (RR-17):1–19. Available at: www.cdc.gov/mmwr/preview/mmwrhtml/00018871.htm. Accessed 28 May 2010.

HIV destroys CD4$^+$ cells—also known as *helper T cells*—that regulate the normal immune response. The CD4$^+$ antigen (cell surface marker) serves as a receptor for HIV and allows it to invade the cell. Afterwards, the virus replicates within the CD4$^+$ cell, causing cell death.

HIV can infect almost any cell that has the CD4$^+$ antigen on its surface, including monocytes, macrophages, bone marrow progenitors, and glial, gut and epithelial cells. The infection can cause dementia, wasting syndrome and blood abnormalities.

Modes of transmission

HIV is transmitted in three ways:

through contact with infected blood or blood products during transfusion or transplantation (although routine testing of the blood supply since 1985 has greatly diminished the risk of contracting HIV this way) or by sharing a contaminated needle

through contact with infected body fluids, such as semen and vaginal fluids, during unprotected sex (especially anal intercourse, because it causes mucosal trauma)

across the placenta from an infected mother to a foetus or from an infected mother to an infant either through cervical or blood contact during delivery or through breast milk.

Although blood, semen, vaginal secretions and breast milk are the body fluids that most readily transmit HIV, it has also been found in saliva, urine, tears and faeces. However, there's no evidence of transmission through these fluids.

What to look for

After initial exposure, the infected person may have no signs or symptoms, or he or she may have a flu-like illness (primary infection) and then remain asymptomatic for years. As the syndrome progresses, the patient may have neurologic symptoms from HIV encephalopathy or symptoms of an opportunistic infection, such as *Pneumocystis carinii* pneumonia, cytomegalovirus or cancer. Eventually, repeated opportunistic infections overwhelm the patient's weakened immune defences, invading every body system. (See *HIV in children*.)

Treatment

Although HIV disease has no cure, several types of drugs are used to prolong life.

Teamwork works

Highly active antiretroviral therapy (HAART) reduces the number of HIV particles in the blood, increasing T-cell counts and improving the immunologic function. HAART protocols combine three or more antiretroviral drugs to produce the maximum benefit with the fewest adverse

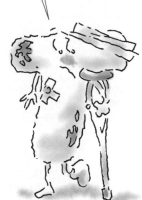

I regulate the normal immune response. When HIV invades me, it gets ugly fast.

reactions. Combination therapy also helps to inhibit the production of mutant HIV strains resistant to particular drugs. Antiretroviral drugs fall into several categories:

• nucleoside reverse transcriptase inhibitors, such as abacavir (Ziagen), didanosine (Videx), emtricitabine (Emtriva), lamivudine (Epivir), stavudine (Zerit), zalcitabine (Hivid) and zidovudine (Retrovir)
• non-nucleoside reverse transcriptase inhibitors, such as delavirdine (Rescriptor), efavirenz (Sustiva) and nevirapine (Viramune)
• nucleotide analogue reverse transcriptase inhibitor, which includes tenofovir (Viread)
• protease inhibitors, such as amprenavir (Agenerase), atazanavir (Reyataz), fosamprenavir (Lexiva), indinavir (Crixivan), lopinavir (Kaletra), nelfinavir (Viracept), ritonavir (Norvir) and saquinavir (Fortovase)
• fusion inhibitors, such as enfuvirtide (Fuzeon).

The selection of an effective combination is a complex process. However, the use of combination therapy has reduced HIV in the blood of infected adults by 98%.

Anti-infective drugs, such as dapsone and rifabutin (Mycobutin), are used to prevent or combat opportunistic infections. Although many opportunistic infections respond to anti-infective drugs, infections tend to recur after treatment ends. Therefore, the patient usually requires lifelong prophylaxis.

Add-ons

Additional treatment may include:
• antineoplastic drugs, such as methotrexate (Trexall), to combat associated cancers
• immunomodulatory agents, such as interferon beta, to boost the immune system weakened by HIV disease and retroviral therapy
• human granulocyte colony-stimulating growth factor to stimulate neutrophil production (retroviral therapy causes anaemia, so patients may receive epoetin alfa)
• supportive therapy, including fluid and electrolyte replacement, pain relief and psychological support.

Nutritional assessment

HIV disease has an overwhelming effect on the patient's nutritional status. Early in the course of the disease, signs of malnutrition are subtle and often overlooked. The patient may be deficient in thiamine, riboflavin, vitamin B_6, vitamin B_{12}, folate, magnesium, zinc and selenium. He or she may also experience minor weight loss. As the disease progresses, symptoms of malnutrition, such as fatigue, depression, diarrhoea and peripheral neuropathy, may be present and may worsen HIV symptoms.

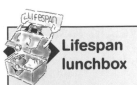

Lifespan lunchbox

HIV in children

In children, the incubation period of human immunodeficiency virus (HIV) averages only 17 months. Signs and symptoms resemble those for adults, except that children are more likely to have a history of bacterial infections, such as otitis media, lymphoid interstitial pneumonia and other types of pneumonia not caused by *Pneumocystis carinii*.

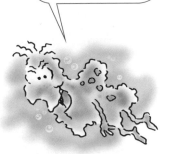

Combination drug therapy helps inhibit production of mutants like me!

Weight-loss woes

As HIV disease worsens, the combined effects of drug therapy, opportunistic infection, cancer and decreased nutritional intake cause profound weight loss. Some patients lose as much as 40% of their pre-HIV weight.

HIV wasting syndrome is diagnosed when involuntary weight loss reaches 10% or more of a patient's baseline body weight. This weight loss differs from weight loss due to dieting because there's a disproportionate loss of lean body mass compared with fat loss. (Lean body mass is defined as body mass minus stored fat and includes muscle, bone, connective tissue, body organs and water.) HIV wasting decreases the patient's quality of life by causing depression, apathy, decreased functional capacity and increased risk of opportunistic infection. If the patient's weight loss equals 40% of lean body mass, death typically ensues from factors such as malnutrition, reduced immune function and organ dysfunction.

Combo therapy: Not without problems

HAART therapy, combining three or more antiretroviral drugs, has greatly reduced the incidence of HIV wasting syndrome. However, some patients experience visceral fat accumulation, which results in hyperlipidaemia and insulin resistance, placing the patients at risk for diabetes mellitus and heart disease.

Multifaceted malnutrition

The cause of malnutrition in patients with HIV disease is multifaceted:
• Metabolic rate is increased by fever, infection, cancer and some medications, increasing nutrition and energy requirements.
• Malabsorption of nutrients may be caused by medications, low serum albumin levels, diarrhoea, cancer and infection.
• Oral intake is inadequate because of anxiety, depression, nausea, vomiting, impaired swallowing, impaired taste, fatigue, infection, shortness of breath and mouth ulcers.

Nutritional intervention is required to help prevent and reverse malnutrition in the patient with HIV disease.

Health history

The first step in assessing the patient's nutritional status is completing a detailed health history. During the interview, ask the patient about weight loss. Ask them to compare their current weight with their typical weight to evaluate their weight-loss pattern. Question the patient about other symptoms, such as nausea, anorexia, altered taste, diarrhoea, mouth pain, difficulty chewing or swallowing, and fatigue.

Ask the patient about allergies, smoking, eating patterns, alcohol or drug use, food choices and vitamin use. Ask about current medications (including over-the-counter medications and herbal preparations). Also ask the patient about his or her ability to prepare medications.

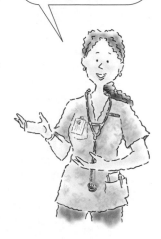

Combination drug therapy has reduced HIV in the blood of infected adults by 98%.

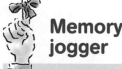

Memory jogger

To remember the four stages in assessing the nutritional status of a patient with HIV disease, think **H**unger **E**nds **A**fter **L**unch:

Health history

Examination

Anthropometric measurements

Laboratory studies.

A day in the life

Have the patient describe his or her typical day. This will give you important information about the patient's routine activity level and eating habits. Ask him or her to recount what and how much he or she ate yesterday, how the food was cooked and who cooked it. This information not only tells you about the patient's usual intake, but also gives clues about food preferences, eating patterns and even the patient's memory and mental status.

Ask the patient about his or her support system, which may include family, friends and volunteers. Assess whether he or she has help with shopping and meal preparation. Socialisation during meals may improve nutritional intake.

Physical examination

The second step in assessing the patient's nutritional status is performing the physical examination. In addition to observing the patient's body structure, do a head-to-toe assessment of his or her body systems.

Skin, hair and nails

When assessing the patient's skin, hair and nails, ask yourself these questions: is the patient's hair shiny and full? Is his or her skin free from blemishes and rashes? Is it warm and dry, with normal colour for that particular patient? Are his or her nails firm with pink beds? Does the skin tent when pinched?

Eyes, nose, throat and neck

Are the patient's eyes clear and shiny? Are the mucous membranes in the patient's nose moist and pink? Is the tongue pink with papillae present? Are the gums moist and pink? Is his or her mouth free from ulcers or lesions? Is the neck free from masses that would impede swallowing?

Cardiovascular system

Is the patient's heart rhythm regular? Are his or her heart rate and blood pressure normal for his or her age? Are the patient's extremities free from swelling? Are his or her jugular veins flat or distended?

GI system

Is the patient's appetite satisfactory? Are GI problems present? Are his or her elimination patterns regular? Is his or her abdomen free from abnormal masses on palpation?

Neurologic system

Is the patient alert and responsive? Are the patient's reflexes normal? Is his or her behaviour appropriate? Are the patient's legs and feet free from paresthesia?

Anthropometric measurements

The third step in assessing nutritional status is taking anthropometric measurements. These measurements can help identify nutritional problems in the patient who's seriously underweight. These measurements include:
- height
- weight
- midarm circumference
- midarm muscle circumference
- skinfold thickness.

Midarm circumference, midarm muscle circumference and skinfold thickness are used to evaluate muscle mass and subcutaneous fat, both of which reflect nutritional status.

Laboratory studies

The fourth step in assessing nutritional status is evaluating the patient's laboratory test results. Make sure to assess:
- *Serum albumin, prealbumin and retinol-binding protein levels*—patients with HIV disease typically have low serum levels, indicating protein deficiency.
- *Serum cholesterol*—levels may be elevated from adverse effects of drug therapy.

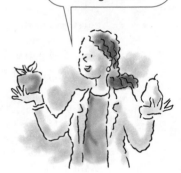

Nutritional therapy may help prevent or delay HIV wasting syndrome if initiated soon after diagnosis.

Dietary management

When a patient is diagnosed with HIV disease, he or she should be referred to a dietitian for assessment and dietary teaching. Nutritional therapy may help prevent or delay HIV wasting syndrome if initiated soon after diagnosis. It should be initiated even if dietary intake appears adequate.

Aiming high

The goals of nutritional support are to:
- provide a well-balanced, nutrient-rich diet
- preserve the patient's independence
- maintain the patient's quality of life
- slow disease progression.

Calorie high

Altered metabolism associated with HIV disease increases caloric needs. The recommended calorie intake for a patient with HIV disease is typically 35 to 45 kcal/kg. These requirements increase in the presence of fever.

Protein provisions

Protein requirements also increase in patients with HIV disease. Daily protein intake should be increased to 1 to 2 g/kg. (See *Increasing dietary intake of protein*.)

NutriTips

Increasing dietary intake of protein

The patient with human immunodeficiency virus disease typically needs to increase his or her intake of dietary protein. Use this list of tips to help the patient increase protein in his or her diet.

Food	Protein content (g)	Suggestions for use
250 ml milk	8	• Add to soup, casseroles, fruit smoothies, pudding, cream sauces, milkshakes and hot or cold cereal. • Substitute for other liquid in recipes.
4 tbls milk powder	7	• Add to milk to make double-strength milk. • Add to any food in which milk is added. • Mix with fruit purees. • Add to milkshakes.
2 tbsp peanut butter	4 to 9	• Spread on celery, apple slices, banana slices, crackers, bagels, bread and muffins. • Mix with apple sauce or yoghurt.
28 g meat, chicken or fish	12 to 19	• Add chunks to salads, casseroles, soup, noodles and stir-fried vegetables.
One portion (62 g) kidney beans	15	• Add to salads, soups or casseroles. • Use pureed chickpeas as a spread.
28 g hard cheese	7	• Melt into soups and casseroles. • Make cheese sauce for vegetables. • Add to salads and sandwiches.
250 ml yoghurt	8	• Combine yoghurt, fruit and milk to make yoghurt drinks. • Make vegetable dip containing yoghurt, dill and lemon juice. • Use as a topping for granola, cold cereal, pancakes, waffles and French toast.
One scoop ice cream	2 to 4	• Make milkshakes. • Mix with fruit. • Use as a creamer for coffee and tea.

Hold the fat

Patients who experience malabsorption may need to limit their fat intake. To make sure that calorie consumption is adequate, the patient may require supplemental medium-chain triglycerides. Medium-chain triglycerides, supplied in the form of oil, don't require lipase or bile for digestion and absorption, so people with impaired digestion or absorption are able to absorb them.

Vital facts about vitamins and minerals

It's recommended that patients with HIV take fat-soluble vitamins according to the Reference Nutrient Intake (RNI). Water-soluble vitamins should be taken in amounts two to five times greater than the RNI value. Patients should avoid large doses of iron and zinc because they can adversely affect immune function. Supplements of trace elements and antioxidants may also be prescribed.

Dealing with adversity

Patients with HIV disease may experience alterations in the sense of taste and problems with appetite and intake similar to patients with cancer. Patients should be encouraged to consume small, frequent meals despite a lack of appetite. Patients should be educated about techniques to improve taste when taste alterations occur. (See *When food doesn't taste good anymore*.)

Medications used to treat HIV disease can also affect nutrition. Many cause food–drug interactions and adverse effects that can impact appetite as well as drug absorption and elimination. Patients must be thoroughly educated about all aspects of their drug therapy. (See *Combating food–drug interactions*.)

Stimulating appetite and combating fullness

Appetite stimulants are sometimes necessary to combat anorexia. Cyproheptadine (Periactin), megestrol acetate (Megace) and mirtazapine (Zispin Sol) are effective in some patients. Other drugs that may help include testosterone, growth hormones and anabolic steroids.

Many patients also complain of feeling full and having heartburn after eating a small amount. Encouraging the patient to take the following precautions may help combat fullness and heartburn:
• Eat foods that are easily digested, avoiding highly spiced and very rich foods if they cause discomfort.
• Consume small meals throughout the day.
• Eat only half a portion at a time, wait 2 hours and then eat the second half.
• Eat slowly.
• Wait at least half an hour after meals before drinking fluids.
• Consume starches, which are easily digested, such as pasta, potatoes, rice, oatmeal, bread, fruit and fruit juices.

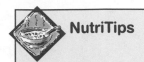 **NutriTips**

When food doesn't taste good anymore

As human immunodeficiency virus disease progresses, patients typically develop alterations in taste. Suggest these tips to help improve taste and increase intake:

• Marinate meat, chicken or fish in sweet fruit juices, beer, Italian dressing, sweet wines, soy sauce or sweet and sour sauce.
• Use seasonings, such as basil, oregano and garlic.
• Add lemon juice, lime juice or vinegar to food.
• Eat a tart apple or lemon wedge just before meals to stimulate saliva.
• Use mouthwash and brush your teeth at least twice per day with a soft toothbrush.
• Eat meat, chicken, fish, tofu or beans cold, instead of hot.

Combating food–drug interactions

Some drugs used to treat HIV disease interact with food. Educate the patient about such interactions and the interventions needed to combat them.

Drug	Interaction	Patient education
Protease inhibitors		
amprenavir (Agenerase)	High-fat meals decrease drug absorption.	• Take drug with or without food but avoid high-fat meals.
atazanavir (Reyataz)	Any food increases drug absorption.	• Take drug with, or immediately after, food. • Take with 8 oz of water.
fosamprenavir (Lexiva)	Food doesn't affect drug absorption.	• Take with or without food.
indinavir (Crixivan)	Any food especially high-fat, high-protein foods substantially decreases drug absorption.	• Take drug on an empty stomach with water 1 hour before or 2 hours after a meal. • Take the drug with other liquids, such as fat-free milk, juice, coffee or tea, if desired. • Meals high in fat, calories and protein reduce the drug's absorption.
lopinavir (Kaletra)	Any food increases drug absorption.	• Take drug with meals.
nelfinavir (Viracept)	Any food increases drug absorption.	• Take drug with a meal or light snack. • Drink plenty of fluids but avoid grapefruit juice. • Monitor for adverse effects or altered plasma drug concentrations if grapefruit or grapefruit juice is consumed. Avoid these foods if an interaction is suspected.
ritonavir (Norvir)	Any food increases drug absorption.	• Take the drug with meals to improve absorption.
saquinavir (Fortovase)	Any food increases drug absorption.	• Take the drug within 2 hours of a meal. • Avoid consuming large amounts of grapefruit juice or grapefruit.
Nucleoside reverse transcriptase inhibitors		
abacavir (Ziagen)	Food doesn't affect drug absorption.	• Take with or without food.
didanosine (Videx)	Any food substantially decreases drug absorption.	• Take the drug on an empty stomach, regardless of dosage form. Giving drug with meals can result in a 50% decrease in absorption. • Drink at least 1 oz (30 ml) of water with each dose.
emtricitabine (Emtriva)	Food doesn't affect drug absorption.	• Take with or without food.

(continued)

Combating food–drug interactions (continued)

Drug	Interaction	Patient education
Nucleoside reverse transcriptase inhibitors (continued)		
lamivudine (Epivir)	Food doesn't affect drug absorption.	• Take with or without food.
stavudine (Zerit)	Food doesn't affect drug absorption.	• Take with or without food.
zalcitabine (Hivid)	Any food reduces absorption.	• Take with or without food, although taking on an empty stomach may improve absorption.
zidovudine (Retrovir)	Food may have variable effects on drug absorption.	• Take with or without food.
Fusion inhibitor		
enfuvirtide (Fuzeon)	Administered parenterally.	• Take with or without food.
Non-nucleoside reverse transcriptase inhibitors		
delavirdine (Rescriptor)	Food doesn't affect drug absorption.	• Take with or without food. • Monitor for adverse effects or altered plasma drug concentrations if grapefruits or grapefruit juice is consumed. Avoid these foods if an interaction is suspected.
efavirenz (Sustiva)	High-fat foods reduce drug absorption.	• Take with or without food, but avoid high-fat foods. • Monitor for adverse effects or altered plasma drug concentrations if grapefruits or grapefruit juice is consumed. Avoid these foods if an interaction is suspected.
nevirapine (Viramune)	Food doesn't affect drug absorption.	• Take with or without food. • Monitor for adverse effects or altered plasma drug concentrations if grapefruit or grapefruit juice is consumed. Avoid these foods if an interaction is suspected.
Nucleotide analogue reverse transcriptase inhibitor		
tenofovir (Viread)	Any food increases drug absorption.	• Take with food.

Encourage the patient to avoid:
- drinking a lot of water or diet cola
- coffee, tea or tonic water
- fatty, fried foods
- spicy foods
- caffeine.

Ways to waste wasting

Several therapies are used to combat HIV wasting. The dietitian should suggest ways to increase calorie and protein intake. Antiemetics such as prochlorperazine (Stemetil) should be prescribed if nausea is a problem. Antidiarrhoeal agents such as loperamide (Imodium) should be prescribed to control diarrhoea. Increasing dietary fibre also helps combat diarrhoea. Such anabolic steroids as nandrolone decanoate (Deca-Durabolin), oxandrolone (Oxandrin) or somatropin (Serostim) may also be prescribed to help build muscle mass.

Enteral nutrition

Enteral nutrition is sometimes necessary for patients who continue with malnutrition and HIV wasting despite other dietary interventions. Patient must be monitored closely for tolerance and symptoms such as diarrhoea. The dietitians will prescribe appropriate feeding regimens.

Total parenteral nutrition

Patients with severe diarrhoea, bowel obstruction or intractable vomiting and those at risk for aspiration sometimes require total parenteral nutrition (TPN). TPN allows the GI tract time to rest while providing the patient calories and other nutrients. However, TPN may not meet the nutritional needs of patients with overwhelming infection. These patients commonly experience HIV wasting despite TPN. TPN also places the patient at risk for infection.

I.V. lipid therapy should be used cautiously in patients with HIV disease because they typically have hyperlipidaemia.

Food safety

Because patients with HIV disease have difficulty fighting infection, extra care must be taken in purchasing, storing and preparing food. The patient should be encouraged to:
- select foods that pose the least risk of causing food poisoning
- use only pasteurised cheese and milk
- check the 'sell by' or 'use by' dates
- examine food packaging for defects
- use plastic cutting boards cleaned in the dishwasher or with sanitising solution after use
- wash hands properly and frequently
- avoid raw foods, such as sushi, Caesar salad and oysters on the half shell
- use a meat thermometer to ensure that adequate internal temperature is reached
- order foods well done when eating in a restaurant
- avoid lightly steamed foods
- refrigerate foods immediately after purchase.

Quick quiz

1. Large doses of which two minerals should be avoided in patients with HIV disease?

    A.   Iron and chromium

    B.   Zinc and iron

    C.   Selenium and zinc

    D.   Iodine and iron

Answer: B. Large doses of zinc and iron can adversely affect immune function.

2. How much protein should a patient with HIV disease consume daily?

    A.   0.5 to 1 g/kg

    B.   1 to 2 g/kg

    C.   25 to 35 g/kg

    D.   35 to 45 g/kg

Answer: B. Patients with HIV disease should consume 1 to 2 g/kg of protein daily to replenish losses and help maintain lean body mass.

3. Safe food preparation by patients with HIV includes:

    A.   drinking unpasteurised milk

    B.   eating lightly steamed foods

    C.   refrigerating foods within 3 hours of purchase

    D.   washing hands properly before preparing foods.

Answer: D. Proper hand washing before handling foods reduces the risk of infection in patients with HIV.

Scoring

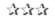 If you answered all three questions correctly, fantastic! You have no knowledge deficiency on this subject.

    If you answered two questions correctly, yippee! There's no need to stimulate your appetite for the facts.

    If you answered fewer than two questions correctly, relax, have a nutritious snack and review the chapter.

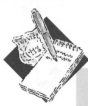

18 Special conditions

Just the facts

In addition to the health problems already presented in this book, various other conditions can also affect a patient's nutritional status. In this chapter, you'll learn:

♦ the effects of severe stress on metabolism

♦ nutritional needs of patients with cancer, traumatic injuries or burns

♦ indications for enteral or parenteral nutrition in cancer, trauma and burn patients

♦ ways to maximise the nutritional status of cancer, trauma and burn patients.

A look at special conditions

Patients with cancer, trauma or severe burns experience changes in nutrient metabolism. Proper nutrition plays an indispensable role in helping these patients cope with changes and avoid or minimise complications.

The importance of being nutritious

In cancer, local disease effects may reduce the patient's oral intake, while systemic effects may increase energy expenditure and speed protein catabolism. Also, some cancerous tumours produce substances that alter nutrient absorption and metabolism.

Severe stress due to trauma and burns leads to hypermetabolism (increased energy expenditure) as well as protein catabolism. Starting nutritional support within the first 24 hours after injury can improve survival, decrease the risk of infection and shorten the length of a hospital stay.

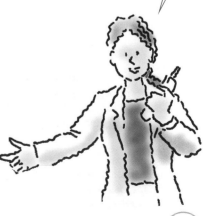

Cancer takes a local and long distance toll on a patient's nutritional needs.

Stress response

In trauma and burns, hormonal and metabolic changes help the body adapt to stressors. This complex stress response has two major phases: ebb and flow. The ebb phase occurs soon after the stress occurs. As the patient's condition stabilises, he or she enters the flow phase. (See *Exploring ebb and flow.*)

Adapting to the environment

After the initial stress response, protein catabolism peaks. During this adaptive phase, levels of stress hormones and blood glucose fall and metabolism returns to normal. Gradually, nitrogen balance is restored.

If adaptation succeeds, the patient recovers. If it fails, the body's inability to adapt to stress results in exhaustion and, possibly, death.

How stress affects nutritional status

Prolonged hypermetabolism and hypercatabolism accelerate the loss of energy and protein stores. As the body breaks down lean mass to meet increased protein demands, acute malnutrition may occur—even in a previously healthy patient.

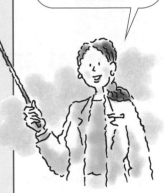

Stress response has its downs and ups— better known as ebb and flow.

Exploring ebb and flow

The body's response to stress can be broken down into two phases: ebb and flow.

Ebb

In the *ebb* phase—the first phase after exposure to severe stress when the patient is haemodynamically unstable—cardiac output, blood pressure, body temperature and oxygen consumption all decrease. As the insulin level drops and catecholamine and glucagon levels rise, hyperglycaemia occurs.

Flow

During the *flow* phase, as the patient's haemodynamic status stabilises, the high metabolic demands of stress force the body to mobilise nutrients. As levels of glucocorticoids, catecholamines and glucagon surge, the patient experiences:

- pronounced hypermetabolism
- accelerated protein catabolism
- persistent hyperglycaemia
- increased urinary losses of potassium and nitrogen
- sodium and fluid retention
- slowed GI motility, possibly leading to abdominal distension, anorexia, nausea, vomiting or constipation.

The body must break down its energy reserves to meet the high-energy demands, and significant loss of protein and fat may occur.

Timing is everything

Once fluids and electrolytes are stabilised, early nutrition intervention, particularly enteral nutrition, can reduce infectious complications. Other early goals of nutrition therapy include minimising nutrient losses and preventing acute malnutrition. After the metabolic rate normalises, nutrition therapy aims to promote a positive nitrogen balance and weight gain.

Nutrition administration methods

In patients with a functioning GI tract, oral or enteral nutrition is preferred because these methods help preserve GI functioning and stimulate GI-associated lymphoid tissue.

Oral feeding is contraindicated if the patient isn't alert enough to eat, is receiving mechanical ventilation or has a nasogastric tube. Enteral feeding isn't administered when conditions such as intestinal obstruction, ileus or perforation are present. Parenteral nutrition may be indicated when enteral feeding isn't appropriate. Intestinal or post-pyloric tube feeding typically can begin sooner than gastric feedings because the intestines regain motility much sooner than the stomach does.

Cancer

Although a cancer patient is more likely than other patients to become malnourished, appropriate nutrition support can maximise the effectiveness of cancer treatments, minimise adverse effects of the disease and treatments, and improve quality of life.

As a cancer patient undergoes treatment, he or she faces many nutritional challenges. The patient is also highly susceptible to claims made by proponents of unproven nutritional therapies.

Effects of cancer on nutritional status

Cancer patients typically have poor appetites, altered metabolism and increased catabolism from direct and indirect tumour effects as well as from treatments and psychological factors (such as anxiety and depression).

Many cancer patients become full after just a few bites. This early satiety may result from:
- poorly understood mechanisms related to the cancer itself
- pressure from the tumour on the abdomen
- ascites (fluid accumulation in the abdomen).

Taste alterations are also common in cancer patients. Many report that food tastes bitter or metallic or that it isn't sweet or salty enough.

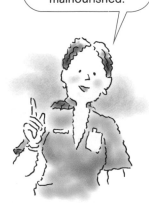

A cancer patient is more likely than any other patient to become malnourished.

Wasting away

Commonly, the cancer patient consumes fewer—and expends more—calories. All too often, weight loss progresses to the point of *cachexia*, a wasting syndrome marked by a maladaptive metabolic rate, anorexia, muscle wasting, severe weight loss and general debility.

Cachexia impairs wound healing and increases the risk of infections and other complications. It's associated with poor quality of life and shorter survival. In fact, cachexia causes more deaths than does cancer itself.

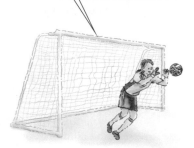

Here's the catch—cachexia causes more deaths than the cancer itself.

Local effects

The tumour itself may directly involve or interfere with GI tract function, causing dysphagia (difficulty swallowing), obstruction, nausea, vomiting and malabsorption. Ovarian, hepatic and genitourinary cancers may lead to ascites, which impairs oral intake by causing early satiety. Brain cancer, on the other hand, may alter the patient's mental status to the extent that oral intake decreases significantly.

Systemic effects

Various metabolic changes may impair the patient's nutritional status. These changes include:
• increased metabolic rate (particularly with lung and gastric cancer and sarcomas)
• increased protein catabolism
• peripheral insulin resistance, possibly caused by cytokines and tumour necrosis factor
• increased fat oxidation.

Effects of cancer treatments on nutritional status

Cancer treatments and their adverse effects commonly cause problems that jeopardise the patient's nutritional status.

Surgery

Effects of cancer surgery on nutrition vary with the surgical site:
• Head and neck surgery may alter chewing and swallowing ability.
• Surgery for oesophageal cancer moves the stomach higher up in the chest. This limits the amount of food the patient can consume at one time and increases the risk of diarrhoea and reflux.
• After gastrectomy, the patient must consume small, frequent meals and may develop severe diarrhoea or dumping syndrome (nausea, weakness, sweating, palpitations and syncope) after eating.
• Pancreatic surgery may alter absorption, gastric emptying and blood glucose levels.

Other potential adverse effects of surgery also can affect nutrition—for example infection, fistulas and short-gut syndrome (malabsorption after removal of part of the small intestine).

To help ensure adequate nutrition during the postoperative period, many patients have feeding tubes placed during surgery.

Radiation therapy

Like cancer itself, radiation may alter the patient's taste perception. Patients commonly complain that foods taste bitter and that they can't distinguish sweet from salty.

Simply radiating

Other adverse effects depend on the radiation dose and site. For instance radiation to the abdominal area damages cells lining the GI tract, causing nausea, vomiting and diarrhoea. When such damage persists and intestinal inflammation becomes chronic, the condition is called *radiation enteritis*. The intestinal lining may remain inflamed for up to 10 years after radiation therapy. Besides vomiting and diarrhoea, enteritis can cause intestinal narrowing, fistula development, poor absorption and bowel obstruction.

Radiation to the head, neck or oesophagus may lead to sore throat, mucositis and taste changes, resulting in anorexia and nausea. Radiation to the chest may cause oesophagitis.

Chemotherapy

Chemotherapy drugs are highly toxic and damage not only cancer cells but also healthy cells. The rapidly growing cells of the GI tract, bone marrow and hair are especially vulnerable.

On the side

Nausea and vomiting are among the most distressing adverse effects of chemotherapy. However, not all chemotherapeutic regimens cause these problems. Nausea and vomiting are more likely to occur with certain drugs and often can be prevented or minimised by administering antiemetics before the chemotherapy session.

Chemotherapy also may cause anorexia, diarrhoea or constipation, malabsorption, mouth sores (stomatitis), mouth inflammation, taste changes and infection. Signs or symptoms lasting more than 2 weeks are likely to significantly affect the patient's nutritional status.

Chemotherapy drugs that affect the bone marrow may lead to anaemia and bleeding. Some also suppress the immune system, increasing the risk of serious infection.

Immunotherapy

Immunotherapy (also called *biologic response modifier therapy*) uses the body's natural defences to fight cancer. Immunotherapies involving certain cytokines and antibodies have become part of standard cancer treatment. Other types of

The healthy cells most likely to be damaged by chemotherapy are those of the GI tract, bone marrow and hair.

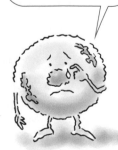

immunotherapy remain experimental. Interferon is the best known and most widely used biologic response modifier.

Depending on the specific agent used, immunotherapy may cause diarrhoea, nausea, vomiting, appetite loss, abdominal pain, stomatitis, taste changes and weight loss. It also may increase the patient's calorie and protein requirements.

Bone marrow transplantation

A patient with leukaemia, lymphoma or breast cancer may undergo bone marrow transplantation. Before transplantation, the patient receives high-dose chemotherapy and total body irradiation to suppress immune function and kill cancer cells. These treatments commonly cause nausea, vomiting, GI tract inflammation, taste changes and anorexia. The transplantation itself may cause mucositis, stomatitis, oesophagitis and intestinal damage (leading to severe diarrhoea).

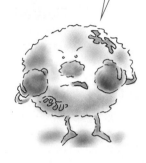

Immunotherapy uses the body's natural defences to fight cancer.

Temporary TPN

Maximising pain management and antiemetic therapy can improve the patient's ability to tolerate an oral diet. If severe GI dysfunction rules out oral or enteral intake, the patient may receive total parenteral nutrition (TPN).

Usually, GI dysfunction resolves about 30 days after transplantation and the patient can resume oral intake or tube feedings (if needed). To optimise nitrogen balance, the patient should receive adequate energy and protein as calculated, based on the individual patient. These will be calculated by the registered dietitian.

What to look for

Weigh the patient and ask if he or she has experienced recent unintentional weight loss. More than 10% weight loss within 3 months indicates severe malnutrition, a greater risk of complications and a poorer prognosis. (At diagnosis, patients with stomach or pancreatic cancer typically show the greatest weight loss. Expect moderate weight loss in patients with lung, colon, oesophageal or prostate cancer.)

Also obtain other relevant history information. (See *Nutritional assessment in cancer patients*.)

Let's get physical

Then, perform a physical examination, checking for classic signs of malnutrition such as:
- oedema
- subcutaneous fat loss
- muscle wasting
- dry, brittle hair
- pale skin
- skin rashes
- poor wound healing.

Also inspect the patient for ascites and for fluid build-up in other body cavities. Be sure to assess for complications of cancer treatments or surgery that may affect nutritional status.

Laboratory data

Serum protein levels may reflect skeletal muscle and visceral protein status. The doctor may request serum albumin, prealbumin and transferrin tests.

Levels of serum prealbumin, which serve as a marker for protein status, reflect the patient's response to stress or nutritional support earlier than do serum albumin levels. A level below 190 mg/dl indicates malnutrition.

It is debatable as to whether laboratory tests are appropriate in managing the chronic malnutrition associated with cancer. Planning nutritional support before there is clear evidence of malnutrition is important in caring for people with chronic disorders.

Interfering with interpretation

When interpreting test results, keep in mind that they can be altered by various factors—the patient's hydration and iron status, infection, stress, other diseases, medications and even bed rest. Ultimately, weight and diet history are the most important elements of nutritional assessment.

Nutritional requirements

Because of hypermetabolism and increased catabolism, the cancer patient has high-protein and energy requirements. To spare protein for vital tissue building, he or she must receive adequate carbohydrates and fats.

Calorie and protein needs vary with the cancer type and stage, presence of metastases, treatments administered and the patient's nutritional status. When determining the patient's specific calorie and protein needs, consider such factors as:
- whether the patient needs to maintain, gain or lose weight
- renal function
- presence of diabetes
- wound status
- patient's activity level.

Calories

A cancer patient who hasn't experienced significant weight loss needs 25 to 35 kcal/kg/day to maintain weight. If the patient needs to gain weight, he or she requires higher calorie levels. A malnourished patient may need 35 to 40 kcal/kg/day. The exact amount of energy required is normally calculated by the registered dietitian.

Be aware that breast cancer patients typically *don't* have a high-calorie requirement. In fact, weight *gain* is relatively common among these patients.

Nutritional assessment in cancer patients

When assessing the nutritional status of a cancer patient, be sure to obtain:

- detailed weight history, although solid tumours can affect reliability of weights recorded
- GI symptoms (such as nausea, vomiting, diarrhoea and anorexia) lasting more than 2 weeks
- functional capacity (whether the patient can function normally, ambulates or is bedridden)
- dietary history, including food preferences (if the patient is receiving oral intake)
- treatments received or scheduled (such as surgery, radiation or chemotherapy)
- medication use
- type of cancer
- emotional status.

Protein

To build tissue, the cancer patient needs nitrogen and essential amino acids, which promote healing and offset tissue breakdown. The patient should receive an optimal ratio of proteins to calories.

Specific protein needs hinge on nutritional status. A patient with a good nutritional status needs roughly 0.8 to 1.2 g/kg/day of high-quality protein to meet maintenance requirements. A malnourished patient needs 1.2 to 1.5 g/kg/day to combat deficits and regain a positive nitrogen balance.

Vitamins and minerals

Certain vitamins and minerals help regulate protein and energy metabolism. The cancer patient should receive optimal vitamin and mineral intake—at least the Reference Nutrient Intake (RNI), but possibly higher.

Each patient's vitamin and mineral needs must be assessed individually. Factors that may influence requirements include the cancer type and stage, nutritional status, medications and presence of such GI complications as malabsorption, diarrhoea and vomiting.

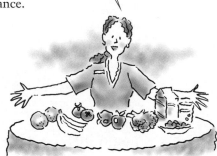

Cancer patients may need more than the Reference Nutrient Intake of vitamins and minerals.

Fluids

Adequate fluid intake is crucial—especially if the patient has been experiencing vomiting, diarrhoea, fever or infection. In addition to replenishing lost fluids, a high fluid intake of 2 L/day or more helps the kidneys eliminate metabolic breakdown products of toxic chemotherapy drugs and destroyed cancer cells.

Certain chemotherapy agents increase fluid needs even further. For instance a patient who's receiving cyclophosphamide (Cytoxan) or ifosfamide (Ifex) may need up to 3 L/day of fluid to avoid haemorrhagic cystitis (bleeding from the bladder).

Dietary management

Nutritional support is essential for combating cancer and boosting the immune system. Early nutritional intervention can improve the patient's tolerance for treatment, minimise adverse effects of treatment and improve quality of life.

Goals of nutritional support are to prevent or reverse catabolism and help relieve side effects of the disease and treatments. In some patients, supplemental nutrition, which is rich in essential nutrients that aid in the metabolism and digestion of food, limits complications and allows completion of a course of chemotherapy or radiation therapy. (In terminally ill patients, however, it hasn't been shown to improve quality of life or outcome.)

Make a plan

For a patient who's receiving oral intake, develop a food plan in collaboration with the patient, family and dietitian. The plan must account for the patient's food preferences and tolerances as well as any eating problems, such as

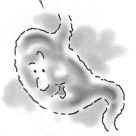

If the GI tract is functioning, enteral nutrition beats parenteral nutrition every time.

anorexia, nausea or vomiting, or stomatitis. The food plan should focus on nutrient density in smaller volumes of food.

The backup plan

A patient who won't be able to receive adequate oral intake for a prolonged period needs nutritional support. If the GI tract is functioning, enteral nutrition is preferable to parenteral nutrition because it's safer, preserves GI function and costs less.

If the GI tract isn't accessible or functional, parenteral nutrition may be given. Despite its risks, TPN can convert the patient's metabolic status from catabolism to anabolism and help prevent cancer cachexia.

Improving intake

If your patient's oral intake is limited by anorexia, nausea and vomiting, stomatitis or other problems, take steps to help him or her overcome these obstacles.

Food fight

Anorexia—the most common cause of malnutrition in cancer patients—may stem from:
- chemicals produced by the tumour
- pain
- early satiety
- depression
- mouth sores
- nausea and vomiting
- altered taste.
  You can help your patient fight anorexia by:
- providing small, frequent meals
- increasing the nutrient density of foods—for instance adding dried milk powder to liquid milk
- encouraging family members to eat with the patient or bring his or her favourite foods from home
- asking the doctor to prescribe an appetite stimulant, such as megestrol acetate (Megace) or dexamethasone (Decadron)—if benefits don't appear after 2 to 6 weeks of drug therapy, the medication should be discontinued.

To help promote adequate intake after discharge, review appropriate eating tips with the patient and family. (See *Overcoming anorexia*, page 364.)

Keep it down

Nausea and vomiting may result from the cancer itself, cancer treatments, pain or certain pain medications. If your patient's undergoing chemotherapy, instruct him or her to take an antiemetic drug 6 hours before chemotherapy starts (if appropriate) and to continue taking it regularly as prescribed.

Here are more suggestions for relieving nausea and vomiting:
- Serve small, frequent meals.
- Instruct the patient to eat slowly.

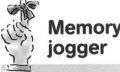

Memory jogger

To help your patient fight anorexia, remember **F**ood **N**ever **G**oes **A**way. Recommend:

Frequent, small meals

Nutrient-dense foods

Gathering family or friends for meals

Appetite stimulants.

NutriTips

Overcoming anorexia

To help your anorexic patient maintain adequate oral intake after discharge, provide the following suggestions to the patient and family:

- Eat small, frequent meals or snacks (every 1 to 2 hours).
- Eat nutrient-dense foods. Avoid low-calorie foods.
- Try to eat when you're feeling best. When not feeling able to eat, consider milky drinks or milkshakes.
- Add extra calories and protein to food by preparing it with butter, cream honey, sugar or dry milk powder.
- Make your eating environment as pleasant as possible.
- Experiment with different recipes, flavourings, spices and food consistencies.
- To avoid strong food odours, which may cause nausea, have someone else prepare meals, cook outdoors on a grill, eat foods cold instead of hot, order take-out meals and take tray covers off early.

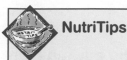

NutriTips

Resuming oral intake

If your patient has been vomiting, instruct him or her not to eat or drink. When the vomiting is under control, advise the patient to try eating small amounts of clear liquids, starting with 1 tsp every 10 minutes and increasing the amount gradually as tolerated.

Once the patient is able to tolerate clear liquids, instruct him or her to eat low-fat, nonspicy foods, such as hot cereal, crackers, pudding and canned fruits. Suggest that the patient continues to take food in small amounts as long as he or she can keep them down. Advise the patient to add new foods gradually.

- Provide liquids for the patient to sip between meals, and advise him or her not to drink fluids with meals.
- Serve beverages cool or chilled.
- Instruct the patient to avoid foods that are fatty, greasy, fried and spicy and foods with strong odours.
- Recommend low-fat foods, which are digested faster and leave less content in the stomach.
- Encourage the patient to eat bland foods, such as toast, crackers, pretzels, rice cakes, hot cereal, popsicles and canned fruits.

For tips on eating after a bout of vomiting, see *Resuming oral intake*.

These are a few of my favourite foods

Some patients develop aversions to foods they ate just before a bout of nausea or vomiting. To prevent food aversions, instruct the patient to avoid favourite foods for 48 hours before and after chemotherapy or radiation therapy.

Fighting fatigue

Fatigue can result from the cancer itself or from radiation, chemotherapy, depression, poor nutrition or dehydration. To counter fatigue, advise the patient to:
- choose healthy foods
- eat small, frequent meals
- use convenience foods and nutritional supplements to decrease energy demands

- drink plenty of fluids
- get adequate sleep and rest
- engage in light exercise, if possible.

A sore subject

Cancer treatment may cause stomatitis (sores in the mouth and throat), which certain foods may aggravate. To make eating less painful, instruct the patient to choose foods carefully and to practise good oral hygiene. To ease discomfort, advise the patient to use a topical anaesthetic. (See *Coping with stomatitis*.)

A change in taste

Chemotherapy, radiation therapy or cancer itself may alter taste perception. Some patients complain of a bitter, metallic taste when eating high-protein foods. Others become sensitive to sweets and prefer unsweetened foods and beverages. With radiation therapy, taste changes typically occur by the third week and resolve within 1 year after therapy ends.

To help your patient maintain adequate intake despite altered taste, advise him or her to:
- eat foods that look and smell good
- eat fish, chicken, turkey, eggs, dairy products or tofu for protein if red meat tastes bad
- use small amounts of seasoning, such as basil, rosemary or oregano

NutriTips

Coping with stomatitis

A patient with stomatitis may experience severe pain when he or she tries to eat. Provide the following tips to help the patient maintain adequate intake:

- Eat soft, mild foods and beverages, such as apple sauce, bananas, canned fruits, cottage cheese, yoghurt, milkshakes, nutritional supplements, milk, mashed potatoes, macaroni and cheese, custard, pudding, scrambled eggs, hot cereals, pureed or mashed vegetables and pureed meats.
- Consume nutrient-dense foods and beverages, such as creamy soups and milk.
- Avoid foods that irritate the mouth, including citrus fruits and juices, spicy or salty foods, and rough, coarse or dry foods.
- Mix food with butter, gravy or sauce.
- Use a straw to drink beverages.
- Eat food cold or at room temperature. Cold foods have a numbing effect, whereas hot or warm foods can irritate mouth sores.
- Practise good oral hygiene to remove food and bacteria and promote healing. If necessary, use an anaesthetic mouthwash.

- consume tart foods and beverages, including oranges, lemonade and lemon custard (unless the patient has stomatitis)
- eat foods at room temperature
- drink liquids throughout the day to moisten the mouth and to flush metabolites from the body
- use plastic utensils rather than metal ones to counter a metallic taste
- rinse the patient's mouth before he or she starts eating.

Zinc deficiency also may lead to taste alterations. Supplemental zinc may help correct this problem.

Trauma

Like other severely stressed patients, trauma patients experience hypermetabolism and protein catabolism. These changes, combined with prolonged bed rest and inadequate nutrition, can lead to drastic loss of lean body mass. Adequate nutrition can minimise catabolic effects, help fight infection and promote wound healing.

Nutritional requirements

Calorie needs vary among trauma patients, whereas protein needs are almost always high.

Calories

The trauma patient should receive only enough calories to promote recovery. Giving excessive calories increases metabolism, oxygen consumption and carbon dioxide production, placing a heavier burden on the heart and lungs.

Specific calorie requirements depend on the patient's condition. A sedated, paralysed patient has very low resting energy expenditure. Other trauma patients, especially those with head injuries, may have high resting energy expenditures.

Ideally, indirect calorimetry should be used to measure the patient's actual energy expenditure. If this technology isn't available or practical, you can use one of several equations, such as the Schofield regression equations, to estimate energy expenditure. (See *Using the Schofield regression equations*.)

It is important that a patient who has suffered trauma is assessed by a registered dietitian who will calculate their individual requirements. Most patients will require adequate energy to conserve their protein mass. Inadequate energy intakes lead to increase protein utilisation, which can compromise the patient's recovery.

Protein

Trauma patients have high-protein requirements because of the presence of wounds, which need protein to heal, and the liver's preferential use of protein for energy during critical illness. Their protein requirements

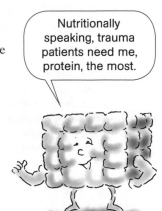

Nutritionally speaking, trauma patients need me, protein, the most.

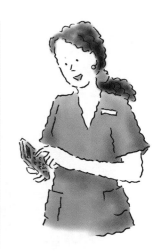

Using the Schofield regression equations

The Schofield regression equations are used to calculate an estimated basal metabolic rate. In clinical practice, stress factors and activity factors are added.

Females (kcal/day)	Males (kcal/day)
10–17 years: 13.4W + 692	10–17 years: 17.7W + 657
18–29 years: 14.8W + 487	18–29 years: 15.1W + 692
30–59 years: 8.3W + 846	30–59 years: 11.5W + 873
60–74 years: 9.2W + 687	60–75 years: 11.9W + 700
Above 75 years: 9.8W + 624	Above 75 years: 8.4W + 820

vary on the degree of hypermetabolic stress of their condition and range from 1 to 2 g protein/kg/day. It is not advisable to give a patient more than 2 g protein/kg/day particularly when he or she is suffering from hypermetabolism.

Vitamins and minerals

Experts aren't sure if trauma patients or other critically ill patients have special vitamin, mineral or trace element requirements. Generally, however, they should receive adequate vitamins and minerals to meet established national standards. To maximise healing, patients with extensive wounds may receive extra zinc, vitamin C and beta-carotene.

Nutrition support

Nutrition support for trauma patients depends on such factors as injury type and severity, the patient's baseline nutritional status and when the patient will be able to take adequate oral nutrition.

Usually, patients with minor injuries and those who can consume adequate oral intake (or are expected to recover within a few days) don't need enteral or parenteral nutrition, but they must receive an appropriate diet with adequate protein to promote healing. They may need liquid nutritionally complete supplements if oral intake is less than optimal.

Severe circumstances

For a trauma patient who's severely malnourished or isn't expected to take adequate oral nutrition for a prolonged period, enteral nutrition should begin as soon as the patient is haemodynamically stable. Starting tube feedings early is associated with fewer infectious complications and a shorter length of stay. (On the other hand, starting parenteral nutrition early probably isn't beneficial.)

Check it out! Starting enteral nutrition early can help trauma patients be discharged sooner.

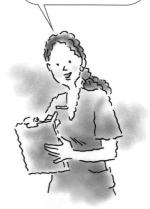

Burns

Severe burns cause a complex and extreme form of hypermetabolism. After a severe burn, energy expenditure increases and catabolism of lean body mass occurs. These changes result in muscle wasting, negative nitrogen balance and depletion of protein and fat stores.

Many factors can influence the extent of these metabolic changes, including:
- burn depth and burn surface area
- evaporative losses from wounds
- fever
- sepsis
- serum catecholamine, glucagon and cortisol levels
- surgery.

Nutritional requirements

Burn patients have altered fluid, protein and calorie requirements. However, energy needs may vary from one patient to the next, and high amounts of calories may be inappropriate for some patients. The hypermetabolic response to a burn injury can continue to increase the nutritional needs of the patients for up to a year postinjury.

Fluids

Patients with burns should be assessed for I.V. fluid resuscitation as soon as possible. The more major the burn is, the more important it is to initiate fluid resuscitation within the first few hours of injury to maintain adequate blood flow to vital organs. Immediate fluid administration helps offset fluid shifts and eliminate waste products produced by the burn injury. Fluids also help prevent gastric distension and paralytic ileus. The amount of fluid given depends on the burn extent, time elapsed since the injury, the patient's weight and his or her response to fluid administration.

Here comes the flood

Once fluid resuscitation is completed, the patient should receive fluids in amounts that produce adequate urine output—30 to 50 ml/h in adults. Fluid requirements remain high for several weeks because water losses may be 10 times greater than normal during this period.

Calories

Hypermetabolism increases the patient's usual calorie needs, but rarely exceeds 180% even in the most severe cases. A high-calorie intake spares the protein essential for tissue rebuilding and meets the dramatically increased metabolic demands. Also, burn patients are at high risk for sepsis—a condition

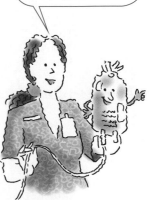

Patients with burns over more than 15% of their bodies need I.V. fluid during the first 48 hours.

Estimating calorie needs in burn patients

The Curreri formula is the most commonly used formula for estimating calorie requirements in adult burn patients.

Here's the formula:

(25 kcal × usual body weight in kg) + (40 × % of total body surface area burned)

This formula yields the number of calories required daily.

Too generous?

Some experts think the Curreri formula overestimates calorie requirements. Overfeeding can lead to hyperglycaemia and hyperosmolality, which, in turn, result in osmotic diuresis, dehydration and ketotic acidosis.

Children

In children with burn injuries, calorie requirements are based on age and burn surface area, as shown here:

Infants <1 year = 2,100 kcal/m² total body surface area (TBSA) + 1,000 kcal/m² burn surface area

Children <12 years = 1,800 kcal/m² TBSA + 1,300 kcal/m² burn surface area

Children >12 years = 1,500 kcal/m² TBSA + 1,500 kcal/m² burn surface area

---

that raises the metabolic rate even further. Most patients continue to have high-calorie needs for several weeks or even longer after the burn injury.

Calorie requirements must be determined individually. Ideally, the patient's actual resting energy expenditure should be measured using indirect calorimetry. However, in the UK, most centres use the Schofield equation or the Ireton–Jones equation (if critically ill). (See *Estimating calorie needs in burn patients*.)

Protein

Burn patients need extremely large amounts of protein to promote wound healing and bolster the immune system. Requirements range from 2 to 3 g/kg of body weight per day, depending on burn extent and catabolic losses. Protein should account for 20% to 25% of total calories.

Much of the increased protein requirement comes from muscle breakdown for use in energy production. Although providing extra protein doesn't stop this breakdown, it provides the materials needed to synthesise lost tissue. Extreme hypercatabolism is compounded by protein losses from wound exudate. Nitrogen losses peak during the first 3 days after the injury, and then taper off slowly until finally ending at about day 16. Even after that time, though, the patient must continue to receive large amounts of protein to promote wound healing and replenish wasted muscle.

Being a protein is hard work! Burn patients need lots of protein to promote healing and boost immune function.

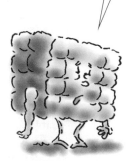

The nitrogen balancing act

Estimating the patient's nitrogen balance can help determine adequacy of protein intake. To estimate nitrogen balance, use this formula:

$$\text{Nitrogen balance} = \text{nitrogen intake} - (\text{total urinary nitrogen} + \text{faecal nitrogen loss} + \text{nitrogen loss from burn wounds})$$

Total urinary nitrogen, faecal nitrogen loss and nitrogen loss from burn wounds are based on a 24-hour period. To achieve nitrogen balance, most adults need 2 to 3 g/kg. (See *Estimating nitrogen loss from wounds*.)

Carbohydrates and fats

The burn patient should get about 50% of daily calories from carbohydrates and roughly 25% to 30% from fat. Because excess fat intake may decrease immune function, fat intake must be monitored closely.

Vitamins and minerals

Many micronutrients are essential for optimal burn wound healing. Although specific requirements after severe burn injury haven't been determined, the patient should receive at least the RNI of each vitamin and mineral. Some vitamins and minerals have been shown to remain at suboptimal levels even when supplemented above this.

Thiamine, riboflavin and niacin requirements may rise because of increased energy and protein metabolism. Some experts also recommend giving additional amounts of vitamins A and C and zinc to promote wound healing and limit oxidative damage.

Dietary management

Without aggressive nutrition therapy, the burn patient is at high risk for malnutrition, weight loss and, possibly, death from tissue destruction and hypermetabolism. Early and aggressive nutritional support reduces the loss of lean body mass, promotes wound healing and helps prevent infection. In many cases, it determines whether the patient will survive.

However, severe burns pose a serious challenge to nutritional support because the patient is likely to have fluid and electrolyte imbalances, pain, anorexia, gastric distension, paralytic ileus, infection and emotional trauma. Also, he or she may need to undergo various medical procedures or surgery.

Nutrition administration routes

During the immediate postburn period, a patient with severe burns may be unable to receive oral intake because of paralytic ileus and other factors.

Experts disagree on the best time to begin feedings of any type. Within the UK, most centres start tube-feeding within 4 to 6 hours of the injury.

Estimating nitrogen loss from wounds

You can estimate nitrogen loss from your patient's wounds, as described here:

- ≤10% open wound: 0.02 g of nitrogen/kg of body weight/day
- >10% to <30% open wound: 0.05 g of nitrogen/kg/day
- ≥30% open wound: 0.12 g of nitrogen/kg/day.

Estimate faecal nitrogen losses at about 2 g/day.

Total urinary nitrogen is determined by collecting a 24-hour urine specimen and determining the number of grams of urinary urea nitrogen present.

Lip service

Whenever possible, oral intake is preferred. But even when oral feedings are possible, they usually must be augmented with oral supplements, and frequently with enteral tube feeding.

To encourage oral intake, provide small, frequent meals and assist in feeding as appropriate. Provide the patient's favourite foods, and encourage the family to bring food from home.

Try to schedule treatments and diagnostic procedures so they don't interfere with meals. (For tips on increasing protein and calorie intake, see *Boosting calorie and protein intake*.)

Enteral versus parenteral nutrition

Enteral nutrition has become the preferred feeding method for all major burns and critically ill patients who can't tolerate oral intake. TPN should be used only when enteral and oral intake fail completely to meet requirements. Due to the nature of a burn injury, TPN is associated with an increased infection risk. Nonetheless, if GI function is absent, parenteral nutrition should be started within 3 to 4 days in severely burned patients.

Formula for success?

Because of the high risk of infection among burn patients, researchers are studying the use of immune-enhancing enteral nutrition formulas. These high-calorie, high-protein formulas contain extra glutamine, arginine, omega-3 fatty acids, ornithine, alpha-ketoglutarate and other related compounds. At this time, though, researchers don't have strong evidence that the formulas improve outcome in burn patients.

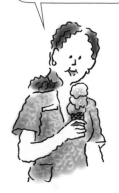

Whenever possible, oral intake is preferred.

Memory jogger

Not sure when a burn patient may require enteral or parenteral nutrition? It's a **SNAP**. Just look for:

Significantly high-calorie and high-protein needs

Neck or facial burns that make swallowing impossible

Anorexia

Paralytic ileus.

When the GI system is functioning, enteral nutrition should be used. When it isn't, choose parenteral nutrition.

NutriTips

Boosting calorie and protein intake

Like other critically ill patients, burn patients have high-protein and high-calorie requirements. To help these patients meet their increased needs, follow these guidelines:

- Add grated cheese to rice, pasta, casseroles and soups.
- Spread raw fruit and vegetable slices with peanut butter.
- Add chopped hard-boiled eggs to soups, sauces and casseroles.
- Use whole or evaporated milk in recipes instead of water.
- Serve egg- or milk-rich desserts, such as puddings, ice cream and custard.
- Add butter to breads, pancakes, waffles, soups, vegetables, rice and pasta.
- Top desserts and hot beverages with whipped cream.
- Provide high-calorie snacks, such as candy, nuts, dried fruit, cheese and ice cream.

Survey the situation

Nutrition therapy for a burn patient must be monitored and, as needed, adjusted continuously—increased if complications occur and decreased as wound healing progresses. Be sure to document daily calories consumed or administered by enteral or parenteral nutrition.

Quick quiz

1. For the trauma patient, which nutritional requirement is the highest?
A. Protein
B. Fat
C. Carbohydrates
D. Vitamin E

Answer: A. Protein needs are the highest requirement for a trauma patient because of multiple physiologic compromises.

2. Which metabolic changes occur in a cancer patient, impairing his or her nutritional status?
A. Decreased metabolic rate
B. Decreased protein catabolism
C. Decreased fat oxidation
D. Peripheral insulin resistance

Answer: D. Peripheral insulin resistance, possibly caused by cytokines and tumour necrosis factor, can adversely affect a cancer patient's nutritional status. Metabolic rate, protein catabolism and fat oxidation all increase in cancer patients.

3. To help make eating less painful for your patient with stomatitis, suggest that he or she eats:
A. hot foods
B. soft, mild foods
C. salty foods
D. dry foods.

Answer: B. Eating soft, mild foods such as applesauce is less irritating to sore mouth tissue.

4. How many grams of protein per kilogram of body weight does a burn patient require each day?
A. 1 to 2 g
B. 2 to 3 g
C. 3 to 4 g
D. 4 to 5 g

Answer: B. A burn patient requires 2 to 3 g/kg/day of protein to boost his or her immune system and promote healing.

5. A malnourished cancer patient may require:
   A.   25 to 35 kcal/kg/day
   B.   20 to 30 kcal/kg/day
   C.   25 to 30 kcal/kg/day
   D.   35 to 40 kcal/kg/day.

Answer: D. A malnourished patient may need 35 to 40 kcal/kg/day to improve his or her nutritional status.

Scoring

☆☆☆   If you answered all five questions correctly, congratulations! One thing is for sure—you're certainly not nutrient dense.

☆☆   If you answered four questions correctly, good job! Your answers weighed in at the top of the class.

☆   If you answered fewer than four questions correctly, keep at it! With a second helping of studying, you'll see that nutrition can be as easy as pie.

Appendices and index

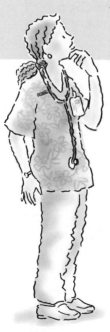

Fad diets

In an attempt to lose weight quickly, some patients try fad dieting. The increased use of the Internet means that people can access diets from across the world, many of which are not supported by research. This chart provides information about many common fad diets, including their pros and cons.

Diet	Description	Pros	Cons
Atkins	• High-protein, low-carbohydrate diet to help body burn fat stores for energy • Initially limits carbohydrates to 20 to 40 g/day • Allows consumption of meat, eggs, cheese, butter and cream	• Produces rapid weight loss (however, after 1 year, patients show no significant difference in weight loss compared to other popular diet plans) • Initially reduces cholesterol levels • Is easy to follow with no counting of calories or complicated meal plans to follow	• Has limited food choices, with carbohydrates being severely restricted • Is extremely high in saturated fat and protein • Limits fruit, vegetable and fibre intake • Restricts foods that fight cancer • May damage the kidneys (due to long-term high-protein intake) • May be difficult to maintain long term • Can cause ketosis, which may lead to nausea and fatigue
Cabbage soup	• Unlimited consumption of cabbage soup and water with limited amounts of other foods for 1 week	• Results in immediate weight loss • Is easy and affordable to follow	• Results in temporary weight loss • Offers little variety in diet • Results in very low intake of calories, protein, vitamins and complex carbohydrates, which can adversely affect health • Can be used only short term
Eat more, weigh less	• High-carbohydrate, low-fat diet	• Emphasises healthy eating, not amounts of foods • Promotes high-fibre intake and limitation of processed foods • Promotes cholesterol and weight reduction • Promotes regular exercise	• Is time consuming to prepare • Limits foods, reducing long-term success • Restricts proteins from dairy and meats

Diet	Description	Pros	Cons
Eat right for your type	• Promotes eating foods that are compatible with blood type • Based on belief that each blood type reacts negatively to certain foods	• Doesn't require calorie counting • Promotes decreased calorie consumption, possibly resulting in weight loss • Provides lists of foods to avoid	• Restricts certain foods • Requires dieter to know blood type • Presents concerns for those eating high-protein, low-carbohydrate diets (recommended for type "O" blood) same as with other similar diets
Glucose revolution	• Promotes foods with a low glycaemic index	• Reduces consumption of refined carbohydrates • Provides lists of foods with high and low glycaemic indexes	• Requires dieter to understand the concepts of 'glycaemic index' and 'glucose load' • Lacks unified glycaemic lists for foods
Grapefruit	• Promotes consumption of grapefruit or grapefruit juice with meals in the belief that grapefruit contains fat-burning enzymes that promote weight loss	• Offers several diet plans • Is easy to follow	• Is based on special fat-burning enzyme in grapefruit that has no scientific basis • May cause drug interactions (grapefruit juice interacts with many medications) • Offers limited choice of foods in small amounts • Results in very low intake of calories, proteins, fibre, and vitamins and minerals, which can adversely affect health • Can be used only short term
Liquid protein	• Replaces breakfast, lunch and snacks with shakes, bars and other special foods	• Encourages portion control • Simplifies portion control by using special products • Provides structured diet plan	• Can be costly for special shakes • Offers limited food choices, making diet hard to maintain • Results in temporary weight loss • Shouldn't be followed long term
Pritikin	• Low-fat, high-carbohydrate diet based on vegetables, grains and fruits • Promotes belief that fat intake shouldn't exceed 10% of total daily calories	• Promotes foods with fewer calories per pound • Encourages exercise	• Requires dieter to calculate caloric density or refer to lists for food choices • Is difficult to maintain and promotes hunger (very low fat diet)

(continued)

Diet	Description	Pros	Cons
Scarsdale	• Rigid low-carbohydrate, low-fat, high-protein diet that's followed for 2 weeks, followed by a maintenance plan	• Requires no calorie counting	• Doesn't allow snacking, except for carrots, celery and low-sodium broth • Encourages use of artificial sweeteners and herbal appetite suppressants to promote weight loss • Requires dieter to follow strict diet plan with very little substitutions and many rules
South Beach	• Initially carbohydrate restriction • After initial phase, refined carbohydrates restricted but wholegrains, fruits and vegetables allowed	• Promotes vegetable, fruit and wholegrain intake after initial ban on carbohydrates • Promotes intake of low saturated fat and high monounsaturated fats • Requires no calorie or carbohydrate counting • Encourages exercise	• Promotes very low carbohydrate intake during initial phase • Results in water loss during initial phase that may result in electrolyte imbalances • Requires dieter to understand glycaemic index
Stop inflammation now	• Promotes a very low fat, low-protein diet	• Encourages intake of fruits, vegetables, wholegrains, beans and legumes • Connects inflammation with heart disease	• May result in insufficient calcium intake • Restricts protein from dairy and animal sources • Is very strict, making compliance difficult
Sugar busters	• Promotes avoidance of simple sugars and refined grains • Promotes high-fibre carbohydrate, lean meat and unsaturated fat intake • Based on the belief that sugar is toxic to the body and leads to excess insulin levels and storage of excess sugar as fat	• Provides clear guidelines on foods to avoid • Uses the glycaemic index to rank food	• Limits food portions • Requires dieter to understand glycaemic index • Is difficult to follow
Volumetrics	• Promotes consumption of high-volume, low-calorie foods to produce feeling of fullness on fewer calories • Promotes portion control of high-density foods	• Allows all types of foods	• May result in slow weight loss • Involves much preparation time

Diet	Description	Pros	Cons
Zone	• Divides meals into portions of 40% carbohydrates, 30% proteins and 30% fats • Based on the belief that 'the zone' is a state in which the body is at peak physical performance, mental focus, increased energy and reduced illness and entering 'the zone' is achieved by maintaining a specific insulin level, leading to a balance of eicosanoids	• Allows lean meats and fats • Emphasises fruits and vegetables • Isn't as restrictive as other diets • Allows for a broad range of foods • Has a simple-to-follow eating plan • Promotes reduced caloric intake, which leads to weight loss	• Results in low fibre intake • Involves difficult 'block' system

Commonly used herbs

If your patient is taking a herbal preparation, you'll need to know its intended use, adverse effects and special considerations for use. Advise the patient to consult with his or her practitioner before taking any herbal preparation and to inform all practitioners and pharmacists about their use.

Herb	Use	Adverse reactions	Practice pointers
Black cohosh	• Menopausal symptoms • Premenstrual syndrome • Dysmenorrhoea	• Headache • GI complaints • Seizures • Weight gain	• Avoid use in pregnant and breast-feeding women and those with breast cancer. • Know that the drug may interact with antidepressants, antihypertensives, anti-platelets, anticoagulants, disulfiram, metronidazole, oestrogen replacement therapy, iron preparations, sedatives, tamoxifen and analgesics. • Avoid confusion with blue or white cohosh.
Chamomile	• Diarrhoea • Anxiety • Restlessness • Stomatitis • Haemorrhagic cystitis • Flatulence • Motion sickness • Wound healing	• Conjunctivitis • Eyelid angioedaema • Nausea • Vomiting • Contact dermatitis • Eczema • Anaphylaxis	• Know that the drug may interact with central nervous system (CNS) depressants, warfarin, alprazolam, atorvastatin, diazepam, ketoconazole and verapamil. • Know that the drug may cause anaphylaxis in patients who are sensitive to ragweed or feverfew and in those with a history of hay fever or asthma. • Avoid use in pregnant or breast-feeding women and those with liver or kidney disorders.

Herb	Use	Adverse reactions	Practice pointers
Echinacea	• Stimulates the immune system • Acute and chronic upper respiratory infection • Urinary tract infection; wound healing • May prevent upper respiratory infection and common cold	• GI complaints • Fever • Taste disturbance • Polyuria • Allergic reactions	• Avoid use in people with autoimmune diseases, human immunodeficiency virus, acquired immuno-deficiency syndrome, tuberculosis and pregnant and breast-feeding women. • Limit use to no more than 8 weeks. • Know that the drug may interact with protease inhibitors, disulfiram, metronidazole, immunosuppressants and alcohol.
Evening primrose oil	• Mastalgia, premenstrual syndrome • Cyclic mastitis • Neurodermatitis • Menopausal symptoms	• Headache • GI disturbances • Allergic reaction	• Know that the drug may interact with phenothiazines and tricyclic antidepressants (TCAs). • Know that the drug may be given with vitamin E to prevent toxic metabolites. • Avoid use in pregnant and breast-feeding women and people with seizure disorder.
Garlic	• Elevated cholesterol and triglyceride levels • Bacterial and fungal infections • Digestive problems • Hypertension	• Heartburn • Flatulence • Fatigue • Headache • Insomnia • Asthma • Shortness of breath • Contact dermatitis • Body odour • Facial flushing • Hypersensitivity reactions • Orthostatic hypotension	• Monitor for increased risk of bleeding. • Know that the drug may interact with anti-inflammatory and nonsteroidal anti-inflammatory drugs. • Avoid use in people following surgery or with diabetes, insomnia, pemphigus, organ transplants or rheumatoid arthritis.

(continued)

Herb	Use	Adverse reactions	Practice pointers
Ginkgo biloba	• Enhances memory • Peripheral vascular disease	• Headache • Dizziness • GI disturbances • Palpitations • Allergic reaction • Bleeding	• Know that the drug may interact with anticoagulants, aspirin, vitamin E, garlic supplements, trazodone, anticonvulsants, disulfiram, metronidazole, monoamine oxidase (MAOI) inhibitors, TCAs, oral antidiabetic agents and thiazide diuretics. • Avoid use in people with diabetes and bleeding disorders. • Explain that the components of ginkgo can vary significantly and should be obtained from a reliable source.
Ginseng	• Mental alertness • Energy enhancement • Atherosclerosis • Bleeding disorders • Colitis • Diabetes • Depression • Cancer	• Dizziness • Headache • Insomnia • Restlessness • Hypertension • Hypotension • Diarrhoea • Vomiting • Oestrogen-like effects, such as vaginal bleeding and mastalgia	• Avoid use in people with untreated hypertension and women with history of breast cancer. • Know that the drug may interact with MAO inhibitors, digoxin, insulin, CNS stimulants, oestrogen, furosemide, ibuprofen, oral antidiabetic agents, warfarin and ticlopidine. • Monitor for ginseng abuse syndrome in those taking large amounts: increased motor and cognitive activity, diarrhoea, nervousness, insomnia, hypertension, oedema and skin eruptions.
Saw palmetto	• Benign prostatic hyperplasia • Congestion from colds, bronchitis or asthma • Mild diuretic • Urinary antiseptic and astringent	• Dizziness • Headache • Hypertension • Urine retention • Abdominal pain • Diarrhoea • Nausea	• Avoid use in people with bleeding disorders or scheduled for surgery and women who are pregnant, planning pregnancy or breast-feeding.

Herb	Use	Adverse reactions	Practice pointers
			• Know that the drug may interact with anticoagulants, adrenergics, aspirin, vitamin E and gingko. • Obtain baseline prostate-specific antigen level in men before starting this herb.
St. John's wort	• Depression • Anxiety • Seasonal affective disorder • Restlessness • Viral infections • Sleep problems	• Dry mouth • Dizziness • GI complaints • Fatigue • Headache • Pruritus • Neuropathies • Hypothyroidism • Delayed hypersensitivity • Photosensitivity	• Avoid use in people with photosensitivity, undergoing ultraviolet treatment, and suffering from bipolar disorder and in women who are pregnant or want to become pregnant and their male partners. • Stop herb several weeks before surgery. • Know that the drug may interact with Ritalin, ephedrine, caffeine, protease inhibitors, digoxin, statins, warfarin, anaesthetics, chemotherapy, hormonal contraceptives, TCAs, olanzapine, clozapine, theophylline, cyclosporine and many over-the-counter drugs.

Toxic herbs

In 2005, the Medicines and Healthcare products Regulatory Agency (MHRA) launched a new registration scheme for herbal medicines—the Traditional Herbal Registration Scheme (THR)—under which herbal medicines have to be made to specific standards of safety and quality. These products have a **THR** number on their labels.

- A herbal remedy without a PL or THR number on its label is unlicensed and has **not** been assessed by the MHRA; therefore, nothing is known about its safety, quality or any potential side effects.
- As herbs are assessed, information about their safety can be found on the MHRA website.

Herbs not listed should not be consumed until safety and quality can be established.

Common name	Botanical name
Arnica	Arnica montana
Belladonna	Atropa belladonna
Bittersweet	Solanum dulcamara
Bloodroot	Sanguinaris canadensis
Broom-tops	Cytisus scoparius
Buckeye	Aesculus hippocastanum
Heliotrope	Heliotropium europaeum
Hemlock	Conium maculatum
Henbane	Hyoscyamus niger
Jimsonweed	Datura stramonium
Lily of the valley	Convallaria majalis
Lobelia	Lobelia inflate
Mandrake	Mandragora officinarum
Mayapple	Podophyllum peltatum
Mistletoe	Phoradendron flavescens
Periwinkle	Vinca major, Vinca minor
Snakeroot	Eupatorium rugosum
Tonka bean	Dipteryx odorata, Coumarouna odorata
Wahoo bark	Euonymus atropurpureus
Wormwood	Artemisia absinthium
Yohimbe	Corynanthe yohimbe

Selected references

Bernstein, H., Cosford, P., and Williams, A. *Enabling Effective Delivery of Health and Wellbeing.* An Independent Report DH, London, 2010.

COMA. *Dietary Reference Values for Food, Energy and Nutrients for the United Kingdom. Report of the Panel on Dietary Reference Values of the Committee on Medical Aspects of Food Policy.* London: HMSO, 1991.

Diabetes UK. *Recommendations for the Provision of Services in Primary Care for People with Diabetes.* London: Diabetes UK, 2005.

DH. *Putting Prevention First Vascular Checks: Risk Assessment and Management.* London: DH, 2008.

DH. *Weaning Starting Solid Food.* London: DH, 2008.

DH. *Delivering Choosing Health: Making Healthier Choices Easier.* London: DH, 2005.

DH. *Five Years on: Delivering the Diabetes National Service Framework.* London: DH, 2008.

Expert Group on Vitamins and Minerals. *Safe Upper Levels for Vitamins and Minerals.* London: FSA, 2003.

Joint National Committee on Prevention, Detection, Evaluation, and Treatment of High Blood Pressure.

"The Seventh Report of the Joint National Committee on Prevention, Detection, Evaluation, and Treatment of High Blood Pressure: The JNC 7 Report," *JAMA* 289:2560–72, 2003.

NICE. *Guidance on the Use of Long-Acting Insulin Analogues for the Treatment of Diabetes. Technical Appraisal Guidance No.53.* London: NICE, 2002.

National Collaborating Centre for Acute Care. *Nutrition Support for Adults Oral nutrition Support, Enteral Tube Feeding and Parenteral Nutrition Methods, Evidence and Guidance.* London: NICE, Royal College of Surgeons, 2006.

National Collaborating Centre for Mental Health. *Eating Disorders. Core Interventions in the Treatment and Management of Anorexia Nervosa, Bulimia Nervosa and Related Eating Disorders. National Clinical Practice Guideline Number CG9.* London: NICE, The British Psychological Society and Gaskell, 2004.

National Collaborating Centre for Women's and Children's Health. *Type 1 Diabetes Diagnosis and Management of Type 1 Diabetes in Children and Young People.* London: NICE RCOG Press, 2004.

National Institute for Health and Clinical Excellence. *Obesity Guidance on the Prevention, Identification, Assessment and Management of Overweight and Obesity in Adults and Children. NICE Clinical Guideline 43.* London: NICE, 2006.

National Institute for Health and Clinical Excellence. *Routine Antenatal Care for Healthy Pregnant Women. NICE Clinical Guideline 62.* London: NICE, 2008.

National Institute for Health and Clinical Excellence. *Diabetes in Pregnancy. Management of Diabetes and its Complications from Pre-conception to the Postnatal Period. NICE Clinical Guideline 63.* London: NICE, 2008.

Food Standards Agency. Eat well be well helping you to make healthier choices. Available at: http://www.eatwell.gov.uk/. Accessed June 2010.

Food Standards Agency. *Saturated Fats Made Simple.* London: Food Standards Agency, January 2009.

Giger, J.N., and Davidhizar, R.E. *Transcultural Nursing: Assessment & Intervention,* 4th ed. St. Louis: Mosby–Year Book Inc., 2004.

Nursing Herbal Medicine Handbook, Springhouse Ed. 3rd ed. Philadelphia: Lippincott Williams & Wilkins, 2006.

Managing Chronic Disorders. Springhouse Ed. Philadelphia: Lippincott Williams & Wilkins, 2006.

Miller, E.R., and Jehn, M. "New High Blood Pressure Guidelines Create New At-Risk Classification: Changes in Blood Pressure Classification by JNC 7," *Journal of Cardiovascular Nursing* 19(6): 367–71, November–December 2004.

National Service Frameworks. Available at: http://www.nhs.uk/ NHSEngland/NSF/Pages/ Nationalserviceframeworks.aspx. Accessed June 2010.

NICE (National Institute for Health and Clinical Excellence). Available at: http://www.nice.org. uk/. Accessed June 2010.

ONS. *The National Diet & Nutrition Survey: Adults Aged 19 to 64 Years.* HMSO London, 2003.

Reeves, R. *A Liberal Dose? Health and Wellbeing – the Role of the State. An Independent Report.* London, 2010.

Swanton, K., and Frost, M. *Lightening the Load: Tackling Overweight and Obesity.* London: National Heart Forum, 2007.

Thibodeau, G.A., and Patton, K.T. *The Human Body in Health and Disease*, 4th ed. St. Louis: Mosby–Year Book Inc., 2005.

Index

A

Abdominal distension, 169
Absence seizure, 309. *See also* Epilepsy
Absorption. *See also* Digestion
    of amino acids, 50
    of carbohydrates, 40
    of fats, 60–61
    of fluids, 90–91
    of gastrointestinal (GI) tract, 21–29
    of minerals, 83
    of proteins, 50
    of small intestine, 22t, 25, 26,
        27–28, 49t, 60
    of vitamins, 76
Acquired immunodeficiency syndrome
    (AIDS), 341, 342. *See also*
    Human immunodeficiency
    virus (HIV) disease
ACS. *See* Acute coronary syndromes
    (ACS)
Active transport, fluid movement and,
    91–92, 92i
Acute coronary syndromes (ACS), 259
Acute kidney failure, 289–292
    dietary management of, 291–292
    pathophysiology, 289–290
    sign and symptoms of, 290–291
    treatment of, 291–292
Adefovir dipivoxil, 241
Adenosine triphosphate (ATP), 4, 91,
    92, 92i
Adolescence
    energy and protein requirements
        during, 142t
    growth and development during,
        145
    healthful diet during, 146
    nutrient needs during, 145–146
    nutritional concerns during, 146–148

Adults, nutrition and, 148–149
AIDS. *See* Acquired immunodeficiency
    syndrome (AIDS)
Albumin
    in fluid movement, 94
    nutritional status and, 119
Alcohol
    adolescents and, 147
    pregnancy and, 131
Alcoholics, vitamin supplements for, 79
Alkaline mucous, 28
Alzheimer's disease, 304–306
    pathophysiology of, 305–306
    sign and symptoms of, 306
    treatment of, 306–307
Amino acids, 46–47
    absorption of, 50
    essential and non-essential, 47t
    tryptophan, 52
Anabolism, 4, 5
Anorexia nervosa, 195–196
    long-term effects of, 198–199
    nutrition therapy for, 199–200
    signs and symptoms of, 197–198
Anthropometric arm measurements,
    116, 117i
Antrum, 25
Argentaffin cells, 26
Artificial sweeteners, pregnancy
    and, 131
Ascending colon, 28–29
Ascorbic acid, 73t, 78t
Aspartame, 44
    in pregnancy, 131
Aspiration pneumonia, 170
Atherosclerosis, 259
Athletes, dietary intake of, 148
ATP. *See* Adenosine triphosphate (ATP)
Auerbach's plexus, 20
Axons, 302

B

Balanced diet, nutrition and, 6–16,
    10i, 13i
BAPEN. *See* British Association for
    Parenteral and Enteral
    Nutrition (BAPEN)
Basophils, 120, 121
Behaviour therapy, for weight
    loss, 190
Bile, 31
Biliary duct system, 30–31
Biliopancreatic diversion, 193i, 195
Binge eating disorder, 196
    long-term effects of, 199
    nutrition therapy for, 201
    signs and symptoms of, 198
Biotin, 73t, 78t
Blood pressure readings, 270–271,
    271t
BMI. *See* Body mass index (BMI)
Body composition measurements, 116
    midarm circumference, 116, 117i
        muscle, 116, 117i
    triceps skinfold measurements,
        116, 117i
Body mass index (BMI), 113–115, 257
    calculation of, 114
    determination of, 115i
Body structure, minerals in, 80, 82
Bolus feedings
    enteral nutrition and, 166–167
Bone mineral density test, 122
Brain, 303
Brain stem, 303
Breast-feeding, 134–135
    advantages of, 135
Breast-feeding woman
    nutritional needs for, 129–130
    vitamin supplements for, 79

t refers to a table; i refers to an illustration

t refers to a table; i refers to an illustration

t refers to a table; i refers to an illustration

t refers to a table; i refers to an illustration

t refers to a table; i refers to an illustration

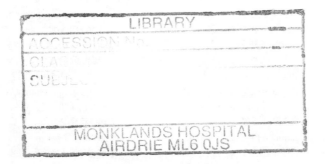

t refers to a table; i refers to an illustration